EMERGENCY CARDIOLOGY

a practical guide

Loukianos S. Rallidis, MD, FESC

Associate Professor of Cardiology
University of Athens Medical School
Second Department of Cardiology
University General Hospital "Attikon"
Athens, Greece

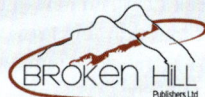

BROKEN HILL
Publishers Ltd

The author would like to thank
Philip Lees and Dimitris Harvatis for their translation work

Science is ever-changing

New research accomplishments and clinical experience has expanded the field of medical knowledge and represent an ongoing process. With this in mind,it is imperative that we make the appropriate changes as far as it concerns the course of action, in the treatment of our patients.

The content of this textbook reflects all the most recent knowledge and internationally accepted techniques as they are analyzed by experienced authors in the field, in each chapter.

Nevertheless, the authors and the editor acknowledge that every medical opinion is under the limitations of the time frame that this book was created, as well as possible mistakes that might have escaped their attention.

Readers of this textbook are encouraged to keep that in mind, while at the same time we hope that the information included will become a starting point for young colleagues or the more experienced ones, for new research projects, clinical trials or maybe an updated version of the book in the near future.

ISBN: 978-9963-716-81-4

9 789963 716814

Print - Binding

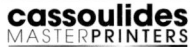

cassoulides
MASTERPRINTERS

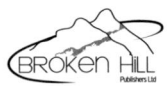

To my late beloved brother Vassilis,

who left us too soon,

my wife Katerina and

my children Maria, Taxiarchoula and Stelios.

Foreword

The diagnostic and therapeutic advances in emergency cardiovascular medicine has created a need for training and education beyond what general cardiology is used to receiving. This demand has, in fact, led to the recognition of acute cardiac care as a legitimate subspecialty. The first European exam for certification in Acute and Intensive Cardiac Care took place approximately 10 years ago. Since then the publication of books and other educational products in this field increased exponentially.

Nevertheless, it is important for the trainee to have a "reference" handbook with practical tips and diagnostic and treatment algorithms for these life-threatening conditions, a book that can be used even when... the computer breaks down.

Before you is an impressive handbook that is different from any other book you have ever read. Professor Loukianos Rallidis is not only one of the most experienced practicing cardiologists but he also has a unique and attractive writing style. That is sure to keep the reader engaged. Although the diagnostic and therapeutic algorithms in this book are based on the guidelines and the current literature Loukianos also used the clinical experience of a very large numbers of experts to give the "true-life" flavor to each chapter. Finally, each and every line in this book has been "tested" extensively in everyday clinical practice by fellows and practicing experts. Throughout the years, I remember Loukianos evaluating the clinical usefulness of all algorithms in everyday clinical practice before considering a chapter as final.

Dr Rallidis has written THE reference handbook for all those who treat patients with cardiac emergencies in the emergency room, in the intensive cardiac care unit or in the ward. It will surely be an enjoyable learning experience for all.

Gerasimos Filippatos, MD, FESC, FHFA
Professor of Cardiology
National and Kapodistrian University of Athens
President
Heart Failure Association ESC

Foreword

Emergency medicine has evolved with galloping paces over the past few years with new methods of treatment and cardiology has been in the forefront of those developments. The result has been the saving of numerous lives. However, it is important for the young doctor in training to be fully aware and develop the skills to recognize, diagnose and treat those conditions that are often life-threatening.

This is an impressive book on cardiac emergencies derived from the author's personal clinical experiences. He produced a unique handbook on diagnosis and management of day-to-day clinical scenarios that will become essential for every junior doctor in training. The unique writing style and medical experiences as lived through the eyes of a practicing cardiologist has taken in consideration existing guidelines and clinical algorithms. He has created an essential reference book for all those who see patients in the clinical emergencies where time and quick thinking are of essence.

Petros Nihoyannopoulos, MD, FRCP, FESC, FACC, FAHA
Professor of Cardiology
First Department of Cardiology
Hippokratio University Hospital, Athens, Greece
and
Professor of Cardiology
Imperial College London, NHLI
Hammersmith Hospital, UK

Author's Preface

The idea for this book came to me about 20 years ago, when I was working in the Accident and Emergency Department of Selly Oak Hospital in Birmingham UK as a senior house officer. Although the theoretical level of my medical knowledge was satisfactory and comparable with that of my English colleagues, I used to lag behind in dealing with the cases. This was a consequence of the fact that I wasn't able within a short time to selectively apply the knowledge that would have allowed me to distinguish the important from the less important, to function in an abstract way and to apply a simple algorithm to solve the diagnostic problem.

This book represents an attempt to decrypt and simplify the way of handling emergency cardiology cases and is directed mainly at the young doctor. At the end of each chapter there is an algorithm that focuses on the basic diagnostic points and the main therapeutic actions for handling the illness. The composition of the text is based for the most part on the existing guidelines of scientific associations. However, in many cases I have used only the most essential information that assists in the management of an emergency case and I have incorporated certain elements from my personal medical experience. For this reason, the algorithms offer only a rough guide to patient management and may need modifications according to the peculiarities of the case and the doctor's judgment.

The text that precedes the algorithm provides the necessary theoretical substrate to allow the reader to assimilate the algorithmic evaluation of the emergency illness. In order to facilitate the young doctor's therapeutic management of the case, the way of preparing and administering intravenous solutions is described, while representative brand names of the main cardiological drugs are included.

It would be remiss of me not to thank my colleagues at the second University Cardiology Department and in particular the doctors in training for their pertinent observations, which have contributed significantly to a simple rendering of the text.

I hope that this book will be a useful tool in the hands of the young doctor for the correct and rapid handling of emergency cardiology cases where the time factor is decisive for the outcome of the cardiac disease.

Loukianos S. Rallidis, MD, FESC
Associate Professor of Cardiology
University of Athens Medical School
Second Department of Cardiology
University General Hospital "Attikon"
Athens, Greece

Contents

Abbreviations

ACE	angiotensin-converting enzyme
ACS	acute coronary syndrome
ACT	activated clotting time
AF	atrial fibrillation
AMI	acute myocardial infarction
aPTT	activated partial thromboplastin time
AV	atrioventricular
AVNRT	atrioventricular nodal reentrant tachycardia
AVRT	atrioventricular reentrant tachycardia
BNP	brain natriuretic peptide
BP	blood pressure
CAD	coronary artery disease
CCR	cardiocerebral resuscitation
cGMP	cyclic guanosine monophosphate
CK	creatine kinase
CP	chest pain
CPAP	continuous positive airway pressure
CPR	cardiopulmonary resuscitation
CrCl	creatinine clearance
CSNRT	corrected sinus node recovery time
CT	computed tomography
cTn	cardiac troponin
CTPA	computed tomography pulmonary angiography
CTV	computed tomographic venography
DAPT	dual antiplatelet therapy
DC	direct current
DES	drug-eluting stent
DVT	deep vein thrombosis
ECG	electrocardiogram
ECT	ecarin clotting time

ELISA	enzyme-linked immunosorbent assay
EMA	European Medicines Agency
FDA	Food and Drug Administration
FFP	fresh frozen plasma
FiO_2	fraction of inspired oxygen
GRACE	Global Registry of Acute Coronary Events
h	hour
HIT	heparin-induced thrombocytopenia
hs-cTn	high-sensitivity cardiac troponin
IABP	intra-aortic balloon pump
ICD	implantable cardioverter defibrillator
ICU	intensive care unit
IMH	intramural hematoma
INR	international normalized ratio
IV	intravenous
J	Joule
LBBB	left bundle branch block
LMWH	low-molecular-weight heparin
MAT	multifocal atrial tachycardia
MD-CTPA	multi-detector computed tomographic pulmonary angiography
MI	myocardial infarction
min	minute
MRA	magnetic resonance angiography
MRI	magnetic resonance imaging
NOACs	non-vitamin K antagonists oral anticoagulants
NSAIDs	nonsteroidal antiinflammatory drugs
NSTEMI	non ST-segment elevation myocardial infarction
NT-proBNP	N-terminal pro-B-type natriuretic peptide
PAU	penetrating aortic ulcer
PCC	prothrombin complex concentrate
PCI	percutaneous coronary intervention
PCWP	pulmonary capillary wedge pressure
PE	pulmonary embolism
PF4	platelet factor 4
po	per os

PPIs	proton pump inhibitors
PRES	posterior reversible encephalopathy syndrome
rFVIIa	recombinant factor VIIa
s	second
STEMI	ST-segment elevation myocardial infarction
TEE	transesophageal echocardiogram
TEVAR	thoracic endovascular aortic repair
TT	thrombin time
UFH	unfractionated heparin
ULN	upper limit of normal
VF	ventricular fibrillation
VKA	vitamin K antagonist
V/Q scan	ventilation/perfusion lung scan
VSR	ventricular septal rupture
VT	ventricular tachycardia
WPW	Wolff-Parkinson-White

Classes of recommendations according to the European Society of Cardiology committee for guidelines

Classes of recommendations	Definition	Suggested wording to use
Class I	Evidence and/or general agreement that a given treatment or procedure is beneficial, useful, effective	Is recommended/is indicated
Class II	Conflicting evidence and/or a divergence of opinion about the usefulness/efficacy of the given treatment or procedure	
Class IIa	Weight of evidence/opinion is in favour of usefulness/effucacy	Should be considered
Class IIb	Usefulness/efficacy is less well established by evidence/opinion	May be considered
Class III	Evidence or general agreement that the given treatment or procedure is not useful/effective, and in some cases may be harmful	Is not recommended

1

Chest pain

Chest pain (CP) is the most common reason why patients come to the emergency cardiology clinic. Failing to recognize the exact cause of the CP and discharging the patient whose pain is due to a cardiovascular cause, such as myocardial ischemia, may have fatal consequences for that patient.

The main causes of CP are shown in Table 1.1. A proper history is the cornerstone of the evaluation of patients with CP. The patient should be asked about the location, the features, the radiations, the causes that trigger the pain, the duration, and the circumstances that worsen or relieve it (Table 1.2). Risk factors for coronary artery disease (CAD) should also be determined. The initial evaluation includes the assessment of vital signs, and auscultation of the heart and lungs.

TABLE 1.1	Causes of chest pain

1) Cardiovascular
a) Ischemic: angina on effort, unstable angina, acute myocardial infarction
b) Nonischemic: acute pericarditis, acute myocarditis, acute aortic dissection, acute pulmonary embolism, pulmonary hypertension

2) Noncardiovascular
a) Gastrointestinal diseases: gastroesophageal reflux, peptic ulcer paroxysm, diffuse esophageal spasm, acute pancreatitis, acute cholecystitis, etc.
b) Lung diseases: pneumothorax, pneumonia, pleurisy, etc.
c) Musculoskeletal: Tietze syndrome, degenerative spondyloarthropathy, herpes zoster, etc.
d) Neuroses: anxiety neurosis

TABLE 1.2	Description of chest pain from cardiovascular causes			
Disease	**Location**	**Character**	**Duration**	**Aggravating or relieving factors**
Stable angina or angina on effort	Retrosternal with radiations to the internal surface of upper limbs (left >right), neck and less often shoulders, lower jaw, back and epigastrium	Constrictive, squeezing, feeling of distress, burning or pressure, progressive establishment and abatement	2–10 min	Triggered by exercise, emotional stress, heavy meal, smoking, or exposure to cold air. Relieved by rest, removal of provocative factors or sublingual nitrates
Unstable angina	As stable angina	As stable angina but usually more severe	Usually >10 min*	As stable angina, but the triggering threshold is lower or the pain occurs at rest
Acute myocardial infarction	As stable angina	As stable angina but more severe	Usually >30 min	Not relieved by nitrates (may be partially resolved) or rest
Acute pericarditis	Retrosternal or precordial with radiation to the left trapezius muscle ridge or similar to angina	Sharp, stabbing, usually sudden onset	Hours or days	Aggravated by supine position, deep breathing, and coughing. Relieved by sitting up and leaning forward
Acute myocarditis	Retrosternal or precordial	As for myocardial ischemia or acute pericarditis		

TABLE 1.2	Description of chest pain from cardiovascular causes *(continued)*			
Disease	**Location**	**Character**	**Duration**	**Aggravating or relieving factors**
Acute pulmonary embolism	Retrosternal in the case of massive embolism or pleuritic in the case of peripheral embolism	Sudden onset with features of myocardial ischemic pain in the case of central obstruction or pleuritic pain in the case of peripheral obstruction		Aggravated by coughing and breathing (pleuritic pain)
Acute aortic dissection	Anterior surface of chest with radiation to the back	Sharp, very intense, sudden onset with maximum intensity at the start. Sometimes migratory	Usually hours	
Pulmonary hypertension	Retrosternal	Pressure, oppressive		Aggravated by effort

*When unstable angina is manifested as resting angina can last >20 min.

Basic examinations for the investigation of chest pain in the Emergency Room

- The electrocardiogram (ECG) should always be obtained even when the manifestation of the pain is atypical. If there is a suspicion of myocardial ischemia, even if the initial ECG is normal, it should be repeated after 1 or 2 h, or even later.
- Markers of myocardial necrosis: the preferred marker is cardiac troponin (cTn) I or T. In particular, if high sensitivity cTn (hs-cTn) assays are used they allow a more rapid "rule in" and "rule out" of acute myocardial necrosis. If cTn assays are not available creatine kinase MB isoenzyme (CK-MB) is determined (see also pages 23-24).
- D-dimers when acute pulmonary embolism (PE) or acute dissection of aorta is suspected.
- Arterial blood gases when there is concomitant dyspnea.
- The chest X-ray is used to rule out cardiomegaly, pulmonary congestion (in case of dyspnea), pneumothorax, pneumonia (in case of fever), pleuritic fluid, or to investigate the mediastinum, etc.
- Echocardiography (transthoracic) should be performed for any patient whose pain is likely to have a cardiovascular etiology:
  - acute myocardial ischemia: disturbances of systolic thickening of the myocardium (usually regional)
  - acute (wet) pericarditis: presence of pericardial fluid
  - acute PE: right ventricular dilation ± dysfunction ± mild (usually) pulmonary hypertension
  - acute myocarditis: disturbances of systolic thickening of the myocardium (usually diffuse)
  - acute dissection of the (proximal) aorta (sensitivity ~70%): distension of the ascending aorta + intimal flap within it ± pericardial fluid ± aortic valve regurgitation. In distal dissection, an intimal flap may be imaged in the aortic arch (suprasternal view) or in the abdominal aorta (subxiphoid view).

> **Warning!** If there are no disturbances of systolic myocardial thickening on the echocardiogram, this does not rule out the presence of myocardial ischemia. Note that if the ischemia is of small extent, there is not usually any visible segmental impairment of systolic myocardial thickening on the echocardiogram.

Special examinations for the investigation of chest pain
- When there is a suspicion (clinical ± echocardiographic) of acute aortic

dissection: transesophageal echocardiogram or computed tomography (CT) of the chest with contrast.
- When there is a suspicion (clinical ± echocardiographic) of acute PE: multi-detector chest CT pulmonary angiography (CTPA).

Differential diagnosis of the patient with chest pain

A) CARDIOVASCULAR CAUSES

1) Stable angina or angina on effort

Angina is due in >90% of cases to atheromatosis of the coronary arteries, that is the formation of atheromatous plaque that causes hemodynamically significant stenosis, leading to insufficient perfusion and myocardial ischemia. When the atheromatous plaque causes 70–90% diameter stenosis of the coronary artery lumen, angina is usually triggered when the myocardial oxygen needs increase, such as during physical exercise (increase in heart rate and systolic blood pressure [BP]), emotional stress (mainly an increase in heart rate), etc. This type of angina is known as stable angina or angina on effort. Coronary artery tone plays an important role in the occurrence of angina. Increased coronary artery tone or spasm can be responsible for causing angina even when the vessel has only a moderate degree of stenosis. Angina may also occur in individuals with "normal" coronary arteries (absence of hemodynamically significant stenoses i.e. <50% luminal stenosis), for example in aortic stenosis or hypertrophic cardiomyopathy, mainly because of the increased oxygen needs of the hypertrophic myocardium and the reduction in coronary flow due to the increase in wall stress during diastole. If there is also concomitant CAD, the threshold for an anginal episode is lowered.

CAD may manifest itself in any of the following forms:
- **Stable angina:** the pathological/anatomical substrate is stable atheromatous plaque that usually causes stenosis of the coronary artery lumen of the order of 70–90%.
- **Unstable angina:** the pathological/anatomical substrate is the rupture of vulnerable atheromatous plaque or superficial plaque erosion that causes severe stenosis (>90% luminal stenosis) of the coronary artery via the formation of a nonocclusive thrombus.
- **Acute myocardial infarction (AMI):** the pathological/anatomical substrate is the rupture of vulnerable atheromatous plaque that causes complete occlusion of the coronary artery via the formation of thrombus.
- **Sudden death:** the pathological/anatomical substrate is the rupture of vulnerable atheromatous plaque and the consequent formation of

TABLE 1.3	Characteristics of pain in stable angina

1) Retrosternal pain that is manifested as pressure, squeezing, burning, tightness, heaviness or discomfort that may be accompanied by nausea and sweating

2) Duration 2–10 min

3) Possible radiations (more rarely may be the only location): upper limbs (left >right), neck, lower jaw, back, etc.

4) Caused by physical exercise, emotional stress, consuming a heavy meal, exposure to cold, or smoking

5) Resolution within 2–5 min by rest or sublingual nitrates

thrombus in the coronary artery, or the presence of myocardial scar leading to fatal ventricular arrhythmias. This is the first manifestation of CAD in 20–25% of cases.

Under the latest classifications, unstable angina and AMI are categorized as acute coronary syndromes (ACSs), either with or without persistent ST-segment elevation. In particular, ACSs without persistent ST-segment elevation include unstable angina without concomitant detectable myocardial necrosis, and "unstable angina" with concomitant myocardial necrosis (elevated cTn), which is referred to as non ST-segment elevation myocardial infarction (NSTEMI). To avoid any confusion, in the current chapter we will refer to the older clinical definition of unstable angina, regardless of the presence or not of myocardial necrosis while AMI is identical to ST-segment elevation myocardial infarction.

Table 1.3 shows the characteristics of the pain of stable angina.

During history taking, the patient should always be asked about risk factors for CAD (Table 1.4). These risk factors do not include diabetes mellitus, because by itself it significantly increases the risk of developing CAD and it is considered to be almost equivalent to CAD. Indeed, the risk is considered to be very high when diabetes mellitus is accompanied by at least one risk factor for CAD and/or by target organ damage (e.g., microalbuminuria). In addition, the risk for CAD is very high in individuals who have peripheral artery disease, carotid disease (symptomatic or with carotid stenosis >50%), abdominal aortic aneurysm, or severe chronic kidney disease (glomerular filtration rate <30 mL/min/1.73 m^2). In general, if ≥2 risk factors for CAD, diabetes mellitus, vascular disease, or severe chronic kidney disease are seen in individuals who come to the Emergency Room with CP that is atypical of myocardial ischemia, then very careful evaluation is needed because of the high risk they run for the development of CAD.

TABLE 1.4	Risk factors for coronary artery disease (CAD)

1) Hypercholesterolemia (cholesterol >200 mg/dL or on hypolipidemic treatment)

2) Low HDL cholesterol (<40 mg/dL). In contrast, high HDL cholesterol (≥60 mg/dL) is a "negative" risk factor for CAD

3) Man aged ≥45 years or woman ≥55 years

4) Hypertension (blood pressure ≥140/90 mm Hg or on antihypertensive medication)

5) Cigarette smoking

6) Family history of premature CAD (CAD in father or brother <55 years or in mother or sister <65 years)

Table 1.5 shows the characteristics of CP that should divert us away from the diagnosis of angina.

Observations about the clinical manifestation of angina

- Sometimes, especially in diabetics and the elderly, the pain may be absent and the ischemia may manifest itself with equivalents to angina, such as dyspnea, fatigue, eructations, etc.
- Radiation of the pain to the upper limbs usually follows an ulnar distribution (inner surface of the arm and forearm, little and ring fingers) and is often described as numbness.
- The pain of angina increases progressively (crescendo pattern) and reaches its maximum intensity in about 30 s.
- Rarely, exertional angina may be reduced or even abolished:
  – with further exercise (walk-through angina) or

TABLE 1.5	Characteristics of chest pain not associated with angina (nonanginal pain)

1) Duration <1 min or many hours

2) Sharp character (like a stab, poke, jab, pinch, pinprick, or skewer)

3) Location in the breast region (usually indicated with one finger while for anginal pain uses a clenched fist)

4) Worsens with body movements or breathing

5) Reproduced when pressure is applied to the chest (local sensitivity)

6) Occurs without being preceded by triggering factors such as physical exercise, eating a heavy meal, exposure to cold, or smoking

 – on second exertion if separated from the first by a brief period of rest (warm-up or second wind angina).
- Sometimes angina is accompanied by epigastric discomfort or the latter may be the only manifestation.
- Concerning the therapeutic criterion for the administration of nitrates:
  a) The abatement of pain after taking sublingual nitrates is not a pathognomonic characteristic of angina, since because of the mechanism of action of nitrates (relaxation of smooth muscle fibers) CP from diffuse esophageal spasm is also relieved.
  b) If the pain does not subside within 5–10 min it is either severe ischemia (unstable angina or AMI) or pain of noncardiac origin.

Warning! In elderly people it is usual for the exertion of pressure on the chest to cause pain, and because of the patient's possible confusion or anxiety it may be described as similar to the pain that brought them to the hospital. Therefore, in these people and in those who have many risk factors, diabetes mellitus, vascular disease, or severe chronic kidney disease, reproduction of the pain during pressure on the chest should not rule out the coexistence of active myocardial ischemia and it is prudent to carry out a careful reevaluation of these patients after at least 1–2 h.

Clinical examination
The clinical findings in the patient with angina are usually poor.
1) Inspection: signs of dyslipidemia may be found, such as:
   - Corneal arcus: a white arc or circle in the periphery of the iris from the deposition of cholesterol in the cornea. When found in individuals <45 years old it is a sign of familial hypercholesterolemia (usually with cholesterol levels >300 mg/dL), an inherited genetic disorder of lipid metabolism causing premature CAD.
   - Xanthelasmas: yellow plaques on the eyelids, most commonly near the inner canthus, from the cutaneous deposition of cholesterol. Although they may be due to hypercholesterolemia, in most cases cholesterol levels are normal.
   - Xanthomas: nodular swellings that usually affect the Achilles tendon and are due to the accumulation of macrophages rich in cholesterol. Their presence is highly specific for familial hypercholesterolemia.
2) Auscultation of the heart: the following may be found:
   - 4th heart sound (increased intensity of the atrial kick due to reduction in left ventricular distensibility).
   - 3rd heart sound (in severe left ventricular dysfunction).

- Transient apical systolic murmur from mitral valve regurgitation (papillary muscle dysfunction caused by ischemia).
- In elderly people, aortic stenosis murmur. Moderate or severe aortic valve stenosis lowers the threshold for the occurrence of angina when there is concomitant CAD, while severe aortic stenosis may cause angina on effort even in the absence of significant CAD.

Warning! The presence of angina in severe aortic stenosis is an indication for valve replacement.

3) Auscultation of the carotid arteries and palpation of the peripheral arteries: atheromatosis is a multifocal disease and the finding of a bruit in the carotids or the absence of pulses in the periphery (peripheral artery disease) increases the probability of the coexistence of CAD in the examinee.

Basic examinations
1) ECG: the most common finding is ST-segment depression, followed by negative T-waves. However the ECG may also be normal during angina.
2) Chest X-ray: mainly to rule out cardiomegaly but also for the differential diagnosis from other causes of CP.
3) Complete blood count (to rule out anemia) and markers of myocardial necrosis (cTn I or T, CK-MB). Note that CK-MB is less sensitive and specific than cTn for the diagnosis of myocardial necrosis and its determination in the Emergency Room is usually unnecessary if it is feasible to determine cTn. We should keep in mind that when there is myocardial necrosis, cTn is usually detected elevated in the blood after the onset of CP within:
   - 1-6 h if hs-cTn assay is used (can be shorter with latest generation hs-cTn assays).
   - 3-12 h if non high-sensitivity cTn assay is used.

Warning! The diagnostic value of cTn should not be misinterpreted or overestimated. If the CP is suggestive of myocardial ischemia a very thorough clinical evaluation is mandatory, even if cTn is negative on repeated measurements, and the possibility of admission should be considered.

General instructions for the management of patients who come to the Emergency Room with angina or angina-like pain
a) In the case of unstable angina the patient is always admitted (see page 12).
b) In the case of angina on effort. The possibility of discharge should be considered if all the following apply:

- The pain has been relieved by taking one or two sublingual nitrate tablets and in general the total duration of the pain is <10 min.
- The patient is known to have CAD and has presented similar angina attacks in the past, which were relieved by taking one or two sublingual tablets.
- The features of unstable angina are absent.
- There are no pathological findings indicative of active ischemia on the initial ECG (or differences in comparison with an older ECG), or on a repeated ECG prior to discharge.
- cTn measurements are negative. If hs-cTn is used and two values measured 3 h apart are both normal, i.e. at presentation and 3 h later (0 h/3 h algorithm), then acute ischemic myocardial necrosis, mainly NSTEMI, can reliably be excluded if the patient remains pain free for the last 3 h. Note that a single negative hs-cTn at presentation is sufficient to rule out acute ischemic myocardial necrosis, if the CP occurred more than 6 h ago and the CP onset can be reliably assessed. We prefer to apply the 0 h/3 h algorithm in the majority of patients who present to the Emergency Room with an angina attack, particularly if the onset, duration and description of the pain are not reliable.

Patients should be advised to increase their antiischemic medication and to be reevaluated as soon as possible by their treating physician. It goes without saying that all patients with CAD, apart from antiischemic medication, should also be taking aspirin (75–100 mg per day) in the absence of any contraindication, statins (LDL cholesterol target is <70 mg/dL [according to the European Guidelines, Catapano AL, et al. Eur Heart J 2016; 37:2999-3058] or LDL cholesterol reduction ≥50% from the untreated baseline [according to the American Guidelines, Stone NJ, et al. Circulation 2014;129:S1-S45]) and should stop smoking if they are smokers. If the LDL cholesterol target is not achieved despite the administration of the maximally tolerated dose of statin, the addition of ezetimibe (10 mg daily) should be considered. In addition, they should also carry sublingual or inhaled nitrates for treating an anginal episode.

The fast action of nitrates when given sublingually is due to their rapid absorption by the rich venous net in the oral mucosa and the avoidance of the first-pass metabolism by the liver (venous drainage from the mouth is to the superior vena cava). In sublingual form there are tablets of isosorbide dinitrate and nitroglycerin. Of these two forms nitroglycerin has the faster action (within 1–2 min) in comparison with isosorbide dinitrate (within 3–4 min). This advantage, however, is significantly offset by the fact that nitroglycerin tablets should not be exposed to light because they spoil, and in addition their effect weakens after 6 months, so that they need to be re-

TABLE 1.6	Instructions for the use of sublingual nitrate tablets* or nitroglycerin spray in a patient with known coronary artery disease

1) For an episode of angina on effort that does not resolve after 2–3 min of rest, a sublingual nitrate tablet should be taken or nitroglycerin spray**applied below the tongue

2) The sublingual tablet is placed under the tongue and left to dissolve (not chewed) and the spray is also applied under the tongue

3) When the sublingual tablets or spray are used, the patient must remain seated for at least 20 min to avoid an episode of orthostatic hypotension that could occur when the patient suddenly stands up straight as soon as the pain recedes

4) During the use of the sublingual tablet or spray a seated posture is preferable to supine. The supine position, because it facilitates the return of venous blood to the heart from the lower limbs, partially counteracts the effect of the nitrates as regards the venostasis and the reduction of blood return to the heart

5) The interval between nitroglycerin (sublingual tablets or spray) doses if the angina does not abate is ~5 min

6) A patient who takes 2 sublingual tablets or 2 puffs in succession to relieve the pain should consult their cardiologist

7) If a patient is obliged to take more than 2 sublingual tablets or 2 sprays in succession because of the intensity of the pain, it is essential that they be transferred to hospital for e-valuation of the pain

8) The patient may take a sublingual tablet or spray as a precaution before activity that usually causes angina in order to prevent this

The term "nitrate tablets" refers to tablets of nitroglycerin or isosorbide dinitrate

**The usual dosage for sublingual medication is one 0.3 mg tablet of nitroglycerin, one 5 mg tablet of isosorbide dinitrate, while for the oral nitroglycerin spray each puff corresponds to 0.4 mg nitroglycerin*

placed. Table 1.6 provides instructions concerning the use of sublingual tablets of nitroglycerin or isosorbide dinitrate, or nitroglycerin given by oral sublingual spray (i.e. Nitrolingual Pumpspray, one puff delivers 0.4 mg nitroglycerin). Usually an anginal episode requires one or two puffs, according to the severity of the angina and the BP levels, into the oral cavity under the tongue during breath hold (should not be inhaled).

c) *In the case of CP that is atypical for angina.* The management of the patient who presents with CP that does not have the typical characteristics of angina, and that at the same time cannot be attributed to an extracardiac cause, is one of the most difficult diagnostic dilemmas and requires particular care. The management must be tailored to the patient and will depend on the experience of the doctor on duty and on the probability that the examinee has CAD based on the known risk factors. The patient should remain in the Emergency Room, preferably in a short-term care unit, for 6–12 h and should be reevaluated at regular intervals with repeated ECGs. If the patient does not exhibit any ECG changes or disturbances of systolic myocardial wall thickening on the echocardiogram, and has negative cTn measurements (i.e. at presentation and 3 h later [0 h/3 h algorithm] if hs-cTn is used or at presentation and 6-12 h later if non high-sensitivity assay is used) — they may be discharged with a recommendation for further investigation on a regular basis. However, the possibility of admission should be considered if:

- the pain continues
- the patient has ≥2 risk factors, suffers from diabetes mellitus, has vascular disease or severe chronic kidney disease, or
- there is even a small suspicion by the doctor on duty that the CP is of cardiac origin.

2) Unstable angina (see Chapter 3)

The definition of unstable angina is mainly clinical. It is very important to take a thorough history, since the decision about admission will be based on this, even in the absence of ECG changes or any increase in markers of myocardial necrosis. Every patient with unstable angina should be admitted to the cardiology department.

Unstable angina includes the following:

- Resting and prolonged (usually >20 min) angina.
- New-onset (<2 months) severe exertional angina.
- Recent deterioration of preexisting stable angina, i.e., more frequent, more intense, and more prolonged episodes of angina, or
- Postinfarction angina appearing within two weeks after the acute phase.

If the unstable angina is accompanied by increased cTn, then it is referred to as NSTEMI.

3) Acute myocardial infarction (see Chapter 2)

The pain from an AMI is typically very intense, constrictive, retrosternal, with a duration usually >30 min, not relieved by sublingual nitrates (or partially resolved), and accompanied by nausea, vomiting, pallor, and sweating. It usually shows radiation to the left or both upper limbs (usually ulnar distribution), the neck, the lower jaw, the shoulders, or more rarely to the epigastrium.

The main task of the doctor on duty is the prompt coordination of efforts that will allow rapid opening of the occluded coronary artery, by primary angioplasty when feasible, or by administration of fibrinolysis. This therapeutic intervention should be carried out as quickly as possible, in order to limit the loss of myocardial mass.

Observations on the clinical manifestations of acute myocardial infarction

- In ~10–20% of cases the pain is atypical. It may be located only in the epigastrium (sometimes observed in an inferior AMI), or may be manifested as dyspnea (left ventricular dysfunction) or confusion (cerebral hypoperfusion).
- The pain may be absent (silent AMI) in ~10% of cases. This most often applies to the elderly and diabetics.
- If the patient has had episodes of angina in the past, the pain from the AMI usually has the same location but is just more intense. This means that if the patient judges that the current pain is similar to that experienced during anginal episodes in the past, it should be taken seriously, even if it is atypical.

4) Acute pericarditis (see Chapter 6)

The pain is retrosternal or precordial, sudden and acute, lasting hours or days, usually radiating to the left trapezius muscle ridge, and exacerbated by inhalation, coughing, or a supine posture, while it is relieved by a seated posture with forward inclination of the body. It is sometimes located in the epigastrium, raising the question of a differential diagnosis from acute abdomen. Acute pericarditis is usually preceded by a viral syndrome.

The clinical suspicion may be confirmed by:
- Auscultation of a pericardial friction rub that is classically triphasic (systolic, early diastolic, and presystolic components), resembles the sound of new leather rubbing on leather, is heard better with the patient in a seated posture with the body inclined forward, and is dynamic (may be lost and reappear during the course of the disease).
- ECG: in the acute phase there is usually upward concave (saddle-shaped) ST-segment elevation in all leads (apart from aVR and V_1), depression of the PR-segment, etc.
- Echocardiography is the examination of choice for the detection and quantification of pericardial fluid (even as little as 15 mL), as well as the estimation of any hemodynamic compromise of the right cardiac chambers. It should be noted that normally the pericardial fluid is <50 mL and does not appear on ultrasound examination during the diastolic phase. In addition, left ventricular function can be evaluated for the possibility of myopericarditis or AMI. It should be stressed that the absence of fluid does not rule out the diagnosis of acute pericarditis, since the latter is often dry.
- Finally, the chest X-ray is of little value in the detection of pericardial fluid, unless there is a large effusion (there is cardiomegaly if the fluid is >250 mL).

The patient should be given nonsteroidal antiinflammatory drugs ±

colchicine, and should be admitted if there are unfavorable prognostic factors, such as temperature >38°C, myopericarditis, immunosuppression, large pericardial fluid accumulation, etc. (see page 107).

5) Acute myocarditis

This is an inflammatory disease of the myocardium, usually caused by a virus (parvovirus B19, enteroviruses, etc.) and more rarely by microbes, drugs, toxic substances, radiation, etc. It is accompanied by CP in ~30% of cases. The pain is usually of similar character to that of acute pericarditis, since in most cases it is due to involvement of the pericardium. Sometimes the pain is constrictive, retrosternal, and requires differential diagnosis from the pain of acute myocardial ischemia.

Acute myocarditis does not show specific clinical manifestations and in most cases the symptoms are absent, or there is a mild symptomatology that escapes diagnosis. Its clinical manifestation may occur during the infection or 2–3 weeks later. The spectrum of clinical manifestations includes fatigue (~80%), dyspnea on exertion (~80%), CP (as mentioned above), palpitations (~50%) [sinus tachycardia or extrasystoles], myalgia and more rarely acute heart failure or sudden death.

From the diagnostic examinations:

- Blood tests: complete blood count (eosinophilia may suggest eosinophilic myocarditis), cTn (variably elevated, in 35-70% of cases, depending partially on the chronicity of the process and on the assay of cTn used) and C-reactive protein (usually elevated but not specific). Measurement of serum viral antibody titers has a limited diagnostic value.
- The ECG (sensitivity <50%) shows sinus tachycardia, nonspecific changes of the ST-segment (sometimes ST-segment elevation without reciprocal ST-segment changes) and T-wave, disturbances of atrioventricular conduction, pathological Q-waves, extrasystoles, etc.
- The echocardiogram may show diffuse (or more rarely localized) hypokinesis of the left ventricle (less frequently of the right ventricle), increased thickness of the left ventricular walls (secondary to interstitial edema), diastolic dysfunction, pericardial effusion, etc.
- Cardiac magnetic resonance imaging (MRI) is the examination of choice. Myocardial tissue edema can be demonstrated by T2-weighted imaging, while gadolinium administration may show late subepicardial (usually) or midwall enhancement (regions of necrosis/fibrosis).
- Endomyocardial biopsy should be performed in selected cases.

Warning! In a young patient (usually <35 years) with a clinical and ECG picture of AMI, always consider in the differential diagnosis acute myocarditis. The possibility of acute myocarditis is high in the setting of virus infection (particularly, parvovirus B19 may cause spasm of coronary arteries and mimic AMI).

Clinical suspicion of this disease mandates the patient's admission under continuous ECG monitoring because of the increased risk of arrhythmias. Note than in ~20% of cases, acute myocarditis will progress to dilated cardiomyopathy.

6) Acute aortic dissection (see Chapter 8)

This is characterized by sudden, very intense pain (greatest intensity at the onset, in contrast to AMI, where the pain worsens progressively), throbbing, in the anterior chest region (proximal dissection), or between the shoulder blades and/or in the lower back (distal dissection), and is sometimes migratory in character during the course of the dissection. It may be accompanied by dyspnea and other symptoms from the extension of the dissection and the causing of stenosis or obstruction of the arteries during the course of the dissection, e.g., hemiplegia from obstruction of the innominate or the left common carotid artery.

Risk factors for acute dissection should be sought, such as hypertension, Marfan syndrome, etc.

The clinical examination should include cardiac auscultation for diastolic murmur suggestive of aortic valve regurgitation, palpation of all peripheral arteries (a lack of peripheral pulse is suggestive of acute dissection), and neurological evaluation.

Basic examinations include the ECG (mainly to rule out AMI), chest X-ray (looking for widening of the mediastinum), and according to the hospital's capabilities a contrast chest CT or transesophageal echocardiogram should be performed as quickly as possible to confirm the clinical suspicion (time delay = large increase in mortality) and arrange immediate referral to the cardiac surgery department.

7) Pulmonary embolism (see Chapter 4)

The clinical picture depends on the extent of the obstruction in the pulmonary arterial tree and the cardiopulmonary reserve. When there is obstruction of:

- A large central pulmonary artery branch, intense constrictive retrosternal CP usually develops (resembles that of AMI), which is associated with dyspnea ± shock. The presence of sustained hypotension (systolic BP <90 mmHg for at least 15 min) is defined as massive PE and has a poor prognosis.
- Moderate or small branches (this is the most usual), there is pain of pleuritic type, with or without concomitant dyspnea. Often the pain is absent and there is only the dyspnea.

From the history and the clinical examination we should be seeking:

- Factors that predispose to deep vein thrombosis: prolonged immobilization, hip or knee replacement, fracture of lower limb, major trauma,

congestive heart failure, previous venous thromboembolism, use of o-
ral contraceptives, etc.
- Signs of deep vein thrombosis of the lower limbs, since usually PE
complicates this disorder. However, clinical signs of thrombosis of
these veins are often absent.

Warning! Acute dyspnea in postoperative orthopedic patients (particularly
after total knee or hip replacement) should raise the suspicion of acute
pulmonary embolism.

The ECG and chest X-ray are of little value in the diagnosis, while for
small PEs arterial blood gases may be normal. In the Emergency Room, of
great assistance are the determination of D-dimers (negative values rule out
the disease when the clinical suspicion of PE is low or moderate), the echocardiogram (the presence of right ventricular dilation ± dysfunction suggests acute PE), and the multi-detector CTPA.

When PE is diagnosed, anticoagulation medication is started, while in
the case of massive PE fibrinolysis is also given.

8) Pulmonary hypertension
The most common symptom of pulmonary hypertension is dyspnea during exercise. Severe pulmonary hypertension may cause CP on effort with
features of angina (probably due to right ventricular ischemia).

From the clinical examination there may be a large a wave in the jugular
venous pulse, a left parasternal heave (from the right ventricle), and accentua-
tion of the 2nd heart sound from reinforcement of the pulmonary element.

From examinations:
- The chest X-ray may show dilation of the conus of the pulmonary artery and a reduction of lung perfusion in the periphery.
- The ECG may show signs of right ventricular hypertrophy (e.g. R-wave
in lead V_1 ≥7 mm, R/S in lead V_1 ≥1, etc.).
- The echocardiogram can estimate the dimensions and function of the
right ventricle and can quantify the degree of pulmonary hypertension
(measurement of the maximal velocity of tricuspid regurgitation).

B) NONCARDIAC CAUSES

1) Gastrointestinal disorders

a) Gastroesophageal reflux
This is a common disorder, affecting 10–20% of the general population.

It is characterized by acidic regurgitation, and epigastric or retrosternal burning pain lasting 10-60 min that is relieved by antacids, H_2-receptor antagonists or protein pump inhibitors and is triggered or worsens during lying down after ingesting food.

Examinations for the diagnosis are esophageal gastroscopy (in ~40% of cases there is damage to the esophageal mucosa) and 24-h pH monitoring in the lower esophagus.

b) Diffuse esophageal spasm

The pain may have clinical features that make it extremely difficult to differentiate it from ischemic cardiac pain. It usually manifests with retrosternal constrictive or burning pain and there may be radiation to the back, neck, and upper limbs. It may be triggered during effort and may also be relieved by sublingual nitrates or nifedipine (through relaxation of the smooth muscle fibers of the esophagus). Evidence to suggest diffuse esophageal spasm is the coexistence of dysphagia, or triggering of the pain on the consumption of very cold or hot beverages.

Examinations for the diagnosis are a barium meal with esophageal fluoroscopy and manometry.

c) Gastrointestinal disorders manifested by epigastralgia

Since an inferior AMI may sometimes be manifested as epigastralgia, it is possible for this pain to be incorrectly attributed to certain gastrointestinal disorders that are manifested as epigastric pain.

This occurs mainly with:

- **Paroxysm of a peptic ulcer.** The history is of great importance. Pain from a peptic ulcer abates in response to antacids, H_2-receptor antagonists, or proton pump inhibitors.
- **Acute pancreatitis,** which is characterized by epigastralgia with radiation to the lumbar region, vomiting, while there may also be hypotension. The basic diagnostic examination is the determination of blood amylase, which increases within 12 h from the appearance of pain and is considered diagnostic when its levels are >3 times the upper normal. Amylase loses its diagnostic value (false negative) in acute pancreatitis that is due to markedly elevated serum triglycerides (>1000 mg/dL). It should be noted that an increase in amylase is also observed in perforation or ischemic necrosis of the bowel.
- **Acute cholecystitis,** which is normally characterized by cramping pain in the right hypochondrium that may also radiate to the epigastrium.

The differential diagnosis may become extremely difficult when the acute pancreatitis or cholecystitis is accompanied by ECG changes such as negative T-waves or ST-segment depression, although these are rarely observed. It is prudent to record an ECG in every case of epigastralgia not typical for gastrointestinal disorder or epigastralgia and coexistent multiple risk factors for CAD. If the ECG is abnormal, then markers of myocardial necrosis should be determined.

Finally, in the case of severe retrosternal pain after intense vomiting, esophageal rupture, a rare condition which requires surgical intervention (Boerhaave syndrome), should be ruled out. In this case careful checking of the chest X-ray is required for the possible presence of air in the mediastinum, and subcutaneous cervical emphysema should also be checked for.

> **Warning!** In every patient with epigastralgia not typical for gastrointestinal disorder or epigastralgia + multiple risk factors for CAD, an ECG should always be performed to exclude inferior AMI.

2) Lung diseases

a) Pneumothorax

This is characterized by sudden unilateral acute pleuritic pain that is usually accompanied by dyspnea. In young males it is usually spontaneous, while in people aged >40 years it is usually a complication of chronic obstructive pulmonary disease.

During lung examination, hyperresonance to percussion and decreased breath and voice sounds are noted in the region of the pneumothorax. A small pneumothorax at the apex of the lungs can easily escape examination.

The diagnosis is made by chest X-ray in expiration, when a nonopacified and nonvascularized region is seen around the collapsed lung with or without mediastinal shift away from the involved side. In case of doubt, a chest CT should be performed.

b) Pneumonia and pleurisy

These two conditions are grouped together because usually pleurisy complicates pneumonia (extension of lung inflammation to the pleura). During inflammation of the pleura there is pain of pleuritic type, which is usually located below the mammary or in the axillary region, is sharp and intensifies during deep breathing or coughing. Lung auscultation reveals a pleural (friction) rub that is produced from the friction of the two inflamed pleural layers. This sound may be continuous (like low-pitched rhonchi) or intermittent (like fine crackles); it is heard during both phases of respiration, becomes louder when strong pressure is applied with the stethoscope to the chest and is not changed by coughing.

In lobular pneumonia, during lung examination, percussion reveals dullness and bronchial (tubular) breath sounds and crackles are heard on auscultation over the affected area. In addition, the patient exhibits fever, dyspnea, and productive cough. The diagnosis is usually confirmed by chest X-ray.

3) Musculoskeletal pain

a) Tietze syndrome (costochondritis)
The pain is long-lasting and is exacerbated by coughing and deep breaths. During chest examination fusiform swelling of the pleural chondra is found together with local sensitivity.

b) Degenerative spondyloarthropathy of the cervical and thoracic spine
This causes zosteroid pain in the anterior or posterior chest wall or in the neck. It often radiates to the upper limbs, is long-lasting, and is exacerbated by body movements or coughing.

c) Herpes zoster before rash eruption
If herpes zoster (shingles) involves thoracic dermotomes, CP can precede (prodromal phase) the eruption of blisters. CP has a unilateral dermatomal distribution (belt-like pattern limited to one side of the chest). There is usually also skin sensitivity. The appearance of the characteristic blisters occurs 4-5 days after the onset of pain.

d) Chest wound
There is a history of injury and during clinical examination there is local sensitivity in the wound region. An appropriate radiological examination is carried out to rule out bone fracture, such as fracture of the ribs, sternum, etc.

4) Neurotic pain
This is a frequent reason, especially in young women, for coming to the Emergency Room. The most common cause is anxiety neurosis. The pain is usually located in the left mammary region (usually pointed out with the forefinger), is acute (like a stab, electric shock, or pinch), lasts for a few seconds, usually occurs at rest, and is not related to effort. Examinees are likely to complain about "gasping for breath" (can't get enough air), numbness, and weakness. Sometimes the pain may last many hours and/or days.

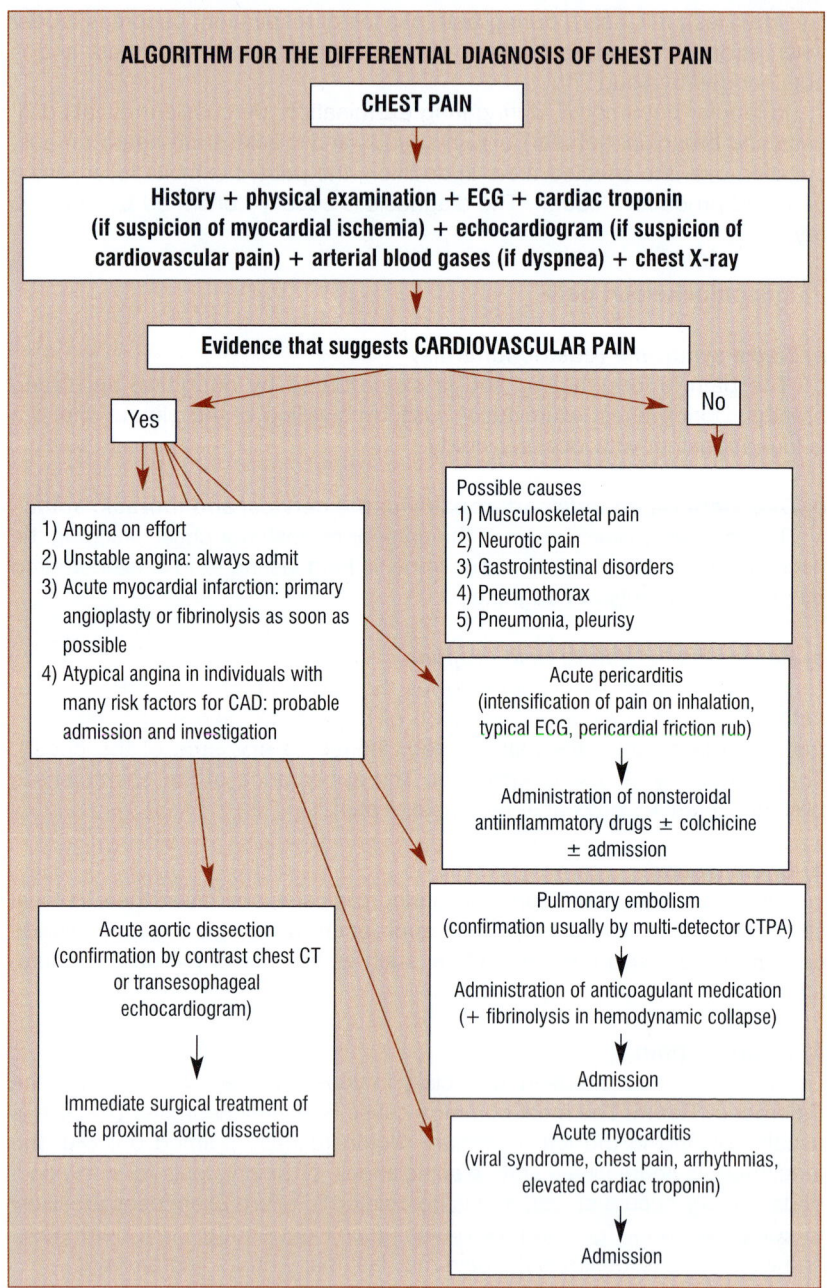

ALGORITHM FOR THE DIFFERENTIAL DIAGNOSIS OF CHEST PAIN

CHEST PAIN

History + physical examination + ECG + cardiac troponin (if suspicion of myocardial ischemia) + echocardiogram (if suspicion of cardiovascular pain) + arterial blood gases (if dyspnea) + chest X-ray

Evidence that suggests CARDIOVASCULAR PAIN

Yes

No

1) Angina on effort
2) Unstable angina: always admit
3) Acute myocardial infarction: primary angioplasty or fibrinolysis as soon as possible
4) Atypical angina in individuals with many risk factors for CAD: probable admission and investigation

Possible causes
1) Musculoskeletal pain
2) Neurotic pain
3) Gastrointestinal disorders
4) Pneumothorax
5) Pneumonia, pleurisy

Acute pericarditis
(intensification of pain on inhalation, typical ECG, pericardial friction rub)

Administration of nonsteroidal antiinflammatory drugs ± colchicine ± admission

Acute aortic dissection
(confirmation by contrast chest CT or transesophageal echocardiogram)

Immediate surgical treatment of the proximal aortic dissection

Pulmonary embolism
(confirmation usually by multi-detector CTPA)

Administration of anticoagulant medication (+ fibrinolysis in hemodynamic collapse)

Admission

Acute myocarditis
(viral syndrome, chest pain, arrhythmias, elevated cardiac troponin)

Admission

CT: computed tomography, CTPA: CT pulmonary angiography, CAD: coronary artery disease

2

Acute myocardial infarction with ST-segment elevation

Acute myocardial infarction (AMI)* is the leading cause of death in developed societies. The mortality from AMI has declined steadily over the past 30 years. This is due to the improvement in therapy, mainly the development of coronary care units and early reperfusion (primary percutaneous coronary intervention [PCI] or fibrinolysis). The in-hospital mortality of patients with AMI is 5-10%, while in patients without comorbidities it is even lower.

According to the current classification, acute coronary syndromes (ACSs) include:

a) ST-segment elevation myocardial infarction (STEMI), 25% of all ACSs.

b) Non ST-segment elevation ACS, which comprises:

- Unstable angina (absence of myocardial necrosis) and
- Non ST-segment elevation myocardial infarction (NSTEMI) [presence of myocardial necrosis].

AMI is usually caused by complete occlusion of an epicardial coronary artery following the formation of thrombus on a vulnerable ruptured atheromatous plaque (Table 2.1). Local arterial spasm usually contributes to the occlusion. After ~20-30 min of acute total coronary artery occlusion, if there is no collateral circulation, myocardial necrosis begins in the subendocardium. If myocardial ischemia persists, necrosis progresses in a wavefront pattern from the subendocardium into the subepicardium resulting in transmural necrosis. The degree of left ventricular dysfunction depends on the extent of myocardial necrosis.

TABLE 2.1	Characteristics of atheromatous plaque vulnerable to rupture

- Usually cause <50% luminal stenosis
- Large lipid core
- Intense inflammatory infiltration
- Thin fibrous cap

---

*Throughout the book the term AMI is identical to the term STEMI. The only exceptions are the section "Notes on the myocardial necrosis markers" on page 27 and page 30

Symptoms

1) Typical: severe, crushing, retrosternal pain/discomfort (described as a squeezing, constricting, compressing or burning sensation) usually lasting >30 min, not relieved by nitroglycerin (or partially resolved) or rest and accompanied by nausea, vomiting, pallor and sweating. The pain may radiate to:
   - Left upper extremity (usually ulnar distribution) or both extremities and may produce a tingling sensation or numbness.
   - Neck.
   - Lower jaw.
   - Shoulders.
   - Interscapular region.
   - Epigastrium (usually in inferior AMI, in which case other diagnoses such as acute cholecystitis, peptic ulcer, etc., must be ruled out).
2) Atypical (in ~10-20% of cases, usually in elderly people):
   - Acute dyspnea with no pain.
   - Profuse weakness.
   - Syncope.
   - Acute confusion.
   - Acute indigestion.
   - Peripheral embolization.
3) Silent (asymptomatic) AMI: usually in diabetic or elderly patients.

Warning! Occasionally in AMI, there may be no pain present in the chest (retrosternal), but only in the radiation areas.

Clinical signs

1) Sinus tachycardia: the degree of tachycardia usually reflects the degree of left ventricular dysfunction. Inferior AMI is an exception, where ~50% of cases are accompanied by sinus bradycardia.
2) Hypotension (systolic blood pressure [BP] <90 mmHg) observed in:
   - Cardiogenic shock, as a consequence of a large AMI or mechanical complications of an AMI (ventricular septal rupture [VSR] or papillary muscle rupture).
   - Inferior AMI, as a consequence of parasympathetic stimulation (Bezold–Jarisch reflex).
   - Inferior AMI with involvement of the right ventricle (especially following administration of nitrates).
   - Dehydration-hypovolemia due to vomiting ± profuse sweating.
3) 3rd heart sound in acute heart failure (usually indicates severe left ventricular dysfunction).

4) 4th heart sound (of no diagnostic value as it is heard in the acute phase of almost all myocardial infarctions).

5) Systolic murmur at the apex of the heart, usually with crescendo to the 2nd heart sound, which indicates mitral valve regurgitation due to ischemic dysfunction of the papillary muscle.

6) Loud holosystolic murmur (weaker in shock) lower left parasternally (± thrill) due to VSR (occurs in <0.5% with reperfusion therapy, usually within 5 days). An immediate echocardiogram is required to confirm this diagnosis. Note that VSR associated with anterior AMI is located in the apical septum while those associated with inferior AMI are located in the basal inferior septum. Therefore, during the emergent echocardiogram, if you do not focus at the apex using color Doppler (4-chamber view), you might miss an apical VSR.

7) Holosystolic murmur of variable intensity at the apex of the heart, usually due to rupture of a papillary muscle head (the posteromedial papillary muscle has 1-3 heads while the anterolateral has 1 head) [occurs in ~1% with reperfusion therapy, usually within 5 days]. The rupture of the head of the posteromedial (single blood supply from posterior descending artery) is more common than that of the anterolateral papillary muscle (dual blood supply from anterior descending and circumflex artery). An immediate e-chocardiogram is required to confirm this diagnosis.

8) In acute left heart failure, crackles at the base (or higher) of both lungs.

9) >24 h, pericardial friction rub (present in ~10%).

Warning! Extreme vigilance is required when in the acute phase of the infarction we have: heart rate <50 or >100 beats/min, >20 breaths/min, systolic BP <90 mmHg, and O_2 saturation <90%.

Serum markers of myocardial necrosis

1) **Creatine kinase (CK).** CK activity is detected at pathological levels within 4-8 h of AMI and returns to normal levels within 3-4 days (Table 2.2). The absence of this type of response (quick rise – quick fall), with high levels maintained for several days (plateau), suggests a musculoskeletal origin for CK or acute myocarditis. There are 3 CK isoenzymes:
   - CK-MM: found in the skeletal (main source) and cardiac muscle.
   - CK-BB: found in the brain, and in the gastrointestinal and urinary systems.
   - CK-MB: found in the cardiac muscle (main source), skeletal muscle (1-3% of total CK), and in small amounts in the small intestine, the tongue, the esophagus, the diaphragm, the uterus and the prostate.

In the past, only CK-MB activity (U/mL) was determined and was considered diagnostic for AMI when it was >5% of the total CK activity. Today it is preferable to determine CK-MB mass (ng/mL), which is considered more specific (immunoenzyme technique) than activity. As CK-MB is found in small amounts in the skeletal muscles, it also increases in muscle injuries, myopathies, electrocution, burns, rhabdomyolysis, and very intense physical exercise. The CK-MB mass limits for AMI diagnosis depend on the method of measurement.

2) **Myoglobin.** This is the earliest detectable marker, but it lacks specificity because of its large concentration in skeletal muscles. It has a high negative predictive value. It appears within 1-4 h of AMI.

3) **Cardiac troponins.** Troponin is a protein complex made up of the units troponin C, troponin I and troponin T. It is bound to the actin molecule and plays a regulatory role in the contraction of skeletal and cardiac muscle cells. There are various troponin isoforms in skeletal and cardiac muscle cells. Using specific antibodies, it is feasible to detect only cardiac troponins (cTn) I and T, which are not normally detected in the blood. They are found in the blood 3-12 h after myocardial necrosis (non high-sensitivity assays), even following minimal necrosis. The threshold for myocardial necrosis is the 99th percentile of the reference population and the cutoff value may differ according to the cTn assay used. Evaluation of cTn values is always performed with reference to the clinical findings. In the case of AMI, the cTn values usually increase within 3-12 h, peak within 12-24 h and gradually recede within a few days (Figure 2.1.A). In certain cases of myocardial ischemia, there may be a mild increase in cTn without a concomitant increase in CK-MB. In this case there is minimal myocardial necrosis and the detection period for cTn in

TABLE 2.2	Times of onset, maximum concentration, and return to normal of myocardial necrosis markers in the blood following acute ischemia		
	Onset (hours)	Maximum concentration (hours)	Return (days)
Myoglobin	1-4	6-12	1
CK (activity)	4-8	12-24	3-4
CK-MB (mass)	3-8	12-24	3
Troponin I*	3-12	12-24	3-10
Troponin T*	3-12	12-24	5-14

*Refers to non high-sensitivity cardiac troponin

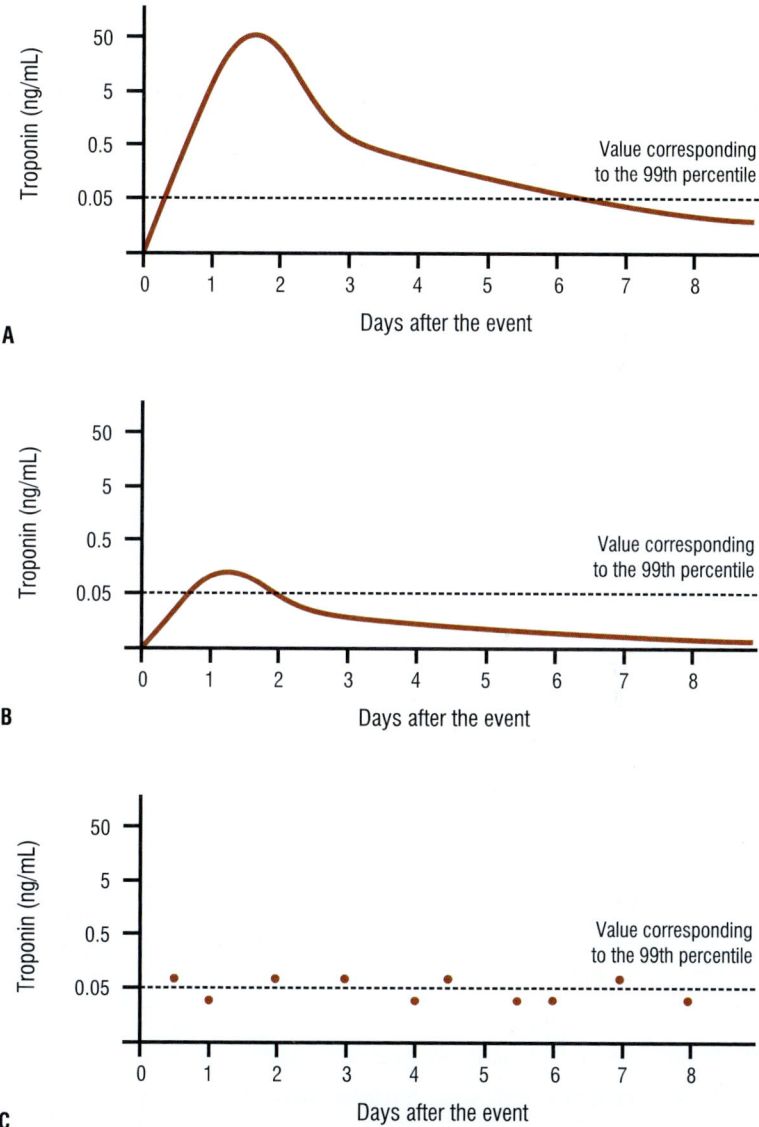

Figure 2.1. Curves displaying onset, peak and reduction of cardiac troponin levels in **A)** acute myocardial infarction, **B)** minimal myocardial necrosis, and **C)** acute myocarditis. (From Melanson SE, et al. Circulation 2007;116;e501-4, with permission).

the blood is shorter than in classical AMI (Figure 2.1.B). It must also be stressed that the detection of cTn in the blood indicates myocardial necrosis but does not determine the mechanism of the necrosis. Thus, the presence of cTn in the blood without concomitant clinical or ECG findings indicative of acute myocardial ischemia mandates a search for other pathological situations that may be accompanied by elevated cTn levels (Table 2.3). In acute myocarditis, cTn levels usually present a mild increase and may remain stable at these levels for days to weeks (Figure 2.1.C). The diagnosis of acute ischemic myocardial necrosis is particularly challenging in patients with chronic kidney disease and chest pain, a population with a markedly high prevalence of coronary artery disease (CAD), because it is common for them to have elevated cTn levels in the absence of an ACS. Reliance on serial cTn measurements is mandatory.

TABLE 2.3	Situations demonstrating increased cardiac troponin levels

1) Myocardial necrosis following ischemia

2) Acute myocarditis or myopericarditis

3) Acute pulmonary embolism

4) Sepsis (~45%)

5) Chronic kidney disease

6) Acute or chronic severe heart failure

7) Takotsubo cardiomyopathy

8) Heart injury (blunt or penetrating)

9) Cerebrovascular accident (ischemic or hemorrhagic stroke) [10-20%]

10) Severe anemia

11) Severe respiratory failure

12) Acute aortic dissection (~15%)

13) Arrhythmias (mainly tachycardia with hemodynamic deterioration)

14) Following open heart surgery

15) Chemotherapeutic cardiotoxic agents (adriamycin, 5-fluorouracil, etc.)

16) Infiltrative heart disease (amyloidosis, hemochromatosis, etc.)

17) Severe burns (>30% of body surface)

18) Electrical cardioversion or radiofrequency catheter ablation

19) Very intense physical exercise

Notes on the myocardial necrosis markers

- For the detection of myocardial necrosis, the test of choice is the determination of cTn. If this cannot be measured, or if there is clinical suspicion of a reinfarction several days ago, CK-MB should be determined because of its shorter half-life in circulation.
- Aspartate aminotransferase (AST or SGOT) and lactate dehydrogenase (LDH) are deprecated today because of their low specificity and the introduction of cTn.
- Myocardial necrosis markers are required for the detection of myocardial necrosis, but in no case should they delay reperfusion therapy, which must be applied as soon as possible if there are clinical and ECG indications of AMI.
- In order to fulfill the criteria for the diagnosis of AMI (type 1, i.e. STEMI and NSTEMI) [Thygesen K, et al. Eur Heart J 2012;33:2551-67] the detection of a rise and/or fall of markers of myocardial necrosis (preferably cTn), with at least one value >99th percentile of the reference population, should be accompanied by at least one of the following:
  - symptoms consistent with myocardial ischemia.
  - new ischemic ECG changes or new left bundle branch block (LBBB).
  - development of pathological Q waves.
  - imaging demonstration (usually echocardiographic, especially in the Emergency Room) of new regional wall motion abnormality.
  - identification of an intracoronary thrombus by angiography or autopsy.
- An AMI complicating a percutaneous coronary intervention (PCI) [type 4a] is defined by an increase in cTn to >5 x 99th percentile of the reference population (within 48 h), when the baseline levels are normal, or a >20% increase if the initial levels are elevated and are stable or falling. Also, at least one of the following must be present:
  - symptoms consistent with myocardial ischemia.
  - new ischemic ECG changes or new LBBB.
  - angiographic findings consistent with a procedural complication.
  - imaging demonstration of new regional wall motion abnormality.
- An AMI complicating a coronary artery bypass grafting (type 5) is defined by an increase in cTn to >10 x 99th percentile of the reference population, when the baseline levels are normal. Additionally, at least one of the following must be present:
  - new pathological Q waves or new LBBB.
  - angiographic findings consistent with new occlusion of a graft or native coronary artery.
  - imaging evidence of new regional wall motion abnormality.

What is type 2 myocardial infarction?

It is a form of myocardial infarction that has come under the spotlight in recent years (Thygesen K, et al. Eur Heart J 2012;33:2551-67) and has an unfavorable prognosis. In type 2 myocardial infarction, the myocardial necrosis (detected as a rule via an increase in cTn) is not due to athe-rothrombotic obstruction of a coronary artery but to a disturbance of my-ocardial oxygen supply and/or demand. Table 2.4 shows the conditions that may be complicated by type 2 myocardial infarction. It is a type of infarction that is encountered not infrequently by the doctor on call in surgical depart-ments, e.g. in postsurgical patients, or in internal medicine departments, e.g. in patients with severe anemia, and its treatment can give rise to many concerns. Note that the differential diagnosis of type 2 myocardial infarction from nonischemic myocardial necrosis (e.g. in sepsis) may sometimes be extremely difficult.

Evidence suggestive of type 2 myocardial infarction includes the following:
1) The presence of conditions that reduce the myocardial oxygen supply and/or increase the demand.
2) The ECG usually shows mild, nonspecific changes, or may be normal. Note that ST-segment elevation is rarely seen.
3) Typical anginal syndrome is usually absent.
4) The increase in cTn is usually small.
5) If cardiac catheterization is performed in these patients, it does not re-veal any culprit ruptured plaque with consequent thrombosis.

TABLE 2.4	Conditions that may lead to the development of type 2 myocardial in-farction.
Reduction in myocardial oxygen supply	**Increase in myocardial oxygen demand**
• Severe anemia (hemoglobin concentration <5.5 mmol/L [~8.9 g/dL] for men and <5.0 mmol/L [~8.0 g/dL] for women) • Sustained hypotension (systolic blood pressure <90 mmHg) • Bradyarrhythmia requiring medical treatment or cardiac pacing • Respiratory failure with severe hypoxemia (partial pressure of oxygen <60 mmHg) lasting ≥20 min • Coronary artery spasm, coronary endothelial dysfunction or coronary embolism	• Tachycardia (>150 beats/min) lasting ≥20 min • Severe arterial hypertension with concomitant left ventricular hypertrophy

The wide use of cTn today, particularly the high-sensitivity assay, has increased the number of patients who are diagnosed with type 2 myocardial infarction. The management of these patients, beyond the treatment of the underlying oxygen supply-demand imbalance, presents a therapeutic dilemma. Depending on the clinical condition coronary angiography may be indicated and if CAD is present, the appropriate treatment should be considered.

High-sensitivity cardiac troponin

A significant advance in the detection of myocardial necrosis is the development of techniques to determine very low cTn levels. Thus, with the high-sensitivity cTn technique (hs-cTn), troponin can be measured at pg/mL levels (note that 1 pg/mL = 1 ng/L), which was unfeasible with previous methods. The role of hs-cTns is essential for the diagnosis of NSTEMI.

The dividing line for detecting myocardial necrosis by hs-cTn is >99th percentile of the healthy population and this value is assay-specific. Determination of hs-cTn allows a quick diagnosis of ischemic myocardial necrosis from plaque rupture and thrombus formation (e.g. peripheral embolization of arterioles/capillaries by detached components from a central nonoclussive thrombus in NSTEMI) and thus rapid treatment. It also allows faster ruling out of ischemic myocardial necrosis. In particular, by applying the 0 h/3 h algorithm (i.e. measurements of hs-cTn at presentation and 3 h later) the "rule-in" and "rule-out" of acute ischemic myocardial necrosis can reliably be performed within 3 h. The recent European Guidelines (Roffi M, et al. Eur Heart J 2016;37:267-315) also recommend the 0 h/1 h algorithm (i.e. measurements of hs-cTn at presentation and 1 h later and reliance mainly on their absolute change) as an alternative to the 0 h/3 h algorithm, provided that the available hs-cTn assay has been validated for this. However, if the patient presents very early (i.e. <1 h from pain onset), the 0 h/3 h algorithm should be preferred. Figure 2.2 presents the main conditions with elevated hs-cTn levels.

The price of detecting minimal or mild myocardial necrosis is:
1) An increase in the number of NSTEMI cases at the expense of unstable angina (diagnostic shift).
2) An "overdiagnosis" of myocardial necrosis in CAD. As there may be a small hs-cTn increase in stable CAD, in some cases this may raise the issue of differential diagnosis from NSTEMI accompanied by minimal myocardial necrosis. In these cases, a study of hs-cTn kinetics is required, which entails repeated measurements.
3) The large increase in the number of patients with small-scale myocardial necrosis due to mechanisms other than acute myocardial ischemia (e.g. heart failure, chronic renal failure, etc.).

A proposed algorithm for the evaluation of hs-cTnT levels, using the cut-off point of 14 ng/L (the 99th percentile of a healthy population, Roche Diagnostic assay), is as follows (White HD. Am Heart J 2010;159:933-6):

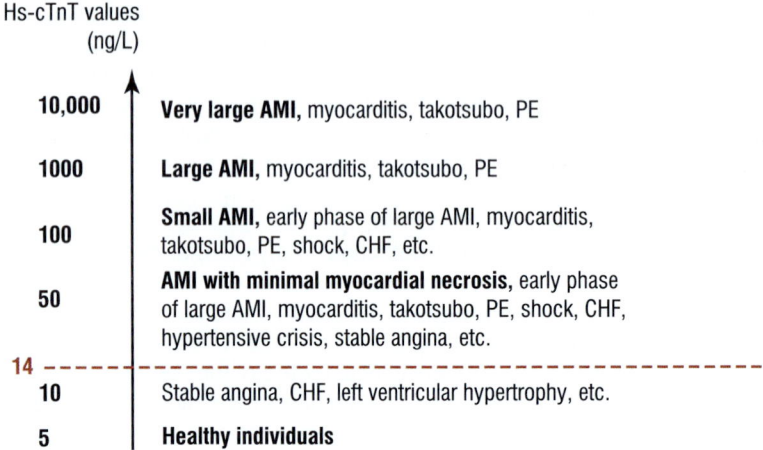

Hs-cTnT values
(ng/L)

10,000	**Very large AMI,** myocarditis, takotsubo, PE
1000	**Large AMI,** myocarditis, takotsubo, PE
100	**Small AMI,** early phase of large AMI, myocarditis, takotsubo, PE, shock, CHF, etc.
50	**AMI with minimal myocardial necrosis,** early phase of large AMI, myocarditis, takotsubo, PE, shock, CHF, hypertensive crisis, stable angina, etc.
14	
10	Stable angina, CHF, left ventricular hypertrophy, etc.
5	**Healthy individuals**

Figure 2.2. The differential diagnosis of high-sensitivity cardiac troponin T (hs-cTnT) depends to a large extent on its levels. (From Twerenbold R, et al. Eur Heart J 2012;33:579-86, with permission). *AMI: acute myocardial infarction, PE: pulmonary embolism, CHF: congestive heart failure*

1) Values <14 ng/L are considered normal. If the clinical setting is consistent with myocardial ischemia, the determination of hs-cTn should be repeated 6 h later. Repeated levels <14 ng/L rule out acute ischemic myocardial necrosis.
2) Values in the range ≥14 to <53 ng/L fall in the gray zone and hs-cTnT determination must be repeated after 3 h. If there is a change (increase or decrease) in the new value of
   a) ≥50%, this confirms acute ischemic myocardial necrosis.
   b) <50%, the test must be repeated after 6, 12 h, etc., if there is a clinical suspicion of myocardial necrosis.
3) Values ≥53 ng/L are pathological. The greater the troponin level, the more likely it is due to an AMI (Figure 2.2). To confirm the AMI, hs-cTnT kinetics must be studied, with measurement repeated after 3 h. If there is a hs-cTnT change of
   a) ≥20%, this confirms acute ischemic myocardial necrosis.
   b) <20%, measurements must be repeated after 6, 12 h, etc., if there is a clinical suspicion of myocardial necrosis.

Warning! Before the doctor on call applies a hs-cTn algorithm, i.e. the 0 h/3 h algorithm, to "rule-in" or "rule-out" an acute ischemic myocardial necrosis, they should know the cutoff values of the particular assay used in their laboratory and interpret hs-cTn levels in conjunction with the clinical assessment and the ECG.

ECG

The ECG presents a succession of changes: peaked T-waves (hyperacute phase) → convex upward ST-segment elevation (persisting for a few hours) → return of the ST-segment to baseline and negative T-waves (T-waves become negative before the return of the ST-segment to baseline) → appearance of pathological Q-waves.

In more detail: the earliest ECG finding (<15 min) is peaked symmetrical T-waves in the AMI region (Figure 2.3) developing into ST-segment elevation, which is the usual picture when the patient comes to the Emergency Room. The elevation is convex upward, it involves ≥2 contiguous leads and is ≥1 mm (0.1 mV)*. In the particular case of leads V_2-V_3, the elevation must

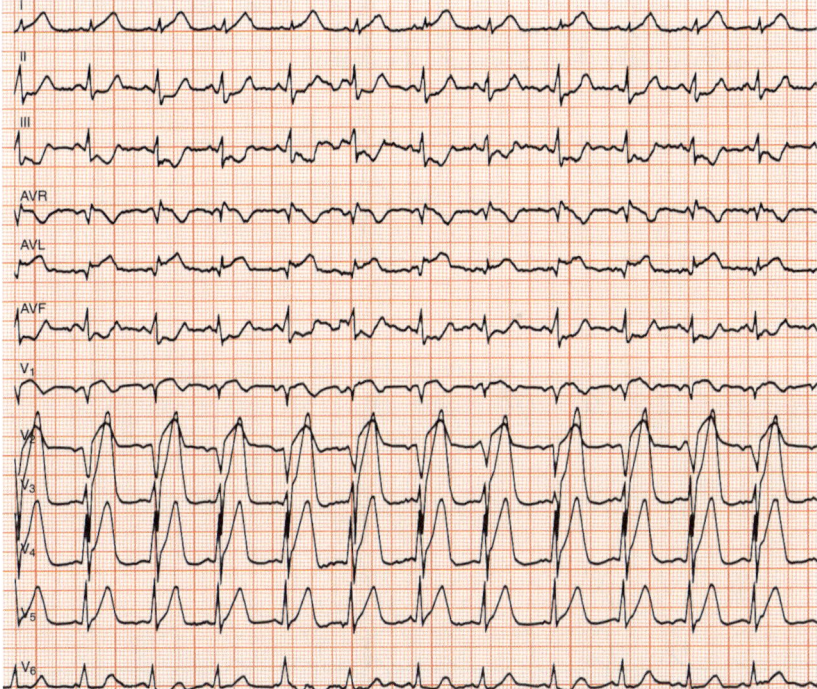

Figure 2.3. The ECG records peaked T-waves in leads V_3-V_5 that indicate a hyperacute phase of myocardial infarction. At the same time, ST-segment elevation (convex upward) is displayed in leads V_1, V_2 and aVL, and reciprocal ST-segment depression in leads II, III and aVF. This is an extensive anterior acute myocardial infarction.

ST-segment elevation is measured at the J-point (junction between the terminal portion of the QRS complex and the beginning of the ST-segment)

be ≥2 mm in men ≥40 years (or ≥2.5 mm in men <40 years) and ≥1.5 mm in women.

The ECG picture shows dynamic variation. ST-segment elevation soon begins to decline progressively towards the isoelectric line (the speed of the decline depends on the promptness and the success of reperfusion). At the same time, the T-wave starts to become negative and Q-waves appear (duration ≥40 ms and Q/R ≥25%). Negative T-waves may persist for a few months, while the Q-waves are often lifelong.

Location of AMI based on ECG findings in the acute phase
- ST-segment elevation in leads V_1-V_6 + I, aVL: **extensive anterior** AMI (proximal occlusion of the anterior descending artery).
- ST-segment elevation in leads V_1-V_4: **anteroseptal** AMI (occlusion in the mid or distal anterior descending artery). In a distal occlusion, lead V_1 does not usually show ST-segment elevation.

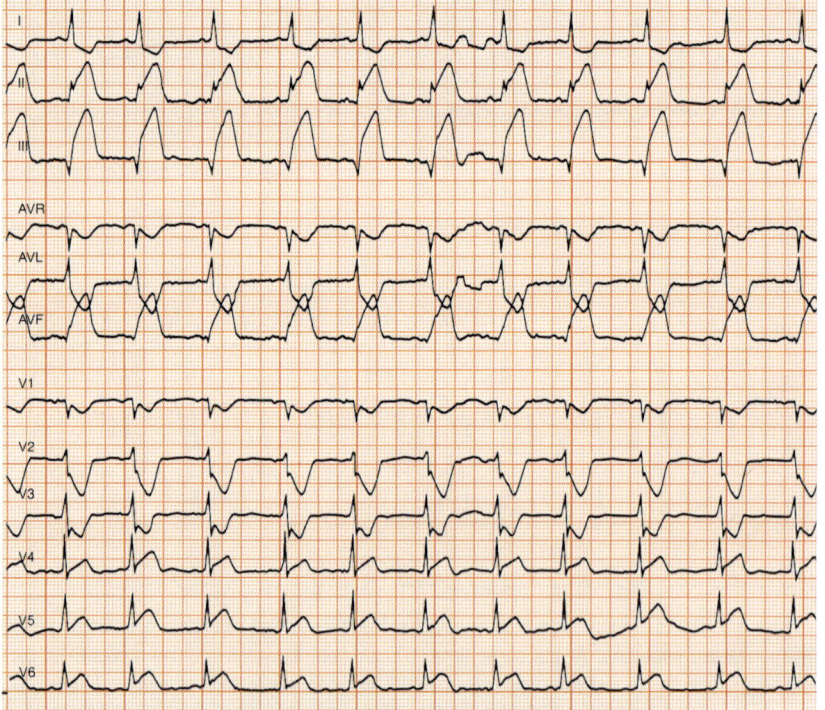

Figure 2.4. The ECG shows ST-segment elevation (convex upward) in leads II, III, aVF, V_5 and V_6, indicative of an acute inferior myocardial infarction with involvement of the lateral wall. There are also reciprocal ST-segment changes in leads V_1-V_3.

- ST-segment elevation in leads II, III and aVF: **inferior** AMI (distal occlusion of the right coronary artery in 85-90% or the left circumflex artery in 10-15% of cases) [Figure 2.4].
- ST-segment elevation in leads I, aVL + V_5, V_6: **lateral** AMI (occlusion of the left circumflex artery or the first [usually] diagonal branch of the anterior descending artery).
- ST-segment elevation in posterior leads V_7-V_9 (≥0.5 mm): **posterior** AMI (occlusion of the left circumflex artery or the right coronary artery and frequently associated with either lateral or inferior AMI, respectively).
- ST-segment elevation in leads V_3R and V_4R ≥0.5 mm (≥1 mm in men <30 years) + ST-segment elevation in leads II, III and aVF: inferior AMI with concomitant **right ventricular** infarction (proximal occlusion of the right coronary artery) [Thygesen K, et al. Eur Heart J 2012;33:2551-67] (Figure 2.5).

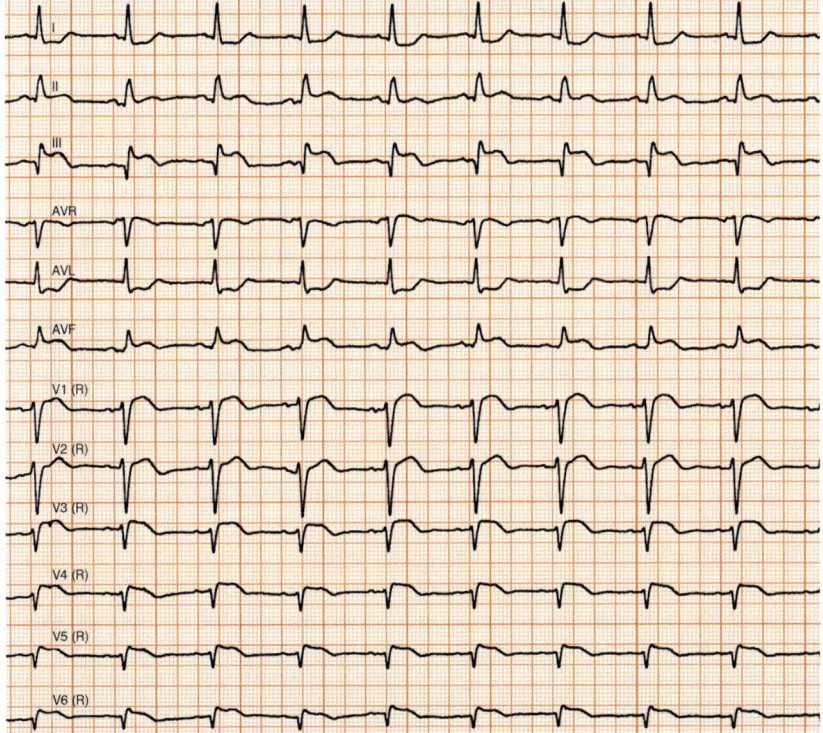

Figure 2.5. The ECG shows ST-segment elevation in leads II, III and aVF, indicative of acute inferior myocardial infarction. The precordial leads that are placed in the right parasternal region, so as to reflect the standard precordial sites, show ST-segment elevation (>1 mm in leads V_3R and V_4R) indicative of right ventricular infarction.

Warning! Acute left main coronary artery occlusion is rarely observed and has a poor prognosis (usually sudden death or cardiogenic shock). ECG findings are: ST-segment elevation in leads aVR and V_1 (aVR >V_1) + ST-segment depression in leads II, aVF, and V_3-V_6 (most evident in V_4) ± right bundle branch block (RBBB).

Notes on ECG findings in AMI

- In posterior AMI, as the precordial leads do not "see" the infarct region, the changes recorded are reciprocal. Thus, ST-segment depression in leads V_1-V_2 of ≥0.5 mm (corresponding to the acute phase of the myocardial infarction and "equivalent" to the ST-segment elevation), or an R/S ≥1 in leads V_1-V_2 (the R wave is "equivalent" to the Q-wave) with a positive, tall and symmetrical T-wave ("equivalent" to the negative T-wave) in the same leads, raises the suspicion of a posterior AMI. In this case, posterior leads V_7-V_9 must also be recorded, so that in the acute phase there will be ST-segment elevation ≥0.5 mm (≥1 mm in men <40 years) in ≥2 leads. It must be noted that the ECG findings of a posterior AMI are usually accompanied by ischemic changes in the lateral or inferior wall.
- Posterior leads V_7-V_9 are recorded at the same level as V_6. More specifically, the electrode for V_7 is placed at the left posterior axillary line, V_8 at the inferior tip of the left scapula, and V_9 left paravertebrally.
- The right-sided precordial leads V_2R-V_6R are recorded by placing the electrodes to the right and parasternally, so as to reflect the corresponding left leads. For every inferior AMI the right-sided precordial leads must be recorded as soon as possible, because elevation in these leads has a much shorter duration than elevation in the inferior wall leads.

Treatment

Before any treatment is started, the patient must be connected to the defibrillator monitor so that the heart rhythm can be observed and defibrillation applied immediately should ventricular fibrillation occur (in 3-5% of cases), or ventricular tachycardia with hemodynamic deterioration. The primary therapeutic target is to institute reperfusion as soon as possible by **fibrinolysis** or **PCI.** The Indications of antithrombotic therapy when PCI is performed are shown on page 46. It should be emphasized that **primary PCI performed in a timely fashion, is the reperfusion therapy of choice.**

The treatment of AMI includes:

1) **Oxygen** in case of dyspnea or arterial oxygen saturation <90%.
2) **Acetylsalicylic acid (aspirin).** This is initially administered in a dose of 150-300 mg immediately after AMI is diagnosed. Aspirin in this ini-

tial dose (nonenteric coated form preferred) is chewed by the patient and remains in the oral cavity for better absorption by the oral mucosa. Thereafter, a dose of 75-160 mg daily (usually 100 mg/day) is taken for life. Aspirin administration reduces mortality by 20% in the first month after the AMI. If there is a history of allergic reaction to aspirin (bronchospasm, anaphylactic shock) only clopidogrel should be given at a loading dose of 300-600 mg, followed by 75 mg daily. If oral administration is impossible, a 300 mg aspirin suppository or a 250 mg IV dose is administered.

3) **Clopidogrel.** In patients aged ≤75 years, a loading dose of 300 mg is administered orally before fibrinolysis followed by a daily dose of 75 mg. In patients aged >75 years or nonreperfused patients, the loading dose of clopidogrel is omitted and 75 mg is administered daily from the start. For newer antiplatelet medications (prasugrel, ticagrelor) there are insufficient data concerning their administration to AMI patients who have not undergone primary PCI. When a protein-pump inhibitor is coadministered, omeprazole should be avoided, because it may impair the antiplatelet action of clopidogrel, or should be administered 12 h after clopidogrel to minimize interaction (more in Chapter 3). The duration of dual antiplatelet therapy is usually 12 months.

4) **Analgesia.** Administration of 2-4 mg of morphine sulfate (reduces preload, anxiety and tachycardia) IV within 5 min with additional 2-4 mg at 5-15 min intervals until the pain is relieved. Morphine is given diluted in 5-10 mL of NaCl 0.9%. An antiemetic (e.g. metoclopramide 10 mg IV) is coadministered for the nausea and vomiting caused by the morphine. In an inferior AMI with bradycardia, instead of morphine it is preferable to administer pethidine hydrochloride in a dose of 20-50 mg IV, because morphine may aggravate the bradycardia, while pethidine has a mild atropinic action.

If morphine administration causes symptomatic bradycardia, atropine is administered in a dose of 0.5-1.5 mg IV, while in the case of respiratory depression naloxone (Evzio, Narcan) is administered in a dose of 0.4 mg IV, repeated at 4-min intervals if necessary (max dose 1.2 mg).

5) **Beta-blockers.** These reduce the rate of reinfarction and ischemia recurrence in AMI patients under fibrinolysis. They are administered orally within the first 24 h (e.g. metoprolol tartrate [Lopressor] at an initial dose of 25-50 mg x 2 daily or carvedilol [Coreg, Dilatrend] at an initial dose of 6.25 mg x 2 daily). They are contraindicated in the acute phase when there are (O'Gara PT, et al. Circulation 2013;127:e362-425):
- Signs of heart failure or low cardiac output.
- An increased risk of cardiogenic shock (systolic BP <120 mmHg,

heart rate <60 or >110 beats/min, age >70 years, delayed admission). The more the risk factors, the greater the risk of cardiogenic shock.

- PR interval >240 ms, 2nd or 3rd degree atrioventricular block.
- History of severe bronchial asthma.
- Suspicion that the AMI has been precipitated by cocaine use (exacerbation of coronary spasm).

IV administration should be preferred during the acute phase when hypertension persists or there is ongoing ischemia, while the above contraindications are absent. Usually, 5 mg of metoprolol tartrate IV (supplied as Lopressor ampoule of 5 mg/5 mL) are administered within 1-2 min x 3 at intervals of 5 min, or until the heart rate drops to <60 beats/min, and after 15 min it is administered orally at a dose of 25-50 mg x 2 daily. Alternatively, infusion of esmolol (Brevibloc), an ultra-short-acting beta1- blocker, can be tried in patients with relative contraindications to beta-blockers.

6) **Nitrates.** The routine use of nitrates has not been shown to be of value and is not therefore recommended. Nitrates reduce myocardial oxygen demand by reducing the preload (venodilation) and to a lesser extent the afterload (systemic arterial dilation) and also improve myocardial blood flow by dilating the coronary arteries. Their administration, usually for 24-48 h, may be useful in patients with hypertension or heart failure. Nitrates are usually administered in a continuous infusion of nitroglycerin solution in an initial dose of 5-10 µg/min, gradually increasing by 5-10 µg/min every 5-10 min, and with the requirement that systolic BP is maintained at >90 mmHg. Nitrates should be avoided in cases of:

- Inferior AMI with right ventricular participation (risk of BP drop).
- Previous use of selective phosphodiesterase type 5 inhibitors, e.g. sildenafil (Viagra, Revatio) within the previous 24 h (risk of sudden BP drop) [see page 59].
- Hypotension (systolic BP <90 mmHg).

Practical guide for the administration of nitrates: 25 mg nitroglycerin (Tridil, Nitro-Bid) are added to 250 mL D/W 5% (making up a solution of 100 µg/mL concentration). Infusion is begun at a rate of 3-6 mL/h (5-10 µg/min), followed by an increase of 3-6 mL/h (5-10 µg/min) every 5-10 min, depending on the patient's response. The mean dosage is ~15 mL/h (25 µg/min), while the maximum is 120 mL/h (200 µg/min).

7) **Fibrinolysis.** The introduction of fibrinolysis about 25 years ago revolutionized the therapeutic treatment of AMI, reducing mortality in the first month by 25-30%. Fibrinolytic agents act by converting plasmino-

gen to plasmin, which degrades fibrin. The aim of the fibrinolysis is to dissolve the thrombus causing the obstruction as soon as possible, so as to restore coronary flow and reduce the extent of the infarction. Fibrinolysis must be started at the hospital within 30 min (<20 min if possible) of the patient's arrival in the Emergency Room (door-to-needle time). The quicker the administration, the greater the benefit. Indications for fibrinolysis are given in Table 2.5.

Prehospital fibrinolysis appears to be superior to in-hospital administration of fibrinolysis, since it is associated with lower short-term cardiac mortality. This benefit is due to the earlier administration of prehospital fibrinolysis (~60 min). Therefore, prehospital fibrinolysis should be considered in patients with AMI in whom a decision has been made to not use primary PCI, the patients are 1 h away from the nearest hospital where fibrinolysis can be given and most importantly, the health-care system provides the facilities for this.

Notes on indications for fibrinolysis in the presence of LBBB
The presence of LBBB when there are typical symptoms of AMI is an indication for fibrinolysis when the LBBB is new or presumed to be new (indicative of proximal occlusion of the anterior descending artery). In practice, however, there are very few cases where the treating physician has the luxury of access to a patient's recent previous ECG in the Emergency Room and can know whether the LBBB is new or not. It is therefore reasonable for any patient with typical symptoms of AMI and LBBB to be a candidate for fibrinolysis or PCI. If, however, the clinical presentation is atypical, then ECG signs suggesting an AMI must be sought indirectly (Table 2.6).

TABLE 2.5	Indications for fibrinolysis in acute myocardial infarction with ST-segment elevation

1) Symptom onset within the previous 12 h with concomitant:
   a) ST-segment elevation ≥1 mm in at least 2 adjacent leads, or
   b) New or presumed new left bundle branch block or
   c) ECG findings consistent with posterior infarction (ST-segment elevation ≥0.5 mm in posterior leads V_7-V_9).

2) Symptom onset within the previous 12 to 24 h, when there is an indication of continuing ischemia (persistence of pain and continuing ST-segment elevation ≥1 mm in at least 2 adjacent leads)

TABLE 2.6	Electrocardiographic criteria for the diagnosis of acute myocardial infarction in the presence of left bundle branch block (total points score ≥3 yields a 90% specificity and a ~90% positive predictive value)

Criteria	Points
ST-segment elevation ≥1 mm in leads with a positive QRS complex	5
ST-segment depression ≥ 1 mm in leads V_1-V_3	3
ST-segment elevation ≥ 5 mm in leads with a negative QRS complex	2

The main fibrinolytic agents are streptokinase, alteplase, reteplase and tenecteplase. Table 2.7 shows the doses at which these are administered for an AMI. Differences among fibrinolytic agents relate to:
- Method of administration (bolus or IV drip infusion).
- Allergic reactions (streptokinase is highly antigenic and is absolutely contraindicated within 6 months of previous administration because of the potential for serious allergic reactions).
- Degree of systemic fibrinolysis (streptokinase causes systemic fibrinolysis because it activates circulating plasminogen, while the others exert a local fibrinolytic action by activating clot-bound plasminogen).
- Half-life (streptokinase ~20 min, alteplase ~5 min, reteplase ~15 min and tenecteplase ~20 min), and
- Cost (streptokinase is the cheapest, with a cost about a quarter that of the other fibrinolytic agents).

The newer fibrinolytic agents (alteplase, reteplase, tenecteplase) have a slight superiority over streptokinase in terms of 30-day mortality, at the expense of a small increase in the risk of intracranial hemorrhage. The 90 min patency rate (TIMI 2 or 3 flow) of the AMI culprit vessel is ~60% for streptokinase, compared with ~80% for the newer fibrinolytic agents. Although the use of streptokinase has been greatly reduced in developed countries in recent years, it is still indicated in low-risk infarction patients (e.g. uncomplicated inferior AMI).

The main complication of fibrinolytic therapy is hemorrhage, which is classified as:
- Minor, usually at the puncture site, or from the mouth or nose. Local pressure is sufficient to treat it.
- Major, either nonintracranial (usually gastrointestinal in ~5%) or intracranial (~1%). To treat severe nonintracranial hemorrhage, packed red blood cells, fresh frozen plasma (15-30 mL/kg) and cryoprecipitate (~10 units) are administered. To counter the action of the unfractiona-

TABLE 2.7	Dose of fibrinolytic agents in acute myocardial infarction	
Fibrinolytic agent	**Dose**	**Coadministration of unfractionated heparin**
Streptokinase (Streptase, Kabikinase)	1,500,000 U within 30-60 min (solution in 100 ml D/W 5% or NaCl 0.9%)	Optional
Alteplase (rtPA) [Activase, Actilyse]	15 mg IV bolus and then: • 0.75 mg/kg (max 50 mg) within 30 min and • 0.5 mg/kg (max 35 mg) within 60 min	60 U/kg (max 4000 U) IV bolus before starting alteplase administration and then continuous infusion 12 U/kg/h (maximum 1000 U/h) for 24-48 h with desired aPTT 50-70 s
Reteplase (rPA) [Retavase, Rapilysin]	10 U IV bolus within 2 min and repeat the same dose after 30 min	As with alteplase, except that continuous heparin infusion is started after the second reteplase dose
Tenecteplase (TNK-tPA) [TNKase, Metalyse]	In one IV bolus administration • 30 mg if BW < 60 kg • 35 mg if BW ≥ 60 - < 70 kg • 40 mg if BW ≥ 70 - < 80 kg • 45 mg if BW ≥ 80 - < 90 kg • 50 mg if BW ≥ 90 kg Note: In patients ≥ 75 years ½ of dose is recommended.	As with alteplase

aPTT: activated partial thromboplastin time, BW: body weight

ted heparin (UFH), protamine sulfate should be administered in a dose of 20-50 mg IV within 10 min. Specifically, 1 mg of protamine sulfate inactivates 100 units of UFH. If <30 min have elapsed since heparin infusion then 1 mg of protamine sulfate is given for every 100 units of UFH. If heparin infusion has been discontinued for >30 min but <2 h then ½ of the dose is administered, while if it has been discontinued for >2 h but <4 h, $^1/_4$ of the dose is administered. If >4 h have elapsed since heparin infusion, then there is no point in administering protamine sulfate, as the half-life of UFH is 1-2 h. Protamine sulfate may cause anaphylactic reactions. It is supplied in a 5 ml vial containing 50 mg of protamine sulfate (1% solution). It should be noted that protamine sulfate has an anticoagulant action when heparin has not previously been administered. However, when it is administered in the presence of heparin, a stable salt is formed, resulting in the inactivation of both.

Risk factors for intracranial hemorrhaging (~60% mortality) are: age >75 years, female gender, low body weight, hypertension on admission, and previous oral anticoagulant therapy. If, during or following fibrinolysis (usually <24 h), there is any mental confusion or any focal neurological sign, the fibrinolytic agents, the heparin and the antiplatelets should be interrupted and a brain computed tomography scan performed to assess the possibility of intracranial hemorrhage. Table 2.8 presents the management of fibrinolysis induced intracranial hemorrhage and Table 2.9 the contraindications for fibrinolysis.

Warning! If placement of a temporary pacemaker is required during or immediately after fibrinolysis it is preferable to use the femoral vein, as pressure can be applied for hemostasis if there is hemorrhage at the puncture site.

8) **Unfractionated heparin** is coadministered with the newer fibrinolytic agents (alteplase, reteplase, and tenecteplase) for 24-48 h (Table 2.7). Initially it is administered at a dose of 60 U/kg (maximum 4000 U) IV bolus and then in continuous IV infusion of 12 U/kg/h with a desired activated partial thromboplastin time of 50-70 s (test every 6 h for the first 24 h and then every 12-24 h). Administration reduces the risk of rethrombosis from the thrombin particles released when the thrombus is dispersed by the action of the fibrinolytic agent. When streptokinase is given, UFH is indicated only if the risk of embolism is great (e.g. atrial fibrillation, large anterior AMI). As an alternative to UFH, enoxaparin,

TABLE 2.8	Management of intracranial hemorrhage caused by fibrinolysis

- Discontinuation of fibrinolytic agent, heparin and antiplatelets
- Protamine sulfate to reverse effect of heparin
- Fresh frozen plasma (15-30 mL/kg)
- Cryoprecipitate (~10 units)
- Consider platelet infusion (6-8 units)
- Consider ε-aminocaproic acid (Amicar) [binds competitively to plasminogen and blocks its conversion to the active plasmin]
- Neurological/neurosurgical consultation

TABLE 2.9	**Contraindications for fibrinolytic treatment in acute myocardial infarction in accordance with the American Guidelines** *(O'Gara PT, et al. Circulation 2013;127:e362-425)*

Absolute contraindications

- History of intracranial hemorrhage
- Malignant cerebral tumor (primary or metastatic)
- Cerebral vessel dysplasia (e.g. arteriovenous malformation)
- Ischemic stroke within 3 months (except acute ischemic stroke within 4.5 h)
- Active hemorrhage or hemorrhagic diathesis (excluding menses)
- Suspicion of acute aortic dissection
- Intracranial or intraspinal surgery within 2 months
- Significant closed-head or facial trauma within 3 months
- Severe uncontrolled hypertension (persistence of systolic BP >180 mmHg or diastolic BP >110 mmHg despite emergency therapy)
- For streptokinase, prior treatment within the previous 6 months
- Noncompressible organ puncture in the past 24 h (e.g. liver biopsy, lumbar puncture)*

Relative contraindications

- History of chronic, severe, poorly controlled hypertension
- Significant hypertension on presentation (systolic BP >180 mmHg or diastolic BP >110 mmHg)
- History of prior ischemic stroke >3 months
- Dementia
- Intracranial pathology not covered in absolute contraindications
- Traumatic or prolonged (>10 min) cardiopulmonary resuscitation
- Major surgery (<3 weeks)
- Recent (within 2-4 weeks) internal hemorrhage. According to European Guidelines, gastrointestinal bleeding within the last month is an absolute contraindication
- Noncompressible vascular punctures
- Pregnancy or within 1 week of delivery*
- Active peptic ulcer
- Oral anticoagulant therapy (the greater the INR, the greater the risk of hemorrhage)
- Severe liver disease*
- Infective endocarditis*

*In accordance with the European Guidelines (Steg G, et al. Eur Heart J 2012;33:2569-619).
INR: international normalized ratio, BP: blood pressure

a low-molecular-weight heparin, may be given (Lovenox, Clexane) in a dose of 30 mg IV bolus, followed 15 min later by 1 mg/kg every 12 h subcutaneously, provided that the patient is <75 years old and has satisfactory renal function (creatinine ≤2.5 mg/dL in men and ≤2 mg/dL in women). For people aged >75 years the initial IV administration is skipped and the subcutaneous dose is reduced to 0.75 mg/kg every 12 h. When creatinine clearance (calculated by the Cockcroft–Gault formula) is <30 mL/min*, the subcutaneous dose is reduced to 1 mg/kg every 24 h. Enoxaparin is continued throughout the patient's hospitalization (5-8 days).

Warning! In all individuals with creatinine levels of >1.5 mg/dL, especially the elderly and thin, creatinine clearance, an estimate of glomerular filtration rate, must always be calculated. A commonly used formula to estimate creatinine clearance is the Cockcroft-Gault formula as follows:

$$\text{Creatinine clearance (mL/min)} = \frac{(140 - \text{age in years}) \times (\text{weight in kgs}) \, [\times 0.85 \text{ for women}]}{72 \times \text{serum creatinine (mg/dL)}}$$

9) **Angiotensin-converting enzyme (ACE) inhibitors.** Administered orally within the first 24 h after the AMI. Although the patients who benefit most are those with anterior AMI, ejection fraction ≤40% and heart failure symptoms, the tendency is to give ACE inhibitors to all AMI patients, provided that systolic BP is >100 mmHg. Initial administration is at low dosages, such as 2.5-5 mg of lisinopril (Prinivil, Zestril) once daily, 2.5 mg of ramipril (Altace, Triatace) every 12 h, or 2.5 mg of enalapril (Vasotec, Renitec) every 12 h, etc. In the case of ACE inhibitor intolerance, e.g. appearance of a dry cough, angiotensin II receptor blockers are given, such as valsartan (Diovan) at an initial dose of 20 mg every 12 h.

10) **Aldosterone antagonists.** Administered if the ejection fraction is ≤40% and there is either symptomatic heart failure or diabetes mellitus. Prerequisites for administration are serum levels of potassium <5 mEq/L, and creatinine <2.5 mg/dL for men and <2 mg/dL for women. Spironolactone (Aldactone) may be given, or the selective aldosterone antagonist eplerenone (Inspra). The starting dose is 25 mg daily.

11) **Rapid-acting insulin** (usually subcutaneously, based on 6-h blood glucose values) in diabetic patients, only if blood glucose levels are >180 mg/dL. In diabetic patients who were taking antidiabetic tablets,

---

Creatinine clearance >90 mL/min denotes normal renal function, while values of 60-90 mL/min, 30-60 mL/min, and <30 mL/min show mild, moderate and severe renal failure, respectively. Note that Cockcroft-Gault formula is less accurate in obese individuals.

these are temporarily discontinued. Although hyperglycemia is an adverse prognostic factor following an AMI, an "aggressive" reduction of blood glucose levels should be avoided, as the onset of hypoglycemia is associated with increased mortality.

12) **Statins.** Given to all AMI patients starting on the first day of hospitalization, with an LDL cholesterol target <70 mg/dL (desired values between 50-70 mg/dL) or reduction of LDL cholesterol by ≥50 if the baseline untreated value is between 70-135 mg/dL (European Guidelines, Catapano AL, et al. Eur Heart J 2016;37:2999-3058). According to the latest American Guidelines (Stone NJ, et al. Circulation 2014;129:S1-S45) an LDL cholesterol reduction ≥50% from the untreated baseline should be achieved by giving high-intensity statin therapy (i.e. 20-40 mg rosuvastatin or 40-80 mg atorvastatin) abandoning the therapeutic target of an LDL cholesterol <70 mg/dL. For patients >75 years an LDL cholesterol reduction in the range of 30-50% from the untreated baseline is recommended by giving a moderate-intensity statin therapy. Immediate administration of statins has rapid clinical benefits, mainly via their pleiotropic effect (antiinflammatory, antithrombotic, etc.). Note that cholesterol determination more than 24 h after an AMI gives artificially lower LDL cholesterol levels, as a result of the drop (~10-15%) caused by the stress of acute myocardial ischemia. Finally, if patients fail to achieve the LDL cholesterol target despite taking the maximally tolerated statin dose, the addition of ezetimibe (10 mg daily) should be considered.

13) **Anxiolytics** in small doses, such as bromazepam at a dose of 1.5 mg x 2 or x 3 daily, or alprazolam at a dose of 0.25 mg x 2 or x 3 daily.

14) **Proton pump inhibitors (PPIs),** during hospitalization (continuation after discharge if there is high risk for gastrointestinal bleeding).

In which cases should primary PCI be preferred to fibrinolysis in AMI?

Primary PCI is defined as angioplasty (+stenting) in the AMI culprit lesion as the initial reperfusion therapy, i.e. without previous or concomitant fibrinolysis, usually <12 h from symptom onset. A prerequisite for this procedure is the existence of a well-organized catheterization laboratory with a wide range of procedural capabilities and the capacity to operate 24/7, staffed by experienced interventional cardiologists. Primary PCI offers faster and more effective reperfusion (restoration of normal TIMI 3 flow in ~90% of cases, compared to ~60% with fibrinolysis). In addition, compared to fibrinolysis it is associated with lower monthly rates of mortality (7% versus 9%), reinfarction (3% versus 7%), and stroke (1% versus 2%). These clinical benefits accrue when primary PCI is carried out within 60-90 min of the patient's arrival at the hospital. The problem, however, with primary PCI is that it is only available in a small percentage of hospitals, whereas fibrinolysis has the advantage of being readily available in all hospitals, or even in primary health care centers. Thus, **reperfusion speed is more important than reperfusion type (mechanical or pharmaceutical).** The recommended reperfusion strategy for treating AMI is as follows:

1) **Hospitals with primary PCI capability:** primary PCI should be performed and initiated within 60 min (preferably) from patients' arrival to hospital (door-to-balloon time ≤60 min) [Steg G, et al. Eur Heart J 2012;33:2569-619]. These time limits for the implementation of a primary PCI are not valid in cases where there is an absolute contraindication for fibrinolysis, or if the patient presents with cardiogenic shock. It should also be noted that primary PCI is not superior to fibrinolysis if the patient arrives <3 h (and especially <2 h) after the onset of symptoms and the AMI is relatively low-risk (uncomplicated inferior or lateral AMI in a patient aged <75 years). In contrast, when the patient presents >3 h after the onset of symptoms, primary PCI should be preferred, irrespective of the type of AMI, since the thrombus is more resistant to lysis. Indeed, if we take into account that cardiac catheterization is routine medical practice in hospitals for all patients treated with fibrinolysis (even those in whom fibrinolysis is successful) then the treatment strategy for AMI in hospitals with primary PCI availability should be primary PCI, not only because of its superiority in relation to fibrinolysis in most cases, but also because of the practical considerations.

2) **Hospitals without primary PCI capability:** primary PCI is preferred provided there is the possibility of transfer to a hospital with a catheterization laboratory to carry out primary PCI within 120 min (total door-to-balloon time) from the time of arrival at the initial hospital, or within 90 min in the case of a large anterior AMI, if the patient's age is <75 years, or the presentation is <2 h from the onset of the symptoms. The patients should also be discharged from the initial non-PCI-capable hospital within 30 min, i.e. the door-in to door-out time should be <30 min. If these criteria are not fulfilled, fibrinolysis must be started as soon as possible (≤30 min or ideally <20 min after arrival at the first hospital). This situation is faced by many provincial hospitals. After the initial fibrinolytic therapy, rapid (ideally between 3 and 24 h) transfer of the patient to a PCI-capable hospital should be pursued.

Warning! It is a mistake to transfer a patient with AMI from a regional center to a PCI-capable central hospital if it is estimated that the PCI will not be started within 2 h. In this case, fibrinolysis should be performed, in the absence of any contraindications, and the patient should be transferred later (ideally between 3 and 24 h).

Transfer of the AMI patient to a hospital with primary PCI capability must also be arranged if there is an absolute contraindication for fibrinolysis (~15-20% of AMIs) or the patient presents with cardiogenic shock. Table 2.10 gives the cases where primary PCI should be preferred over fibrinolysis in the treatment of AMI.

Problems that also limit the benefits of reperfusion (primary PCI or fibrinolysis) are:

- Delay in calling the doctor or ambulance (patient delay). In many countries the arrival of an ambulance does not also entail a diagnosis of AMI, because ambulances are not provided with a cardiologist or a telemetry/telemedicine system for the ECG diagnosis of AMI. As a result, the patient's first medical contact is in the hospital's Emergency Room.
- Delay in transportation of the patient to the hospital by ambulance, depending on the organization of the healthcare system and the traffic congestion.

Ideally, the ambulance should be called within 5 min after symptom onset of the AMI and the transfer to hospital completed within 30 min in order for the reperfusion therapy to have the greatest possible benefit.

As regards the concomitant antiplatelet and anticoagulant treatment when primary PCI is performed, there are small differences compared to the case of fibrinolysis (Table 2.11). More information about prasugrel, ticagrelor, glycoprotein IIb-IIIa inhibitors, and bivalirudin (a direct thrombin inhibitor) may be found in Chapter 3.

Treatment of a patient with cardiogenic shock as a consequence of extensive myocardial ischemia

Cardiogenic shock complicates 5-10% of AMIs and is associated with high in-hospital mortality (~50%). The most usual cause (>80%) is extensive

TABLE 2.10	Primary percutaneous coronary intervention (PCI) versus fibrinolysis in the treatment of acute myocardial infarction

1) Hospital with primary PCI capability
- Primary PCI should be performed ≤60 min after the patient's arrival at the hospital (door-to-balloon time).

2) Hospital without primary PCI capability. The patient must be transferred to another hospital for PCI when:
- the total time for transfer and PCI initiation (total door-to-balloon time) is estimated to be ≤120 min (or ≤90 min in cases where there is a large anterior AMI, the patient's age is <75 years, or presentation is <2 h after the onset of symptoms)
- the patient is in cardiogenic shock
- there is an absolute contraindication for fibrinolysis

TABLE 2.11	Antiplatelet and anticoagulant treatment when primary percutaneous coronary intervention (PCI) is performed in acute myocardial infarction	
Antiplatelet treatment	• Acetylsalicylic acid	• 150-300 mg po, or 80-150 mg IV if oral administration is impossible, then 75-160 mg/day
	• $P2Y_{12}$ receptor inhibitors: – Clopidogrel – Prasugrel or – Ticagrelor	• 600 mg po, then 75 mg/day • 60 mg po, then 10 mg/day • 180 mg po, then 90 mg x 2 /day Notes on $P2Y_{12}$ receptor inhibitors: 1) Duration of administration at least 12 months 2) Given the faster action of prasugrel and ticagrelor, they should be preferred over clopidogrel in the acute phase 3) Absolute contraindication for prasugrel is prior cerebrovascular event and relative contraindication is age ≥75 years. Maintenance dose is 5 mg in patients <60 kg.
	• Abciximab (alternatively eptifibatide or tirofiban)	• 0.25 mg/kg bolus IV, then 0.125 µg/kg/min (maximum dose 10 µg/min) x 12 h. Glycoprotein (GP) IIb/IIIa inhibitors are used in selected patients (massive thrombus, inadequate $P2Y_{12}$ receptor inhibitors loading, etc.)
Options of anticoagulant treatment	• Unfractionated heparin (UFH)	• 70-100 U/kg bolus IV (or 50-60 U/kg if GP IIb /IIIa inhibitors are coadministered). The recommended activated clotting time (ACT) is 250-300 s (HemoTec device) or 200-250 s if a GP IIb/IIIa inhibitor is given. Administration is stopped on completion of PCI
	• Enoxaparin (alternative to UFH)	• 0.5 mg/kg IV bolus
	• Bivalirudin (alternative to heparin)	• 0.75 mg/kg bolus IV followed by IV infusion of 1.75 mg/kg/h for up to 4 h after the procedure as clinically warranted. Dose titration based on ACT is not necessary. It is preferred as monotherapy over the combination of UFH and GP IIb/IIIa inhibitors in patients at high risk of bleeding

myocardial ischemia, followed by mechanical complications of the AMI (rupture of papillary muscle head or ventricular septum). Fewer than 1% of AMI patients exhibit cardiogenic shock in the Emergency Room; most who develop it do so during their subsequent hospitalization. Consequently, it is very important to recognize the precursors of cardiogenic shock, such as the presence of persistent sinus tachycardia and a low systolic BP (90-100 mmHg), which will necessitate a thorough clinical and laboratory investigation. It is essential to perform an emergency echocardiographic study to identify the underlying cause of the shock.

When cardiogenic shock is due to extensive myocardial necrosis, coronary angiography must be pursued as soon as possible with a view to carrying out primary PCI in the culprit vessel, or complete reperfusion in the presence of multiple critical stenoses (multiple PCIs or coronary artery bypass grafting, depending on the anatomy). Note that ~70-80% of patients with cardiogenic shock have significant stenoses/occlusions in more than one vessel. If the hospital does not have a catheterization laboratory, emergency transfer must be arranged to a hospital that does. If transfer is delayed or the patients are unsuitable for invasive therapy they should be treated with fibrinolytic therapy in the absence of contraindications. It should be noted, however, that fibrinolysis has low efficacy and is greatly inferior to invasive therapy, which is the only intervention that improves survival. Until the patient is catheterized, an intra-aortic balloon pump (IABP) is placed (improvement of coronary perfusion and reduction of myocardial oxygen consumption), and efforts are made to increase systolic BP to at least 80 mmHg with the administration of fluids and noradrenaline (vasoconstriction effect), at the lowest effective dose, possibly followed by coadministration of dobutamine (inotropic effect). Table 2.12 shows the hemodynamic and clinical parameters on which the diagnosis of cardiogenic shock is based. It

TABLE 2.12	Hemodynamic and clinical signs in the diagnosis of cardiogenic shock

1) Hemodynamic signs
- Systolic blood pressure <90 mmHg for >30 min (absence of hypovolemia)
- Cardiac index <1.8 L/min/m^2 (or <2.0-2.2 L/min/m^2 on support)
- Elevated filling pressure of left (end-diastolic pressure >18 mmHg), right (end-diastolic pressure >10-15 mmHg), or both ventricles

2) Clinical signs of tissue hypoperfusion
- Oliguria (urine output <0.5 mL/kg/h) or anuria
- Confusion (cerebral hypoperfusion)
- Cool extremities

should be noted that right cardiac catheterization is not always necessary for the diagnosis of cardiogenic shock. Regarding the usefulness of IABP in patients with cardiogenic shock there are conflicting data. In general, IABP can be useful for patients who do not quickly stabilize with pharmacological therapy.

Repeat fibrinolysis or rescue PCI following failed fibrinolysis in AMI

Failed fibrinolysis is defined as persistence of chest pain coupled with <50% resolution of ST-segment elevation and absence of typical reperfusion arrhythmias at 60-90 min after the start of fibrinolytic treatment. This occurs in ~30% of cases. The preferred treatment is to perform PCI (rescue) urgently and not to repeat the fibrinolysis. The benefits from rescue PCI are greater when cardiogenic shock, significant hypotension, severe heart failure, or a large AMI is present.

Special notes on the treatment of right ventricular infarction

Suspicion of right ventricular infarction arises when a patient with an inferior AMI presents:
- A sudden drop in BP upon administration of nitrates
- Distended jugular veins, hypotension, and "clear lungs"
- ST-segment elevation ≥0.5 mm in leads V_3R and V_4R.

This is usually a complication of an inferior AMI when there is proximal occlusion of the right coronary artery. Approximately 25-50% of patients with inferior AMI and accompanying right ventricular infarction will have hemodynamic compromise. Right ventricular dysfunction leads to a reduction in its stroke volume, thus reducing left ventricular filling and causing hypotension. It is very important to maintain satisfactory right ventricular filling (to avoid reducing preload) so as to maintain a satisfactory cardiac output.

The therapeutic strategy in hypotensive patients includes:
- Performing primary PCI as soon as possible. If not available, administration of fibrinolysis, but with clearly less efficacy. It is obvious that antiplatelets (aspirin + a $P2Y_{12}$ receptor inhibitor) and heparin are given in a manner similar to those with acute STEMI.
- Avoiding administration of vasodilators (e.g. nitrates), diuretics, and opiates.
- Performing right heart catheterization to measure pulmonary capillary wedge pressure (PCWP), mainly to guide IV fluid administration.
- A judicious volume challenge in the absence of pulmonary congestion. Usually 200-400 mL of NaCl 0.9% are infused within 10-15 min through a central line. If PCWP increases to 15-18 mmHg but rapid flu-

id infusion fails to improve BP, no further volume challenge should be attempted.

- Administration of inotropes (dobutamine), if the patient remains hypotensive despite the initial volume loading and the achievement of a PCWP between 15-18 mmHg.
- Temporary atrioventricular sequential pacing (preferred over ventricular pacing) if advanced heart block develops.
- Cardioversion of atrial fibrillation (occurs in up to 30% of cases).
- Placing an IABP or reducing afterload by administration of nitroprusside, in the case of concomitant severe left ventricular dysfunction and pulmonary congestion.

Warning! In all inferior AMIs, irrespective of the degree of clinical suspicion regarding right ventricular involvement, the right precordial leads must be included in the initial ECG recorded in the Emergency Room.

Key points

- Clinical indications of AMIs are atypical in ~10-20% of cases (dyspnea, profuse weakness, syncope, epigastric pain, etc.)
- In the treatment of AMI, the three primary actions include administration of dual antiplatelet treatment (aspirin and a $P2Y_{12}$ receptor inhibitor), analgesia and rapid reperfusion (primary PCI or fibrinolysis).
- In the choice between primary PCI or fibrinolysis, the time needed to achieve reperfusion is more important than the type of reperfusion. The faster the occluded vessel is opened, the greater the benefits for the patient. However, it should be emphasized that PCI performed in a timely fashion, is the reperfusion therapy of choice.
- In a hospital:
  - a) with primary PCI capability, primary PCI should be performed ≤60 min of patient's arrival (door-to-balloon time ≤60 min)
  - b) with no primary PCI capability, the patient must be transferred to another hospital with PCI capability when the total time for transfer and PCI initiation (total door-to-balloon time) is estimated to be ≤120 min (or ≤90 min in the case of a large anterior AMI, when the patient's age is <75 years, or presentation is <2 h after the onset of symptoms).
- Irrespective of the capabilities of the hospital to which the patient is admitted, primary PCI must be pursued when the patient is in cardiogenic shock or there is an absolute contraindication for fibrinolytic treatment.
- Every patient with symptoms typical for AMI and LBBB is a candidate for primary PCI or fibrinolysis.
- ST-segment elevation in leads aVR and V_1 (aVR >V_1) + ST-segment depression in "many leads" raise the suspicion of acute left main coronary artery occlusion.
- If there are clinical findings suggestive of AMI and the only ECG finding is ST-segment depression in leads V_1 and V_2, posterior leads V_7-V_9 must also be recorded to rule out a posterior AMI. This is a case for rapid reperfusion with ST-segment depression on the 12-lead ECG.
- In every case with epigastric pain, especially in individuals with multiple risk factors for coronary artery disease, it is prudent to record an ECG.
- In every inferior AMI the right-sided precordial leads should always be recorded to rule out a right ventricular infarction.
- In inferior AMIs, when a sudden drop in BP is noted on administration of small doses of nitrates, this should raise the suspicion of right ventricular involvement, or the recent use of phosphodiesterase type 5 inhibitors.

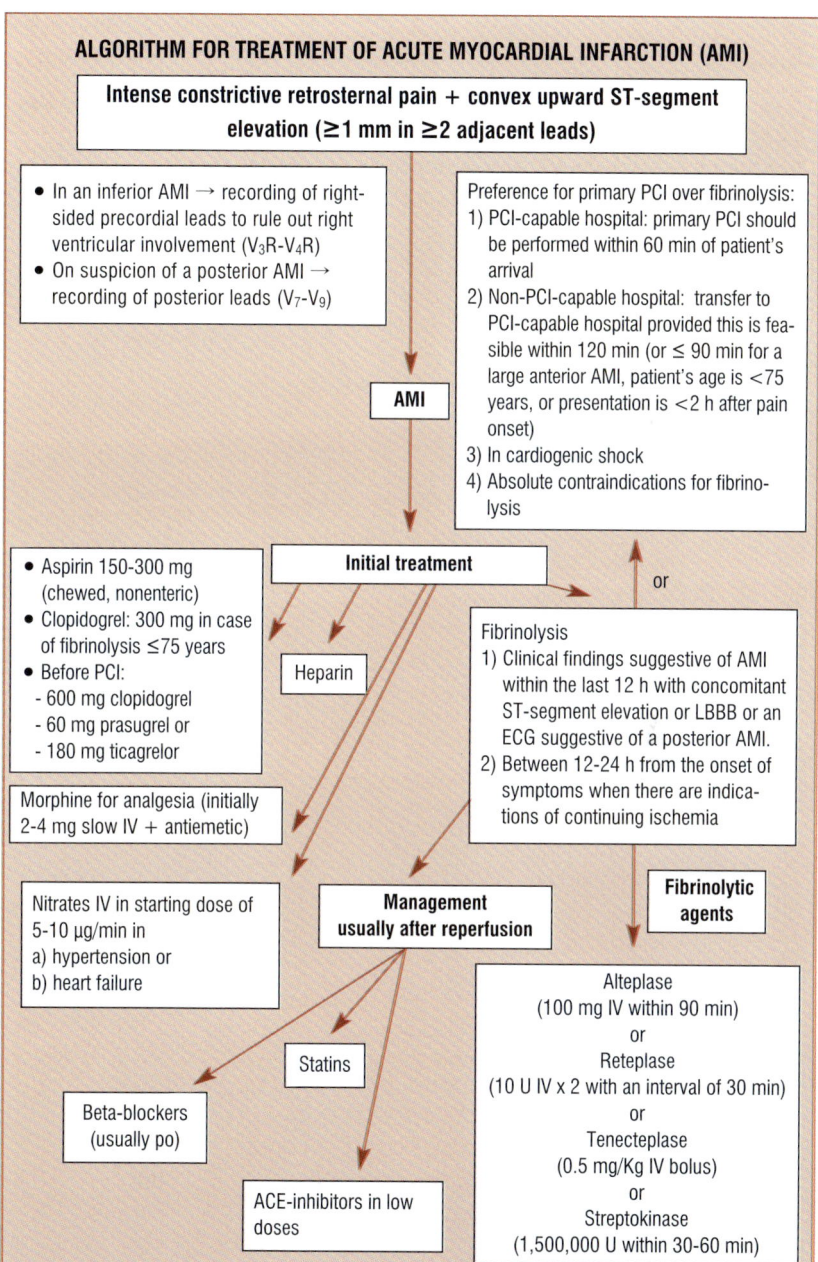

ALGORITHM FOR TREATMENT OF ACUTE MYOCARDIAL INFARCTION (AMI)

Intense constrictive retrosternal pain + convex upward ST-segment elevation (≥1 mm in ≥2 adjacent leads)

- In an inferior AMI → recording of right-sided precordial leads to rule out right ventricular involvement (V_3R-V_4R)
- On suspicion of a posterior AMI → recording of posterior leads (V_7-V_9)

Preference for primary PCI over fibrinolysis:
1) PCI-capable hospital: primary PCI should be performed within 60 min of patient's arrival
2) Non-PCI-capable hospital: transfer to PCI-capable hospital provided this is feasible within 120 min (or ≤ 90 min for a large anterior AMI, patient's age is <75 years, or presentation is <2 h after pain onset)
3) In cardiogenic shock
4) Absolute contraindications for fibrinolysis

AMI

Initial treatment

- Aspirin 150-300 mg (chewed, nonenteric)
- Clopidogrel: 300 mg in case of fibrinolysis ≤75 years
- Before PCI:
  - 600 mg clopidogrel
  - 60 mg prasugrel or
  - 180 mg ticagrelor

Heparin

or

Fibrinolysis
1) Clinical findings suggestive of AMI within the last 12 h with concomitant ST-segment elevation or LBBB or an ECG suggestive of a posterior AMI.
2) Between 12-24 h from the onset of symptoms when there are indications of continuing ischemia

Morphine for analgesia (initially 2-4 mg slow IV + antiemetic)

Nitrates IV in starting dose of 5-10 μg/min in
a) hypertension or
b) heart failure

Management usually after reperfusion

Fibrinolytic agents

Alteplase
(100 mg IV within 90 min)
or
Reteplase
(10 U IV x 2 with an interval of 30 min)
or
Tenecteplase
(0.5 mg/Kg IV bolus)
or
Streptokinase
(1,500,000 U within 30-60 min)

Statins

Beta-blockers
(usually po)

ACE-inhibitors in low doses

ACE: angiotensin-converting enzyme, PCI: percutaneous coronary intervention, LBBB: left bundle branch block.

3

Non ST-Segment Elevation Acute Coronary Syndrome
(unstable angina and non ST-segment elevation myocardial infarction)

The definition of acute coronary syndrome (ACS) without (persistent) ST-segment elevation includes two clinical entities that constitute 75% of all ACSs:

    a) Unstable angina without detectable myocardial necrosis ("negative" cardiac troponin), and

    b) "Unstable angina" with indications of myocardial necrosis (elevated cardiac troponin), called "non ST-segment elevation myocardial infarction (NSTEMI)".

Unstable angina has a better prognosis than NSTEMI.

Table 3.1 presents the Braunwald classification of ACS without (persistent) ST-segment elevation.

Pathophysiology

It is usually caused by rupture or erosion of a vulnerable atheromatous plaque in an epicardial coronary artery, with or without vasoconstriction, and the subsequent formation of a nonocclusive thrombus. **Platelets** play a major role in the formation of the thrombus (adhesion to the endothelium promoted by endothelial injury → activation → aggregation → formation of a platelet thrombus), as does **thrombin** (factor IIa), which is produced from prothrombin (factor II) through the effect of activated factor X. The main trigger to the thrombin pathway is tissue factor (factor III) that is exposed on the damaged endothelium. Thrombin plays a central role in the activation of the coagulation cascade and the formation of its end product, fibrin, which stabilizes the clot. Thrombin is also one of the strongest platelet activators. Note that in non ST-segment elevation ACS the thrombus is mainly **platelet-rich** while in acute MI with ST-segment elevation it is **fibrin-rich.**

Other mechanisms that might be responsible for non ST-segment elevation ACS are coronary vessel spasm (cocaine use, etc.), severe coronary artery stenosis due to advanced disease, restenosis after percutaneous inter-

TABLE 3.1	Braunwald classification of acute coronary syndromes without (persistent) ST-segment elevation	
Grade of severity	**Definition**	**Death or MI in the 1st year (%)**
I	New onset of severe angina or accelerated angina; no pain at rest	7.3
II	Angina at rest within the past month but not within the preceding 48 h	10.3
III	Angina at rest within 48 h	10.8
Grade of clinical instance		
A (secondary angina)	Develops in the presence of extracardiac causes that have intensified ischemia	14.1
B (primary angina)	Develops in the absence of an extracardiac condition that has intensified ischemia	8.5
C (postinfarction angina)	Develops within 2 weeks of acute MI	18.5

MI: myocardial infarction

vention in the coronary vessels, coronary artery dissection, etc. Lastly, in patients with stable coronary artery disease (CAD) or, more rarely without CAD, ACS can be produced by other causes, unrelated to the coronary arteries, that increase oxygen consumption (fever, thyrotoxicosis, aortic stenosis, etc.) or reduce oxygen supply (anemia, hypoxemia, hypotension, etc.).

Symptoms

Since the diagnosis of the syndrome is usually established clinically, all clinical manifestations of unstable angina must be sought. The usual tetrad of clinical manifestations is listed in Table 3.2. Atypical presentations are quite common in the elderly (>75 years), in young adults (25-40 years), in diabetics, in women and in patients with kidney disease or dementia.

Clinical signs

These are poor. Usually, a 4th heart sound is present. The possibility of aortic valve stenosis and hypertrophic cardiomyopathy, which often manifest with angina attacks, should be excluded.

ECG

An ECG during the pain is valuable. Possible findings are:
- Normal, in ~25% of cases.

TABLE 3.2	Clinical manifestations of unstable angina

1) Resting and prolonged (usually >20 min) angina

2) New-onset (<2 months) severe exertional angina (e.g. triggered when climbing one flight of stairs)

3) Recent worsening of preexisting stable angina (more frequent, intense and prolonged attacks)

4) Postinfarction angina occurring within 2 weeks of an acute myocardial infarction

- ST-segment depression with horizontal or downward slope (Figure 3.1). ST-segment depression $\geq$0.5 mm in $\geq$2 adjacent leads is associated with worse prognosis. Note that, unlike ST-segment elevation, ST-segment depression does not localize ischemia.
- Inverted or flattened T waves. T-wave changes are not specific, with the exception of deep inverted symmetrical T waves in precordial leads, which often indicate proximal stenosis in the left anterior descending artery or left main CAD.
- Transient (<20 min) ST-segment elevation in ~10% of cases.

Warning! The diagnosis of non ST-segment elevation ACS is mostly clinical. Therefore, a normal ECG should not exclude this diagnosis if it is consistent with the clinical symptoms.

Markers of myocardial necrosis

Of the cardiac markers, the most valuable is the determination of cardiac troponins (cTns) for the detection of myocardial necrosis and for prognostic risk stratification. Creatine kinase MB isoenzyme (CK-MB) is less sensitive and specific for detection of myocardial injury than cTns and is no longer recommended if cTns are available.

Myocardial necrosis in non ST-segment elevation ACS is caused by embolism of peripheral coronary vessels (arterioles or capillaries) by small platelet thrombi or thrombus components detaching from the central non-occlusive thrombus forming over the ruptured atheromatous plaque.

Warning! If high-sensitivity cTn is used and it is normal on admission, the test should be repeated 3 h later (0 h/3 h algorithm) to "rule-in" or "rule-out" acute ischemic myocardial necrosis. If a non high-sensitivity assay is used the measurement should be repeated 6-12 h later.

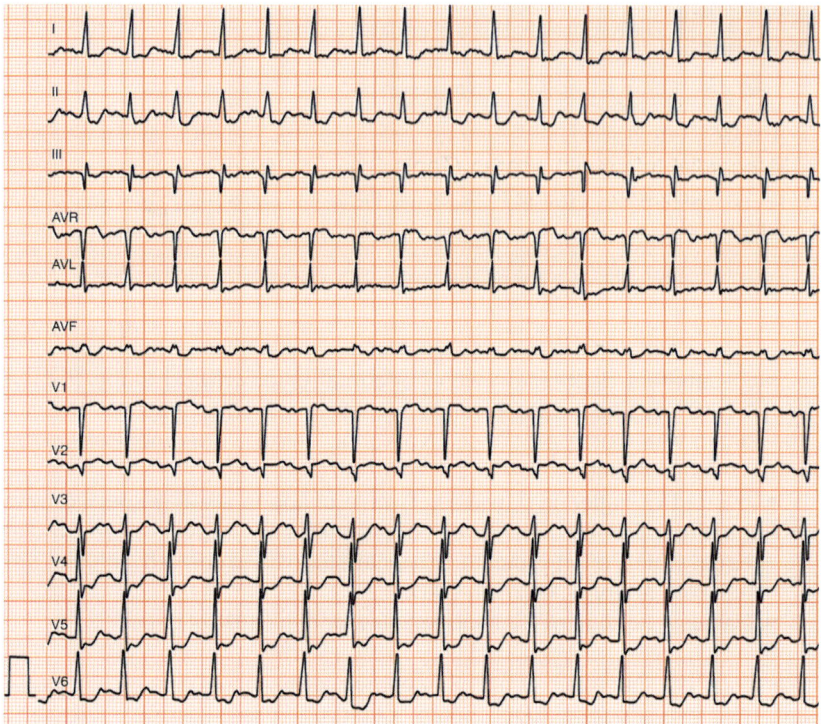

Figure 3.1. The ECG shows sinus tachycardia and ST-segment depression in leads I, II, aVF, V$_4$, V$_5$ and V$_6$. The ECG was recorded during an episode of angina at rest.

Angiographic findings
- ~15% of patients show no hemodynamically significant lesions (i.e. <50% stenosis of the luminal diameter) in the coronary vessels (more frequently in women).
- ~30% have single-vessel CAD.
- ~50% have multi-vessel CAD (2- or 3-vessel CAD).
- ~5% have left main CAD.

Indications for cardiac catheterization during hospitalization
Patients with non ST-segment elevation ACS are classified into three categories with regard to the timing of cardiac catheterization during hospitalization:
- Very high risk (catheterization in <2 h).

- High risk (catheterization in <24 h), and
- Moderate risk (catheterization in <72 h) [Table 3.3].

Various risk scores are also used for risk stratification; these include the GRACE (Global Registry of Acute Coronary Events) and TIMI (Thrombolysis In Myocardial Infarction) scores (Table 3.4). The GRACE score is considered more accurate but, due to its complexity, it usually requires a computer (alternatively, it can be calculated online, at http://www.outcomes-umassmed.org/grace). For the calculation of in-hospital mortality, the GRACE score takes into account 8 factors: the patient's age, clinical picture (Killip classification), systolic blood pressure (BP), heart rate, serum creatinine levels, cardiac arrest at admission, ST-segment deviation and increase in markers of myocardial necrosis. Based on the GRACE score, the in-hospital mortality is:

- Low (<1%) when the score is ≤ 108.
- Intermediate (1-3%) when the score is 109-140 and
- High (>3%) when the score is >140.

TABLE 3.3	Patients with non ST-segment elevation acute coronary syndrome in whom cardiac catheterization during hospitalization is indicated

A) Very high risk: catheterization in <2 h (urgent)
  1) Persistent or recurring angina despite full antiischemic therapy, with or without changes in the ST-segment
  2) Symptoms of heart failure
  3) Hemodynamic instability
  4) Life-threatening tachyarrhythmias (ventricular fibrillation, ventricular tachycardia)

B) High risk: catheterization in <24 h
  1) Changes (rise/fall) in cardiac troponins
  2) Dynamic changes in the ST-segment or the T-wave (with or without symptoms)
  3) GRACE score >140

C) Moderate risk: catheterization in <72 h
  1) Diabetes mellitus
  2) Renal impairment (estimated glomerular filtration rate <60 mL/min/1.73 m^2)
  3) Left ventricular ejection fraction <40%
  4) Percutaneous coronary intervention within 6 months
  5) Previous coronary artery bypass graft surgery
  6) Early postinfarction angina
  7) GRACE score 109-140

TABLE 3.4	TIMI risk score for risk stratification in unstable angina/non ST-segment elevation myocardial infarction	
TIMI risk factors	**Points**	**Comments**
Age ≥65 years	1	The greater the score the higher the event rate.
≥3 risk factors for coronary artery disease (CAD)*	1	Risk for death, new or recurrent myocardial infarction or severe recurrent ischemia requiring urgent
Known CAD (≥50% stenosis)	1	revascularization at 14 days according to score is:
Use of aspirin in prior 7 days	1	• score 0 or 1: 4.7%
≥2 episodes of angina within the past 24 h	1	• score 2: 8.3%
		• score 3: 13.2%
ST-segment deviation ≥0.5 mm on admission ECG	1	• score 4: 19.9%
		• score 5: 26.2%
Increased markers of myocardial necrosis	1	• score 6 or 7: 40.9%
Total score	0-7	

Arterial hypertension, hypercholesterolemia, diabetes mellitus, smoking and family history of premature CAD

Depending on the anatomy observed, the following procedures are performed:

- Percutaneous coronary intervention (PCI) with concurrent dual antiplatelet therapy and possible administration of glycoprotein IIb/IIIa inhibitors (see page 65 for more details), or
- Coronary artery bypass graft surgery, particularly in cases of left main or 3-vessel CAD, and particularly with concomitant impairment of left ventricular function.

Low-risk patients (without the risk factors listed in Table 3.3) undergo noninvasive ischemia testing (e.g. exercise test under antiischemic medication) before being discharged and, depending on the findings, cardiac catheterization is scheduled or conservative treatment is chosen.

Treatment

1) **Oxygen** in case of dyspnea or arterial oxygen saturation <90%.
2) **Nitrates:** Given mainly for pain relief (beginning even before hospital arrival if sublingual nitroglycerin is available in patients without hypotension). They are also beneficial in patients with heart failure and hypertension. Nitrates reduce the myocardial consumption of oxygen by reducing the preload (venodilation) and to a lesser extent the afterload (sys-

temic arterial dilation), while also increasing myocardial perfusion by vasodilation of the large coronary arteries (+ collaterals and arterioles with >100 μm diameter).

If the patient presents with persisting ischemic symptoms (i.e. despite prior administration of up to 3 sublingual nitroglycerin tablets at 5-min intervals) in the Emergency Room and/or the patient is hypertensive or in heart failure, nitroglycerin is administered IV. It is given initially at a dose of 5-10 μg/min, which is gradually increased (5-10 μg/min every 5-10 min) until the pain is controlled or until the systolic BP drops to <90 mmHg [maximum dosage 200 μg/min]. Nitroglycerin (Tridil, Nitro-Bid), is administered IV, usually for 48 h, and is discontinued if the patient remains asymptomatic for 24 h. For the solution preparation and the method of infusion, see Chapter 23.

Warning! If sildenafil (Viagra, Revatio) or vardenafil (Levitra) has been administered during the previous 24 h, then nitrates are not given because of the risk of a precipitous fall of the BP due to profound vasodilation. The same applies when tadalafil (Cialis) has been administered during the previous 48 h.

3) **Beta-blockers:** Should be administered po within the first 24 h in the absence of contraindications (signs of heart failure or low cardiac output, increased risk for cardiogenic shock [systolic BP <120 mmHg, heart rate >110 beats/min, age >70 years], atrioventricular conduction disturbances, history of severe bronchial asthma, etc.). The target is to achieve a heart rate of 50-60 beats/min at rest. Beta-blockers are associated with lower in-hospital mortality.

In high-risk patients (evidence of ongoing ischemia, especially with associated tachycardia or hypertension), the IV route is preferred (e.g. 5 mg of metoprolol tartrate [supplied as Lopressor ampoule of 5 mg/5 mL] over 1-2 min x 3 at intervals of 5 min, and, 15 min after the last IV dose, begin oral administration at a dose of 25-50 mg x 2 daily with gradual dosage increase to 100 x 2 daily). Metoprolol is a cardioselective beta-blocker. Alternatively, carvedilol (Coreg, Dilatrend) can be administered po (non cardioselective beta-blocker which also inhibits α_1-receptors) at an initial dose of 6.25 mg x 2 daily. In cases of suspected contraindications to beta-blockers (e.g. bronchial asthma), esmolol (Brevibloc) IV (cardioselective beta1-blocker) can be tried because of its short elimination half-life (~9 min), and the patient's tolerance to beta-blockers can be monitored. If the patient is not considered high risk, then beta-blockers are administered po. Therefore, beta-blockers are given po in most cases.

4) **Calcium antagonists (calcium channel blockers):** Administered when pain persists despite the administration of a full dose of nitrates and be-

ta-blockers (dihydropyridine-type, e.g. nifedipine, amlodipine, etc.) or if there are contraindications to beta-blockers (non-dihydropyridine type, e.g. verapamil or diltiazem). They are also the drugs of choice for vasospastic angina. The usual initial dosage regimen for nifedipine (Adalat, Feramon) is 20 mg x 2, for diltiazem (Cardizem, Tildiem) 60 mg x 3, and for verapamil (Calan, Isoptin) 80 mg x 3 daily. There is no definite evidence for a benefit of calcium antagonists on prognosis. Verapamil and diltiazem should be avoided in patients with heart failure or evidence of severe left ventricular dysfunction.

> **Warning!** A dihydropyridine-type calcium antagonist (e.g. nifedipine) should never be administered if a beta-blocker is not coadministered to counteract the undesirable reflex tachycardia caused by the calcium antagonist.

5) **Morphine:** Administered in cases of persistent pain despite therapy with nitrates and beta-blockers at doses of 1-5 mg IV. An antiemetic (e.g. metoclopramide 10 mg IV) is also administered concurrently. Antidotes to morphine side effects:
   - In case of respiratory depression: naloxone (Evzio, Narcan) at a dose of 0.4-1.2 mg IV, and
   - In case of bradycardia: atropine at a dose of 0.5-1.5 mg IV.

6) **Acetylsalicylic acid (aspirin):** The first dose (150-300 mg, nonenteric-coated form) must be chewed and held in the oral cavity for fast action (onset of action in 15 min). Thereafter, treatment is continued at a dose of 75-150 mg daily (usually 100 mg/day). Aspirin irreversibly inactivates the platelet enzyme cyclooxygenase-1 (COX-1), which is responsible for the formation of thromboxane A_2, an activator of platelet aggregation. Its antiplatelet action lasts throughout the platelets' life span (7-10 days).
   Aspirin reduces the risk of myocardial infarction (MI) and cardiac death by ~50%. The benefit is apparent from the first day. Absolute contraindications are allergy to aspirin, active bleeding and hemophilia. If the patient is unable to take aspirin because of allergy or major gastrointestinal intolerance only clopidogrel should be given (loading dose followed by a daily maintenance dose).

7) **$P2Y_{12}$ receptor inhibitors:** They inhibit the binding of adenosine diphosphate (ADP) to the platelet $P2Y_{12}$ receptors, thus preventing further platelet activation and aggregation. They are coadministered with aspirin (dual antiplatelet therapy [DAPT]) for 12 months after an ACS. Specifically for patients with drug-eluting stents (DES), the duration of DAPT is at least 12 months. The currently available oral $P2Y_{12}$ receptor inhibitors are:
   - **Clopidogrel** (Plavix, Iscover): A prodrug that is converted to the active metabolite in the liver by cytochrome P450 (CYP450 [isoenzymes

CYP3A4 and CYP2C19]). Clopidogrel is administered at an initial loading dose of 300 or 600 mg and thereafter at a dose of 75 mg/day. When PCI is performed, the loading dose is 600 mg, followed by 75 mg/day. Side effects include gastrointestinal problems (at a lower rate than aspirin) and rash. Also, the presence of clinical factors (e.g. diabetes mellitus) and certain genetic polymorphisms are associated with attenuation (resistance) of clopidogrel action. Resistance is tested *in vitro* and, in certain cases, may be complicated by a thrombotic episode. Of the genetic factors, the one best studied is the CYP2C19 polymorphism, which is associated with reduced CYP450 enzyme activity and with development of resistance to clopidogrel. Also, the administration of proton pump inhibitors (PPIs), especially omeprazole, which are metabolized by CYP2C19 and cause competitive inhibition of clopidogrel activation, leads to attenuation of the antiplatelet action of clopidogrel, at least *in vitro*. Until the interaction between PPIs and clopidogrel is elucidated, it is prudent to avoid the administration of omeprazole in patients receiving clopidogrel or, if coadministered, it should be given 12 h apart so that their interaction can be minimized.

- **Prasugrel** (Effient): A prodrug that is converted to the active metabolite through 2 metabolic steps: plasma esterases and CYP450. It has a faster onset of action than clopidogrel and its activity is not significantly affected by CYP2C19 polymorphisms. It has been approved by the American Food and Drug Administration (FDA) for patients with ACS (with or without ST-segment elevation) who are scheduled for PCI. In particular, prasugrel should be given promptly and no later than 1 h after PCI once coronary anatomy is defined and a decision is made to proceed with PCI (Anderson JL, et al. Circulation 2013;127:e663-e828). It is administered at an initial loading dose of 60 mg po and thereafter at 10 mg daily (5 mg for patients with a body weight <60 kg). The TRITON-TIMI 38 study (Wiriott SD, et al. N Engl J Med 2007; 357:2001-15), which compared it to clopidogrel in patients with moderate-high risk ACS subjected to PCI, showed that it reduces cardiovascular events (including stent thrombosis) to a greater degree, but at the cost of a slight increase in major hemorrhagic complications. The benefits were somewhat greater for diabetic patients. An absolute contraindication for prasugrel use is a history of cerebrovascular event and a relative contraindication is age ≥75 years.

- **Ticagrelor** (Brilique, Brilinta): A nonthienopyridine reversible inhibitor of $P2Y_{12}$ receptors. In contrast to clopidogrel and prasugrel, it is an active drug that does not need metabolic activation. It has a faster onset of action than clopidogrel. It is administered at a loading dose of 180 mg and thereafter at 90 mg x 2/day. In the PLATO study (Cannon CP, et al. Lancet 2010;375:283-93) in patients with ACS without (moderate-high risk) or with ST-segment elevation treated with PCI, it was superior to clopidogrel as regards the occurrence of cardiovascular events, with no increase in the risk of major hemorrhagic complications. With regard to side effects, a greater rate of dyspnea (mostly mild or moderate) was noted in patients receiving ticagrelor compared to those receiving clopidogrel (14.5 versus 8.7%). This side effect might be due to the chemical similarity of ticagrelor to adenosine. The FDA has approved ticagrelor for ACS, with the warning that it should not be coadministered with aspirin at doses >100 mg/day (recommended dose 81 mg/day) because it reduces its effectiveness. Table 3.5 compares the pharmacological properties of the three $P2Y_{12}$ receptor inhibitors.

According to the recent European Guidelines (Roffi M, et al. Eur Heart J 2016;37:267-315):

- Ticagrelor should be preferred in all patients with non ST-segment elevation ACS who present a moderate-high risk for ischemic cardiac episodes (e.g. they are troponin-positive or present ST-segment depression ≥1 mm in at least 2 leads, etc.), regardless of any previous use of clopidogrel (if given, it should be replaced by ticagrelor).
- Prasugrel is recommended for patients with non ST-segment elevation ACS who were not receiving $P2Y_{12}$ receptor inhibitors (especially diabetics), whose coronary anatomy is known, and who are scheduled for PCI. Contraindications: previous cerebrovascular event or ongoing bleeds. It is also avoided in patients ≥75 years of age or with a body weight <60 kg.
- Clopidogrel is a 3rd-choice antiplatelet drug and is recommended only for patients who cannot receive ticagrelor (1st choice) or prasugrel (2nd choice) or who require oral anticoagulation.

TABLE 3.5	Pharmacological properties of $P2Y_{12}$ receptor inhibitors		
	Clopidogrel	**Prasugrel**	**Ticagrelor**
Reversible inhibitor	No	No	Yes
Prodrug	Yes	Yes	No
Onset of loading dose effect*	2-4 h	30 min	30 min
Duration of action	3-10 days	7-10 days	3-5 days
Cessation before major surgery	5 days	7 days	5 days

*50% inhibition of ADP-induced platelet aggregation

We have to mention, that in our clinical practice, clopidogrel continues to play a significant role in the treatment of non ST-segment elevation ACS. However, a preference for newer antiplatelet drugs, especially ticagrelor, is justified in cases of:

- High risk of thrombosis: diabetes mellitus, need for multiple PCIs, history of intracoronary stent thrombosis, or
- Resistance to clopidogrel.

Finally, we should add that the recent American Guidelines do not embrace the enthusiasm of the European Guidelines with regard to newer antiplatelet drugs: in most cases it is recommended that the choice of the second antiplatelet drug should be between clopidogrel, ticagrelor, or prasugrel, with no preference for the new antiplatelets over clopidogrel (Amsterdam EA, et al. Circulation 2014;130:2354-94).

8) **Heparin:** The addition of unfractionated heparin (UFH) to treatment with aspirin reduces even further the risk of death or MI compared to aspirin only. UFH is administered at a dose of 60-70 U/kg bolus IV (maximum dose 5000 U) followed by continuous infusion of 12-15 U/kg/h (maximum dose 1000 U/h) with a target activated partial thromboplastin time (aPTT) between 50-70 s. Until this target is achieved, aPTT is measured every 6 h and then every 12-24 h thereafter.

The primary effect of heparin is to bind and potentiate antithrombin III, which then binds to thrombin and inactivates it (indirect thrombin inhibitor). Inactive thrombin cannot catalyze the formation of fibrin, the end product of the coagulation cascade, from fibrinogen. The complex heparin-antithrombin III also inhibits factor Xa.

Today, there is a trend towards replacing UFH with low-molecular-weight heparins (LMWHs), particularly enoxaparin (Lovenox, Clexane), as it appears to provide a greater clinical benefit. The advantages of enoxaparin include greater bioavailability, which allows subcutaneous administration every 12 h, and a more stable anticoagulant action, which does not need monitoring with blood tests (Table 3.6). Enoxaparin is administered in a dose of 1 mg/kg x 2/d subcutaneously for the duration of hospitalization or until an uncomplicated PCI is performed. In high risk patients an initial loading dose of 30 mg IV may be given for immediate anticoagulation.

Warning! In patients with severe chronic kidney disease (creatinine clearance <30 mL/min) the dose of enoxaparin is reduced to 1 mg/kg once daily subcutaneously.

TABLE 3.6	Major characteristics and differences of low-molecular-weight heparins (LMWHs) from unfractionated heparin (UFH)

1) Lower molecular weight than UFH (~1/3)

2) Inhibit factor Xa (leading to reduced thrombin production) more effectively than factor IIa (factor IIa = thrombin, which acts on fibrinogen [factor I] to produce fibrin); so anti-Xa/anti-IIa >1, whereas UFH has similar activity against factors Xa and IIa, i.e. anti-Xa/anti-IIa = 1

3) Bound to a smaller extent with plasma proteins, longer elimination half-life (4-5 h), better bioavailability

4) Primarily cleared by the kidneys while UFH is metabolized mainly through the reticuloendothelial system

5) Usually no laboratory tests are necessary for monitoring their effectiveness, as opposed to the frequent aPTT tests for UFH because of its "unpredictable" action

6) Cause thrombocytopenia (HIT) [platelet drop ≥50% of baseline platelet count] less frequently than UFH

7) More practical administration regimen: administered subcutaneously once or twice daily

8) Of the LMWHs, enoxaparin is associated with a greater clinical benefit than UFH in the treatment of non ST-segment elevation acute coronary syndromes

9) Protamine sulfate only partly inhibits their activity, since it neutralizes only their anti-IIa activity

10) In cases of renal failure, their dose must be reduced

11) Higher cost than UFH

aPTT: activated partial thromboplastin time, HIT: heparin-induced thrombocytopenia

In patients under heparin therapy, the occurrence of venous thrombosis or a drop in platelets by ≥50% of baseline (usually <100,000/mm^3) raises suspicion of heparin-induced thrombocytopenia (HIT). For laboratory confirmation, the patient is tested for antibodies to the heparin/platelet factor 4 complex and, if the diagnosis is confirmed, heparin is replaced by a direct thrombin inhibitor (lepirudin, available in a 50 mg Refludan vial) or by fondaparinux [more information in Chapter 4].

9) **Nonheparin anticoagulants**

   a) **Fondaparinux** (Arixtra): A synthetic polysaccharide that selectively inhibits coagulation factor Xa (indirect inhibitor by binding to antithrombin III). It has no effect on thrombin already produced, which might explain the greater risk of catheter thrombosis when PCI is performed on a patient who has received only fondaparinux for anticoagulation. It has 100% bioavailability after subcutaneous administration and is cleared by the kidneys (contraindicated when creatinine clearance is

<20 mL/min). It has an elimination half-life of ~17 h and it is adminis-tered subcutaneously at a dose of 2.5 mg daily. The advantages are that it does not need blood tests for activity monitoring, it is adminis-tered once daily, and it is not complicated by HIT (does not interact with platelet factor 4). Compared to the LMWHs, it presents at least e-qual clinical effectiveness and a lower risk of hemorrhagic complica-tions. In cases of serious hemorrhage, there is no specific antidote that reverses its action. Recombinant factor VIIa can be given to control any bleeding events. According to the recent European Guidelines (Roffi M, et al. Eur Heart J 2016;37:267-315), fondaparinux is recom-mended as the anticoagulant of first choice in patients with non ST-segment elevation ACS, and only if this is not available is enoxaparin (2nd choice) or UFH (3rd choice) recommended. This recommenda-tion is based on the better effectiveness/safety ratio (mostly with re-gard to the risk of bleeding) that fondaparinux presents compared to enoxaparin and UFH. Patients on fondaparinux undergoing PCI, should be given UFH (70-85 U/kg IV bolus) during the procedure.

b) **Bivalirudin** (Angiomax, Angiox): A direct inhibitor of thrombin. It is ad-ministered IV and has an elimination half-life of ~25 min. It acts on both free and clot-bound thrombin. It is not complicated by HIT. Its activity is monitored by determination of the activated clotting time (ACT) or the aPTT. Bivalirudin is recommended in high-risk patients with non ST-segment elevation ACS during PCI as an alternative to the combination of UFH + glycoprotein IIb/IIIa inhibitors, particularly in patients with a high risk of bleeding. It is administered initially at a dose of 0.75 mg/kg bolus IV, followed by 1.75 mg/kg/h for up to 4 h after the PCI (Windeker S, et al. Eur Heart J 2014;35:2541-619). In cases of serious hemorrhage there is no specific antidote. However, it is rarely needed because of its relatively short half-life.

10) **Glycoprotein IIb/IIIa inhibitors:** They inhibit the activated IIb/IIIa recep-tors found in the platelet membrane, thus preventing their binding to the fibrinogen that bridges the platelets. Remember that fibrinogen, by bind-ing to the IIb/IIIa receptors, leads to formation of the platelet clot, which is the last step in platelet aggregation. The action of glycoprotein IIb/IIIa inhibitors is independent of the stimuli that have activated the platelets (ADP, thrombin, serotonin, etc.).

The indications for administering glycoprotein IIb/IIIa inhibitors to patients with non ST-segment elevation ACS who are already receiving DAPT are limited to those patients who are undergoing high-risk PCI for periopera-tive MI (elevated troponin, visible thrombus) and also have a low risk of bleeding. The emerging trend is to begin administration in the catheteri-zation laboratory (downstream selective/periprocedural administration) and not sooner (upstream administration), which would have the theoretical advantage of "cooling" the culprit lesion, since the latter practice is associated with a greater risk of bleeding without any clinical benefit.

Available glycoprotein IIb/IIIa inhibitors
- **Abciximab** (ReoPro): monoclonal antibodies. Administered at a dose of 0.25 mg/kg IV bolus 10-60 min prior to PCI and thereafter by infusion of 0.125 μg/kg/min (no more than 10 μg/min) for up to 12 h. Abciximab is approved only for patients undergoing PCI.
- **Eptifibatide** (Integrilin): synthetic heptapeptide. Administered at a dose of 180 μg/kg IV bolus, the initial dose is repeated after 10 min, and thereafter by infusion of 2 μg/kg/min for 12-18 h.
- **Tirofiban** (Aggrastat): nonpeptide substance. Administered at a dose of 25 μg/kg IV bolus and then by infusion of 0.15 μg/kg/min for up to 18 h.

The dosage regimens for glycoprotein IIb/IIIa inhibitors are based on the American Guidelines (Jneid H, et al. Circulation 2012;126:875-910) which express a preference for eptifibatide and tirofiban. The antiplatelet action of abciximab lasts 24-48 h after the end of the infusion, whereas eptifibatide and tirofiban last 4-8 h. Their administration can be complicated by acute thrombocytopenia (0.5-5.6%); this risk is higher with abciximab. In case of serious bleeding, platelets are transfused.

The contraindications to the administration of glycoprotein IIb/IIIa receptor inhibitors are similar to those of fibrinolytic agents. Table 3.7 presents the "antidotes" to antithrombotic drugs used in cases of serious hemorrhagic events.

Warning! In cases of renal failure, the dosage of eptifibatide and tirofiban should be reduced.

11) **Statins:** Administered to all patients, from the first day of hospitalization, regardless of cholesterol levels on admission, with a target LDL cholesterol level of <70 mg/dL, desired levels 50-70 mg/dL, or reduction of LDL cholesterol by ≥50 if the baseline untreated value is between 70-135 mg/dL (European Guidelines, Catapano AL, et al. Eur Heart J 2016;37:2999-3058) or a reduction of LDL cholesterol ≥50% from the untreated baseline by giving high-intensity statin therapy (American Guidelines, Stone NJ, et al. Circulation 2014;129:S1-S45). The main advantage of immediate administration of statins is the rapid clinical benefits achieved mainly through their pleiotropic effects (antiinflammatory, antithrombotic, improvement of endothelial function, etc.). Finally, the addition of ezetimibe (10 mg daily) should be considered if patients

TABLE 3.7	"Antidotes" to antithrombotic drugs (direct action reversal or indirect correction of severe hemorrhagic events)

Anticoagulants

1) Vitamin K antagonists	• Vitamin K_1: 10 mg IV over 30 min • Fresh frozen plasma: 15-30 mL/kg (~4-6 units) IV • Four-factor prothrombin complex concentrate (II, VII, IX and X): 25-50 U/kg IV • Recombinant factor VIIa: 10-90 µg/kg IV
2) Unfractionated heparin (UFH)	• Protamine sulfate: 1 mg (IV)/100 U of UFH administered during the previous 30 min, ½ of the dose if the infusion of UFH was interrupted at >30 min but <2 h, $^1/_4$ of the dose if interrupted >2 h but <4 h
3) Low-molecular-weight heparins (LMWHs)	• Protamine sulfate*: 1 mg (IV)/1 mg of LMWH administered during the previous 4 h
4) Fondaparinux (no specific antidote)	• Recombinant factor VIIa**: 90 µg/kg IV • Fresh frozen plasma: 15-30 mL/kg IV
5) Bivalirudin (no specific antidote)	• Recombinant factor VIIa**: 90 µg/kg IV • Fresh frozen plasma: 15-30 mL/kg IV • Hemodialysis (drug removal)

Antiplatelet drugs

1) Aspirin, P2Y$_{12}$ receptor inhibitors	• Platelet transfusion
2) Glycoprotein IIb-IIIa inhibitors	• Platelet transfusion

* *Achieves only partial reversal of LMWH action*
** *Limited experience*

fail to achieve the LDL cholesterol target despite taking the maximally tolerated statin dose.

12) **Angiotensin-converting enzyme (ACE) inhibitors:** administered to patients with diabetes mellitus, heart failure, ejection fraction ≤40% or hypertension. However, the trend today is to give them to all patients who have suffered non ST-segment elevation ACS. If not tolerated, angiotensin II receptor blockers are administered.

13) **Anxiolytics** at low doses.
14) **Proton pump inhibitors (PPIs)** [preferably not omeprazole]. Continuation after discharge in patients with a history of gastrointestinal bleeding or peptic ulcer, in the elderly and in the setting of triple antithrombotic treatment.

 Key points

- The diagnosis of non ST-segment elevation ACS in the case of unstable angina is mainly clinical, as ischemic changes on the ECG may be absent and markers of myocardial necrosis are not elevated.

- Non ST-segment elevation ACS includes a heterogeneous group of clinical syndromes (resting and prolonged angina, new-onset [<2 months] severe exertional angina, recent aggravation of preexisting stable angina, and postinfarction angina within 2 weeks of MI).

- In the management of non ST-segment elevation ACS, it is very important to perform risk stratification. Depending on the risk, coronary angiography and reperfusion will be performed according to the findings. So:
  a) Very high-risk patients (persistent or recurrent severe ischemia, heart failure, hemodynamic instability, life-threatening tachyarrhythmias) undergo urgent coronary angiography (<2 h).
  b) High-risk patients (cardiac troponin changes, dynamic changes on the ECG, GRACE score >140) undergo coronary angiography at <24 h.
  c) Moderate risk patients (diabetes mellitus, renal failure, ejection fraction <40%, postinfarction angina, PCI <6 months or coronary artery bypass grafting, GRACE score 109-140) undergo coronary angiography at <72 h.
  d) Low-risk patients (not belonging to the previous categories) undergo elective coronary angiography only if noninvasive investigation indicates significant myocardial ischemia.

- As soon as the diagnosis of non ST-segment elevation ACS is established, DAPT (aspirin and a $P2Y_{12}$ receptor inhibitor), anticoagulation therapy (fondaparinux or enoxaparin subcutaneously), IV nitrates (in case of pain), IV morphine (if pain does not resolve with nitrates), beta-blockers (usually po), statins, and ACE inhibitors must be administered.

- Glycoprotein IIb/IIIa inhibitors are administered only to patients undergoing high-risk PCI for perioperative MI (elevated troponin, visible clot) who also have a low risk of bleeding.

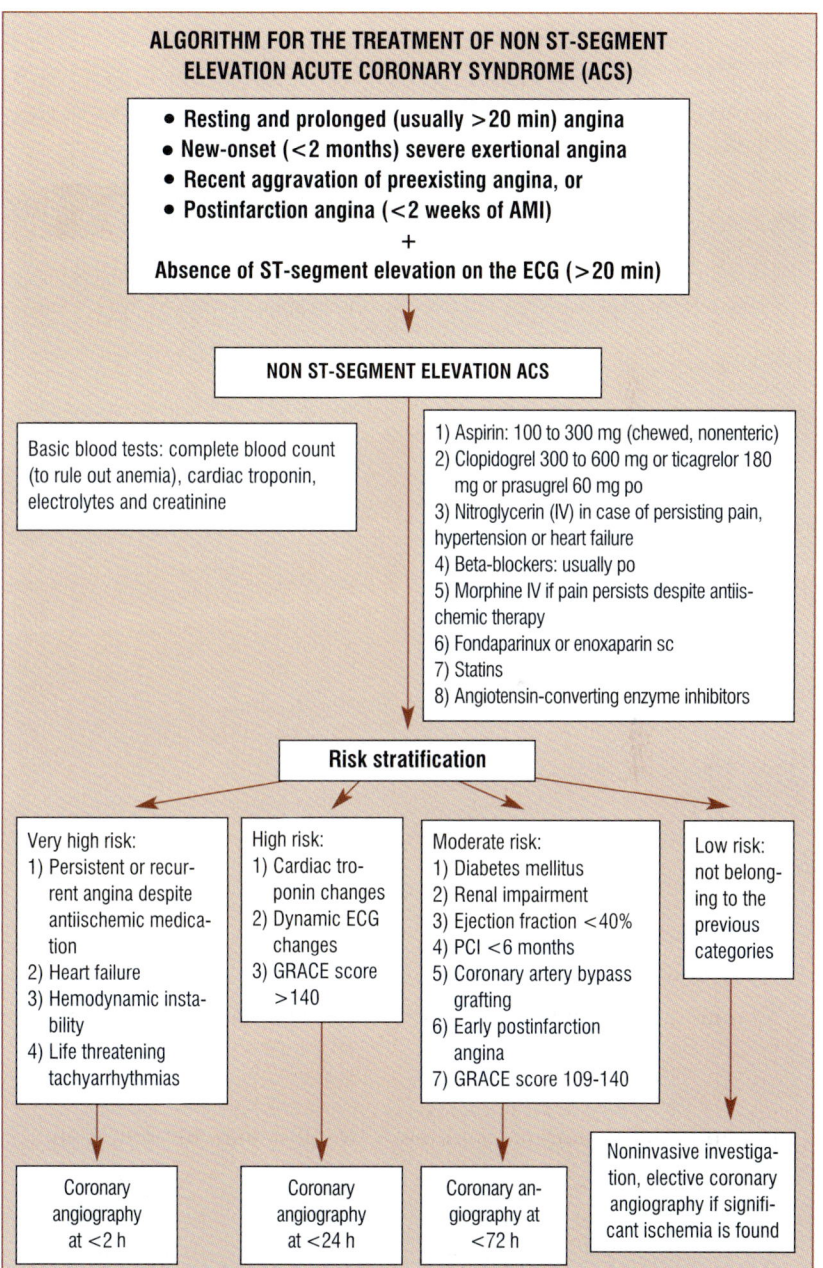

ALGORITHM FOR THE TREATMENT OF NON ST-SEGMENT ELEVATION ACUTE CORONARY SYNDROME (ACS)

- Resting and prolonged (usually >20 min) angina
- New-onset (<2 months) severe exertional angina
- Recent aggravation of preexisting angina, or
- Postinfarction angina (<2 weeks of AMI)

+

Absence of ST-segment elevation on the ECG (>20 min)

NON ST-SEGMENT ELEVATION ACS

Basic blood tests: complete blood count (to rule out anemia), cardiac troponin, electrolytes and creatinine

1) Aspirin: 100 to 300 mg (chewed, nonenteric)
2) Clopidogrel 300 to 600 mg or ticagrelor 180 mg or prasugrel 60 mg po
3) Nitroglycerin (IV) in case of persisting pain, hypertension or heart failure
4) Beta-blockers: usually po
5) Morphine IV if pain persists despite antiischemic therapy
6) Fondaparinux or enoxaparin sc
7) Statins
8) Angiotensin-converting enzyme inhibitors

Risk stratification

Very high risk:
1) Persistent or recurrent angina despite antiischemic medication
2) Heart failure
3) Hemodynamic instability
4) Life threatening tachyarrhythmias

High risk:
1) Cardiac troponin changes
2) Dynamic ECG changes
3) GRACE score >140

Moderate risk:
1) Diabetes mellitus
2) Renal impairment
3) Ejection fraction <40%
4) PCI <6 months
5) Coronary artery bypass grafting
6) Early postinfarction angina
7) GRACE score 109-140

Low risk: not belonging to the previous categories

Coronary angiography at <2 h

Coronary angiography at <24 h

Coronary angiography at <72 h

Noninvasive investigation, elective coronary angiography if significant ischemia is found

AMI: acute myocardial infarction, PCI: percutaneous coronary intervention, Sc: subcutaneously

4 Pulmonary embolism

Pulmonary embolism (PE) is one of the most difficult conditions to diagnose in the Emergency Room, since it can mimic a number of other diseases; in addition, the standard diagnostic tests (ECG, chest X-ray, arterial blood gases) are of little help in its diagnosis. PE shows a tendency to recur and with the exception of low-risk PE, it is characterized by high in-hospital mortality.

Pathophysiology

PE is caused by the obstruction of one or more branches of the pulmonary artery by an embolus, which in >90% of cases originates (detaches) from a primary thrombus formed in the deep veins of the lower limbs or the minor pelvis. Predisposing factors that promote the development of deep vein thrombosis (DVT) and, consequently, the occurrence of PE, are listed in Table 4.1. Specifically, DVT above the knee is associated with a 50% risk of PE, whereas DVT limited to the calf is associated with smaller risk. The presence of two or more risk factors for venous thromboembolism multiplies this risk: for example, a mutation in factor V (factor V Leiden) triples the risk of DVT, while the use of oral estrogen-containing contraceptives by patients with factor V Leiden increases the DVT risk by at least 10-fold, which significantly increases the consequent risk of PE.

The degree of hemodynamic compromise caused by PE depends on the extent of the obstructed arterial pulmonary vasculature (and therefore on the degree of pulmonary hypertension), on the existing cardiopulmonary reserve and on the intensity of pulmonary vasoconstriction. The increase in pulmonary arterial pressure distends the right ventricle, which results in the production of B-type natriuretic peptide (BNP) or its precursor, N-terminal-proBNP (NT-proBNP). There is also the possibility of right ventricular ischemia, development of microinfarcts with cardiac troponin release (due to

TABLE 4.1	Predisposing factors for venous thromboembolism

1) Recent hip or knee replacement

2) Fracture of lower limbs

3) Postoperative immobilization or recent major injury

4) Previous pulmonary embolism or deep vein thrombosis

5) Spinal cord injury

6) Malignancy (higher risk in metastatic disease), chemotherapy

7) Congestive heart or respiratory failure

8) Use of oral contraceptives (particularly by smokers)

9) Hormone replacement therapy

10) Blood transfusion and erythropoietin-stimulating factor

11) Paralytic stroke

12) Acute infection

13) Pregnancy, postpartum period (associated with higher risk than pregnancy)

14) Obesity, advanced age, prolonged sitting (e.g. air travel)

15) Patients bedridden for >3 days

16) Hypercoagulable states

    a) Factor V Leiden (found in 3-5% of the population)

    b) Prothrombin 20210 gene mutation

    c) Protein C, protein S or antithrombin III deficiency (rare)

    d) Antiphospholipid syndrome

    e) Hyperhomocysteinemia

increased oxygen demand and decreased oxygen supply of the pressure overloaded right ventricle), and finally cardiogenic shock. Right ventricular distension also produces a paradoxical shift of the interventricular septum to the left, which results in impaired diastolic filling of the left ventricle and a fall in cardiac output.

Symptoms (nonspecific)
- Acute dyspnea, which is the most common symptom (>70%).

Warning! The onset of dyspnea in a patient with congestive heart failure with no evident decompensation factors should raise the suspicion of PE.

- Chest pain (~65%): pleuritic in cases of peripheral embolism, retrosternal in cases of massive PE.
- Cough (~20%).
- Syncope (~10%) due to a transient fall in cardiac output, caused by acute right ventricular failure, vasovagal stimulation or arrhythmias.
- Hemoptysis (~10%).

Clinical signs
- Tachypnea (≥20 breaths/min), which is the most common sign (~70%), tachycardia (>100 beats/min), low-grade fever, distended jugular veins, hypotension and signs of low cardiac output in case of massive PE.
- Heart auscultation: right-sided 3rd heart sound (from the right ventricle), systolic murmur in the left parasternal region which increases during inspiration (tricuspid valve regurgitation), and a loud pulmonary component of the 2nd heart sound.
- Localized crackles in the lungs.
- Signs of DVT in the lower limbs,* such as edema, redness and pain in the calf or the thigh, rather infrequently (~20%).

Evaluation of the clinical probability of pulmonary embolism
Since the clinical symptoms and signs have relatively low sensitivity and specificity in the diagnosis of PE, a combined evaluation has been suggested for predicting the probability of PE. This combined evaluation is based on validated tables of clinical scales, such as those of Wells and Geneva. The Wells score system is given below (Table 4.2).

Clinical syndromes of pulmonary embolism
- *Massive PE* (5-10% of cases) is defined as acute PE with:
  - sustained hypotension: systolic blood pressure (BP) <90 mmHg for at least 15 min, if not caused by other causes, such as new onset arrhythmia, hypovolemia, sepsis, or left ventricular dysfunction (Jaff MR, et al. Circulation 2011;123:1788-830),
  - requirement for inotropic support, not because of other causes, or
  - pulselessness, or persistent profound bradycardia (heart rate <40 beats/min with signs or symptoms of shock).

Massive PE corresponds to the high-risk PE defined in the latest European Guidelines for PE (Konstantinides S, et al. Eur Heart J 2014;35:3033-69). Dyspnea is usually the most prominent symptom, while chest pain is un-

---

*The Homans sign (pain in the calf during passive dorsiflexion of the foot) has low sensitivity and specificity for diagnosing DVT in the lower limbs.

TABLE 4.2	Clinical prediction of acute pulmonary embolism (PE) according to classic Wells criteria

Criteria	Points
Clinical signs of deep vein thrombosis (DVT)	3
Alternative diagnosis less likely than PE	3
Heart rate ≥100 beats/min	1.5
Previous PE or DVT	1.5
Surgery or immobilization within the past 4 weeks	1.5
Hemoptysis	1
Active cancer	1

Clinical probability of PE*	Total score
Low (6±2%)	0-1
Intermediate (23±5%)	2-6
High (49±6%)	≥7

*Ceriani E, et al. J Thromb Haemost 2010;8:957-70

usual. The in-hospital mortality is ~30%. If massive PE manifests as cardiac arrest the mortality rate is very high (70-95%).

- *Submassive PE* (20-25% of cases) is defined as acute PE without systemic hypotension (systolic BP ≥90 mm Hg) but with either right ventricular dysfunction or myocardial necrosis. Dyspnea is a common presenting symptom.

- *Low risk PE* (~70% of cases) is acute PE without systemic hypotension, right ventricular dysfunction or myocardial necrosis. Symptomatology is mild (usually manifests with unexplained mild dyspnea) and often escapes diagnosis. It has a short-term mortality rate of <2%.

- *Pulmonary infarction:* the embolus occludes a peripheral branch near the pleura, causing necrosis of the corresponding segment of the lung. It is characterized by dyspnea, pleuritic chest pain and hemoptysis. Infarction develops in the peripheral circulation because the peripheral bed of the bronchial arteries, which are the main arteries supplying the lung, is poor. Conversely, an obstruction of more central branches does not lead to ischemic necrosis of the pulmonary parenchyma because of the abundant bronchial artery bed. The chest X-ray shows a triangular shadow (with the base towards the periphery), usually 3-7 days after PE.

Differential diagnosis

This includes primarily the acute coronary syndromes, pneumonia, acute pulmonary edema, pneumothorax, exacerbation of chronic obstructive pulmonary disease, acute aortic dissection, pericarditis, and lung cancer.

Diagnostic techniques

1) **D-dimer determination by enzyme-linked immunosorbent assay (ELISA):** Endogenous fibrinolysis results in fragmentation of fibrin into D-dimers. D-dimer levels >500 ng/mL have high sensitivity (>95%) but low specificity (~40%) for diagnosing PE. Table 4.3 lists conditions in which D-dimers are elevated. Low levels (<500 ng/mL) are more significant since they rule out PE (negative predictive value >95%) in cases of low to moderate clinical probability. In contrast, if there is high clinical probability of PE, a concomitant "negative" D-dimer test does not exclude PE. In general, D-dimers are useful for screening patients in the Emergency Room who have suspected PE but not coexistent acute systemic illness. Since D-dimer levels increase with age, for individuals aged >50 years the following formula is suggested for determining a

TABLE 4.3	Conditions with elevated D-dimer levels
1) Acute pulmonary embolism	
2) Deep vein thrombosis	
3) Acute myocardial infarction	
4) Infection (e.g. pneumonia)	
5) Malignancies	
6) Sepsis	
7) Postoperative period (one week at least)	
8) Disseminated intravascular coagulation	
9) Cerebrovascular accident	
10) Acute aortic dissection	
11) Congestive heart failure	
12) Renal failure	
13) Atrial fibrillation (~20%)	
14) Severe hepatic disease	
15) Preeclampsia / eclampsia	
16) Pregnancy (particularly 2nd and 3rd trimester)	

cutoff value: **age x 10 ng/mL;** i.e. for a patient aged 80 years pathological levels are considered to be those >80 x 10 = 800 ng/mL.

2) **Arterial blood gases:** They have little diagnostic value. Typically, hypocapnia with or without hypoxemia is found. In ~20% of cases, the partial pressure of O_2 is normal. Therefore, the absence of hypoxemia does not rule out PE. In the setting of shock, however, a normal O_2 partial pressure practically excludes PE.

3) **Cardiac troponin:** Elevated levels are associated with worse prognosis.

4) **BNP:** Elevated levels are associated with worse prognosis.

5) **ECG:** Of little diagnostic value. Its primary use is in ruling out an acute myocardial infarction (AMI). It usually shows sinus tachycardia, incomplete or complete right bundle branch block (RBBB), negative T waves in leads V_1-V_4, and less commonly atrial fibrillation and the $S_1Q_3T_3$ pattern (the most specific but relatively rare sign).

6) **Chest X-ray:** Of little diagnostic value. Its primary use is in ruling out other causes of dyspnea (pneumonia, pneumothorax, etc.). Nonspecific findings include pleural effusions, atelectasis and consolidation. Classical signs, such as the **Westermark sign** (focal oligemia distally to the obstruction) and **Hampton's hump** (peripheral wedge-shaped opacification which indicates pulmonary infarction), although specific, are rare.

7) **Ventilation/perfusion lung scan (V/Q scan):** The only findings of diagnostic value are normal scans, which rule out the disease with almost absolute certainty, and scans showing a segmental perfusion defect ("cold" area) with associated good ventilation (ventilation-perfusion mismatch) which indicate PE with a high degree of probability. However, in many cases the findings are not diagnostic because they do not fall into either category. As an imaging technique, it has now been replaced by computed tomography (CT) and is reserved only for patients with contrast allergy (anaphylaxis that cannot be suppressed by high corticosteroid dose), renal failure or pregnancy (lower radiation exposure to the fetus if only perfusion scan is performed).

8) **Chest CT pulmonary angiography (CTPA):** This technique (requires the IV administration of iodinated contrast) images an intravascular filling defect (distal to the obstruction) and can directly detect the intravascular clot. Generally, the detection of segmental or more proximal thrombus confirms PE. CTPA is poor at imaging distal thrombi-emboli. With the latest generation multi-detector-row scanners (multi-detector-CT, MDCT) and the administration of contrast medium (MD-CTPA) it is now feasible to image distal emboli. MD-CTPA is nowadays the main imaging technique for the diagnosis of PE. The advantages of the method, apart from its high diagnostic accuracy, include its rapid performance and the ability to evaluate right ventricular function and demonstrate other causes of

dyspnea or chest pain (e.g. pneumonia, acute aortic dissection, etc.) when the examination is negative for PE. Its disadvantages include radiation exposure (substantially higher breast radiation compared to V/Q lung scan) and nephrotoxicity from the iodinated contrast media. MD-CTPA may be combined with CT venography (CTV) of the pelvis and lower limbs at the same time, without requiring a second contrast infusion. Note that CTV has about the same diagnostic accuracy as venous ultrasonography for the diagnosis of DVT. However, because of the greater radiation exposure, venous ultrasonography is preferred in most cases for DVT diagnosis. Normal MD-CTPA safely excludes PE in patients who have a low or intermediate clinical probability of PE. However, if it is normal in patients who have a high probability of PE further testing is needed, although the optimum examination has not been established. This testing should include: a) repetition of the MD-CTPA ($\pm$ CTV) if the initial examination is considered to be of poor quality; b) venous ultrasonography; c) V/Q lung scan; or d) pulmonary angiography.

9) **Lower-limb venous ultrasonography:** This is a noninvasive technique for the diagnosis of DVT. The primary diagnostic criterion is the non-compressibility of the affected veins when slight pressure is applied to the overlying skin with the transducer. It shows good diagnostic accuracy for DVT in the thigh, but is less accurate for venous thrombosis in the calf or the pelvis, or in cases of obesity or lower limb edema. In general, venous ultrasonography (also called compression venous ultrasonography) detects a DVT in 30-50% of patients with PE. If venous ultrasonography shows a proximal DVT in a patient with clinical suspicion of PE, it confirms the diagnosis of PE, while if it shows only distal DVT (below the popliteal vein), additional testing is required. Note that the diagnostic gold standard for DVT is venography, but this is rarely used today as it is invasive and requires injection of contrast medium.

Warning! A normal venous ultrasonography does not rule out DVT or PE. In fact, if there is a moderate or high degree of clinical suspicion for PE then the patient should be investigated further despite a normal venous ultrasonography.

10) **Echocardiogram:** Nonspecific findings. It evaluates the function of the right ventricle (for risk stratification and treatment selection) and rules out other causes of dyspnea (AMI, acute aortic dissection, cardiac tamponade). It can show:
   - Right ventricular dilation.
   - Right ventricular wall hypokinesia, characteristically sparing the apex (McConnell's sign).

- Paradoxical interventricular septal motion towards the left ventricle.
- Pulmonary artery dilation (main pulmonary artery diameter >25 mm).
- Tricuspid regurgitation (maximum regurgitant flow velocity usually >2.6 m/s and <3.5 m/s if there is no preexisting chronic pulmonary hypertension).
- Inferior vena cava distension (>21 mm) with lack of at least 50% collapsibility during inspiration.
- Free thrombi within the right chambers. This rare finding (<5%) is associated with an unfavorable prognosis.
- Occasionally, a transesophageal echocardiogram can image clots inside the pulmonary artery trunk or the proximal segments of the pulmonary arteries.

11) **Pulmonary angiography:** This was the standard method prior to the introduction of newer-generation CT scanners. Today it is performed rarely, usually before an embolectomy.

Pregnancy and pulmonary embolism

Pregnancy has some special features as regards the occurrence and the diagnosis of PE, as follows:

- Pregnancy is associated with an increased risk of DVT and PE. Note that the risk is higher in the postpartum period.
- D-dimers are often elevated in a normal pregnancy (in the 2nd trimester >50% and in the 3rd trimester >90% of pregnant women have elevated D-dimers).
- One criterion for the selection of the diagnostic technique should be the avoidance or minimization of radiation exposure for the fetus and mother.

According to the European Guidelines (Regitz-Zagrosek V, et al. Eur Heart J 2011;32:3147-97), when there is clinical suspicion of PE in a pregnant woman, D-dimers are elevated, and in addition lower-limb venous ultrasonography is pathological (particularly if it shows proximal DVT), this is an indication for starting anticoagulant medication. Additional imaging is needed only where there is suspicion of PE, D-dimers are elevated, but venous ultrasonography is normal. As regards the choice of imaging technique in relation to fetal radiation exposure, the fetus receives about the same amount of ionizing radiation with either CTPA or V/Q lung scan*. Of course, if the chest X-ray is normal, a ventilation lung scan is unnecessary and only a perfusion lung scan needs to be performed. In this case, the fetal radiation exposure is even low-

---

*The radiation absorbed by the fetus during a perfusion lung scan with technetium-99m is 0.11-0.60 mSv, during a ventilation lung scan 0.10-0.30 mSv, and during a CTPA 0.24-0.66 mSv. For comparison reasons note that the radiation delivered to the fetus during a posteroanterior chest X-ray is <0.01 mSv (Konstantinides S, et al. Eur Heart J 2014;35:3033-69).

er, and the mother's breast region also has significantly lower radiation exposure than with CTPA. Do not forget that CTPA increases the lifetime risk for
breast cancer. The European Guidelines for PE (Konstantinides S, et al. Eur
Heart J 2014;35:3033-69) give precedence to perfusion scintigraphy, rather
than CTPA, when the mother's chest X-ray is normal.

Treatment

1) **General measures:** administration of oxygen, placement of a peripheral
   line, and analgesia. In cases of low cardiac output and normal BP,
   dobutamine and/or dopamine may be administered. In cases of shock,
   adrenaline or noradrenaline might be beneficial (limited data), while the
   benefits of fluid loading (e.g. low-molecular-weight dextran) are disputed
   (if administered, it should not exceed 500 mL).
2) **Anticoagulants:** These constitute the mainstay of treatment.
   - First, 5-10,000 U of unfractionated heparin (UFH) are administered by
     IV bolus (80 U/kg body weight), followed by a continuous infusion of
     1200-1500 U/h (18 U/kg/h), with a target activated partial thromboplas-
     tin time (aPTT) equal to 1.5-2.5 times the control value. Table 4.4 pres-

TABLE 4.4	Continuous IV administration of unfractionated heparin at a dose of 18 U/kg/h, from a 50 U/mL solution (12,500 U added to 250 mL of D/W 5%)		
Body weight (kg)	**Heparin, U/h**		**Solution, mL/h**
50	900		18
55	990		20
60	1080		22
65	1170		23
70	1260		25
75	1350		27
80	1440		29
85	1530		31
90	1620		32
95	1710		34
100	1800		36
105	1890		39
110	1980		40

TABLE 4.5	Protocol for the IV administration of unfractionated heparin (Raschke nomogram). The initial rate of continuous infusion is 18 U/kg/h (an 80 U/kg bolus has been given previously); any further actions are determined based on the aPTT values

*aPTT	Infusion rate adjustment, U/kg/h	Further action
<35 s (<1.2 x control)	+4 (i.e. 22 U/kg/h)	Repeat bolus 80 U/Kg
35-45 s (1.2-1.5 x control)	+2	Repeat bolus 40 U/Kg
46-70 s (1.5-2.3 x control)	0	0
71-90 s (2.3-3 x control)	-2	0
>90 s (>3 x control)	-3	Discontinue infusion for one hour and then reduce the rate of infusion by 3 U/kg/h

*The aPTT is measured every 6 h for the first 24 h, and once daily thereafter unless it is found to be outside the therapeutic range
aPTT = activated partial thromboplastin time

ents the rate of continuous infusion of a 50 U/mL heparin solution by body weight, and Table 4.5 describes the IV heparin administration protocol by therapeutic result.

- Alternatively, low-molecular-weight heparin (LMWH) [enoxaparin, tinzaparin or dalteparin] or fondaparinux may be given. Generally, for patients who are hemodynamically stable, do not suffer from severe renal failure (i.e. creatinine clearance <30 mL/min) and do not present a high risk of bleeding, LMWHs or fondaparinux are preferable to UFH (Table 4.6).

- Administration of vitamin K antagonists (VKAs) from the first day of parenteral anticoagulation treatment and concomitantly with it. When international normalized ratio (INR) levels between 2.0-3.0 have been achieved on at least 2 consecutive days (usually 4-5 days are necessary), heparin or fondaparinux is discontinued. VKA treatment continues for 3-6 months or more in case of thromboembolic episode recurrence or underlying malignancy. If PE is considered "provoked", i.e. there is a reversible risk factor at the time of diagnosis, anticoagulation treatment is recommended for 3 months. The initial dose is 5-7.5 mg for warfarin (Parwarfin, Coumadin) and 4-6 mg for acenocoumarol (Si-

TABLE 4.6	Dose of low-molecular-weight heparins and of fondaparinux given subcutaneously for the treatment of acute pulmonary embolism
Anticoagulant	**Dose**
Enoxaparin (Lovenox, Clexane)	1 mg*/kg x 2/day or 1.5 mg/kg x 1/day (approved for in-hospital treatment in the USA)
Tinzaparin (Innohep)	175 U**/kg x 1/day
Dalteparin (Fragmin)	100 U**/Kg x 2/day or 200 U/Kg x 1/day
Fondaparinux (Arixtra)	5 mg x 1/day (body weight <50 kg) 7.5 mg x 1/day (body weight 50-100 kg) 10 mg x 1/day (body weight >100 kg)

*For enoxaparin 1 mg=100 anti-Xa units
** 1 U=1 anti-Xa unit

ntrom); it is later adjusted based on the INR (therapeutic range: 2.0-3.0).
- In the special case of cancer patients who suffer from PE, for the first 3-6 months LMWH is given (preferably dalteparin), followed by VKA or LMWH indefinitely or until the malignancy is treated. Note that cancer patients run a high risk of PE recurrence. In particular, dalteparin is given in a dose of 200 U/kg x 1/day (maximum dose 18,000 U) for the first month and then 150 U/kg x 1/day subcutaneously for 5 months or until the cancer is considered cured.

Remarks on heparin therapy
- aPTT is "useless" for monitoring the anticoagulant effect of LMWH. The only reliable test is by measuring anti-Xa activity, 4 h after the subcutaneous administration of LMWH. The target range is 0.6–1.0 IU/mL for twice-daily administration, and 1.0–2.0 IU/mL for once-daily administration. This is only required in selected cases, such as patients with renal failure, the morbidly obese, and pregnant women.
- The American Food and Drug Administration (FDA) and the European Medicines Agency (EMA) gave approval for the use of rivaroxaban

and apixaban (direct factor Xa inhibitors) and for dabigatran (direct thrombin inhibitor) for the treatment of acute PE and the prevention of its recurrence. Recently, edoxaban (direct factor Xa inhibitor) received similar approval from the FDA and the EMA. A precondition for their use is the absence of hemodynamic instability or severe kidney failure. More specifically:

- **Rivaroxaban** (Xarelto): may be given as an alternative to the combination of parenteral anticoagulation and VKA in a dose of 15 mg x 2/day for the first 3 weeks and then 20 mg x 1/day for at least 3 months.
- **Apixaban** (Eliquis): may be given as an alternative to the combination of parenteral anticoagulation and VKA in a dose of 10 mg x 2/day for the first 7 days and then 5 mg x 2/day for at least 3 months.
- **Edoxaban** (Savaysa, Lixiana): may be given as an alternative to VKAs in a dose of 60 mg x 1/day for at least 3 months, following 5 to 10 days of initial therapy with a parenteral anticoagulant.
- **Dabigatran** (Pradaxa): may be given as an alternative to VKAs in a dose of 150 mg x 2/day or 110 mg x 2/day in patients aged >80 years for at least 3 months, in patients who for the first 5-10 days have taken parenteral anticoagulation.

• In cases of life-threatening hemorrhagic complications from the administration of UFH, administration is discontinued and protamine sulfate is administered IV within 10 min (see page 39). If more than 4 h have passed since the administration, an antidote is not necessary because the effect of UFH has expired (its half-life is 1-2 h).

• The administration of heparin can be complicated by a fall in the platelet count, a disorder called heparin-induced thrombocytopenia (HIT). In HIT, the platelet count drops by ≥50% of the baseline (usually <100,000/mm^3 and almost never <20,000/mm^3). This is a very serious condition, which develops between the 5th and the 14th day in 1-3% of cases after administration of UFH, and less commonly after administration of LMWH. If the patient has been exposed to heparin during the previous 100 days then HIT may develop sooner, even within 24 h of repeat administration. The risk of HIT is correlated with the duration of heparin administration: if given for <6 days, HIT is extremely rare (~0.2%). Prior to administering heparin, the platelet count should always be checked and this measurement should be repeated every 2-3 days between the 5th and the 14th day of administration.
HIT has an immunological basis and is caused by the formation of IgG antibodies against the heparin-platelet factor 4 (PF4) complex. The interaction of the antibodies with the heparin-PF4 complex leads to platelet activation and the development of thrombosis in ~50% of ca-

ses, either in the arterial (AMI, stroke, etc.) or the venous circulation (DVT, PE, etc.). Venous thrombosis is 4 times more common than arterial thrombosis. This syndrome includes the paradoxical occurrence of thrombotic complications despite the low platelet count; in fact, the hypercoagulable state remains for almost one month after heparin discontinuation.

If there is clinical suspicion of HIT, heparin is discontinued immediately and, after the diagnosis is confirmed by testing for antibodies against the heparin-PF4 complex, alternative (nonheparin) anticoagulation therapy is given for 1-2 weeks. This therapy can include direct thrombin inhibitors (e.g. lepirudin, argatroban or bivalirudin) or fondaparinux (indirect inhibitor of factor Xa). Platelet transfusion is contraindicated. **Lepirudin** (Refludan, 50 mg vial) is administered initially by rapid IV infusion at a rate of 0.20 mg/kg and by continuous infusion at a rate of 0.10 mg/kg/h thereafter. The target aPTT value is 1.5-2.5 times the control value. Lepirudin has a half-life of ~80 min and is eliminated through the kidneys. Its dosage is reduced in patients with renal failure. **Argatroban** (Novastan, Acova) is administered as a continuous IV infusion of 2.0 μg/kg/min adjusted to maintain aPTT 1.5–3.0 times the control value. Argatroban has a half-life of ~45 min and is eliminated mainly through the liver. Its dosage is reduced to 0.5 μg/kg/min in patients with hepatic dysfunction. Although the use of **fondaparinux** (Arixtra) in the treatment of HIT is less well documented (not approved), it can be considered because of its simpler dosage (administered subcutaneously at a dose of 5-10 mg daily, depending on body weight; page 81); also, no blood tests are needed to monitor its effectiveness. After heparin is discontinued, the platelet count gradually recovers and reaches its baseline in 4-5 days. After the platelet count reaches > 100,000/mm^3, a VKA is started with a target INR of 2.0-3.0. Concurrent administration of the alternative anticoagulant and the VKA continues for ~4-5 days, after which only the VKA is given. The duration of VKA administration depends on the underlying disease and on the occurrence, location and severity of thrombotic episodes. The use of heparin is prohibited for the next 100 days, which is the time needed for the autoimmune complex to disappear. Repeated administration of heparin should be avoided, but if done after 100 days then the recurrence of HIT is not inevitable. Table 4.7 summarizes the treatment of HIT.

3) **Fibrinolysis:** This may dissolve the lung embolus as well as the thrombotic source of the emboli in the pelvic or deep leg veins. The early resolution of obstructing pulmonary arterial thrombus may lead to a prompt reduction in pulmonary artery pressure and resistance, with a concomi-

TABLE 4.7	Treatment of heparin-induced thrombocytopenia (HIT)

1) Immediate discontinuation of heparins (even in cases of clinical suspicion only) and avoidance of platelet transfusion

2) Alternative anticoagulation for 1-2 weeks
   - Lepirudin (Refludan): 0.20 mg/kg IV bolus followed by 0.10 mg/kg/h
   - Argatroban (Novastan, Acova): 2.0 µg/kg/min (no bolus) [0.5 µg/kg/min in patients with liver disease] or
   - Fondaparinux (Arixtra): 5-10 mg daily subcutaneously, depending on body weight

3) Withhold vitamin K antagonists (VKAs) until platelets rise to >100,000/mm³, provided that the alternative anticoagulant is coadministered for ~4-5 days

4) Continued administration of VKAs, depending on the underlying disease and on the occurrence and location of thrombotic complications

tant improvement in right ventricular function. Indications for fibrinolytic therapy include (Jaff MR, et al. Circulation 2011;123:1788-830):

- Massive acute PE (systolic BP <90 mmHg for at least 15 min): fibrinolysis is reasonable (class IIa recommendation) if the bleeding risk is acceptable. In general, the contraindications for the administration of fibrinolysis are the same as those for AMI (see page 41). According to the latest European Guidelines for PE (Konstantinides S, et al. Eur Heart J 2014;35:3033-69), the role of fibrinolysis has been reinforced, so that it now has a class I recommendation: fibrinolysis is recommended for high-risk PE (shock or sustained hypotension). The guidelines also mention that absolute contraindications for fibrinolysis might become relative in a patient with immediately life-threatening high-risk PE.

- Submassive acute PE (systolic BP ≥90 mmHg): fibrinolysis may be considered when it is accompanied by clinical evidence of adverse prognosis (new hemodynamic instability, worsening respiratory insufficiency, severe right ventricular dysfunction, or major myocardial necrosis) [class IIb recommendation]. A low risk of hemorrhagic complications is a precondition for the administration of fibrinolysis. The latest European Guidelines suggest that fibrinolysis should be considered for patients with intermediate-high risk PE and clinical signs of hemodynamic decompensation (class IIa recommendation).

The FDA has approved the use of urokinase, streptokinase and alteplase for the treatment of PE. Alternatively, reteplase and tenecteplase can also be given (Table 4.8). According to the FDA, when alteplase is

TABLE 4.8	Dosage of fibrinolytic agents in acute pulmonary embolism
Fibrinolytic agent	**Dose**
Streptokinase (Streptase, Kabikinase)	250,000 U over 30 min and then 100,000 U/h for 12-24 h
Urokinase (Abbokinase)	4400 U/kg over 10 min and then 4400 U/kg/h over 12-14 h
Alteplase (rtPA) [Activase, Actilyse]	100 mg IV over 2 h
Reteplase (rPA) [Retavase, Rapilysin)	10 U IV bolus over 2 min and repeat this dose after 30 min
Tenecteplase (TNK-tPA) (TNKase, Metalyse)	0.5 mg/kg bolus (max 50 mg)

administered then UFH is suspended. After alteplase administration is completed, the aPTT is determined and if it is <80 s then heparin is restarted without a bolus dose. If the aPTT is >80 s then the test is repeated after 4 h, and if it is <80 s at that time then heparin is restarted without a bolus dose. However, according to the latest European Guidelines for PE the administration of UFH can be continued during alteplase infusion.

In contrast to an AMI, the therapeutic window for fibrinolysis is quite wide in the case of PE: it can be given as late as 2 weeks after PE is established. However, the greatest benefit is achieved when fibrinolysis is given within 48 h of symptom onset. In cases of cardiac arrest where there is strong suspicion that the cause is acute massive PE, an IV bolus of 50 mg alteplase or 20 U reteplase may be given directly.

4) **Surgical pulmonary embolectomy** is performed in cases of massive PE where fibrinolysis has failed or is absolutely contraindicated. As an alternative to surgical embolectomy, percutaneous embolectomy and fragmentation of the clot through a catheter may be attempted for centrally located emboli.

✓ Key points

- PE is difficult to diagnose and usually constitutes a common entity with DVT of the lower limbs or the minor pelvis. It is usually caused by a thrombus detaching from these areas and obstructing a branch (or branches) of the pulmonary arterial vasculature.

- Hemodynamically stable patients with no signs of right ventricular dysfunction on imaging tests (echocardiography or CTPA) and normal markers of myocardial injury (i.e. cardiac troponin) or of heart failure as a result of right ventricular dysfunction (i.e. BNP), have an excellent prognosis.

- Despite the frequent coexistence of PE with lower-limb DVT, clinical signs of DVT are usually absent.

- Unexplained dyspnea in patients with risk factors for PE or with a "normal" chest X-ray should always raise suspicion of PE.

- Patients with congestive heart failure treated in the Emergency Room as acute pulmonary edema with no improvement after vasodilator and diuretic therapy may be suffering from PE.

- In patients with low or intermediate clinical probability for PE and no hemodynamic compromise, the first diagnostic test should be the determination of D-dimers. Low levels will rule out the condition.

- MD-CTPA is today the imaging study of choice for the diagnosis of PE, having to a large degree replaced the V/Q lung scan. The latter is preferred in renal failure, contrast allergy, and pregnancy.

- If PE is suspected in a person with hypotension or shock, echocardiography or MD-CTPA should be performed immediately (depending on the availability of these methods and the patient's condition).

- In cases of shock, if echocardiography does not indicate right ventricular dilation with dysfunction then PE is ruled out as a possible cause of the hemodynamic collapse.

- Treatment for PE includes anticoagulation therapy (UFH or LMWH or fondaparinux + VKA) and fibrinolysis in the case of massive PE.

- Nowadays, the non-VKA oral anticoagulants (NOACs) can be used for the treatment of acute PE and the prevention of its recurrence:
  - Rivaroxaban, apixaban: as immediate treatment (monotherapy)
  - Edoxaban, dabigatran: after 5-10 days of initial treatment with parental anticoagulants.

- Fibrinolysis has a relative indication in cases of submassive PE with clinical evidence of adverse prognosis (new hemodynamic instability, worsening respiratory insufficiency, severe right ventricular dysfunction, or major myocardial necrosis)

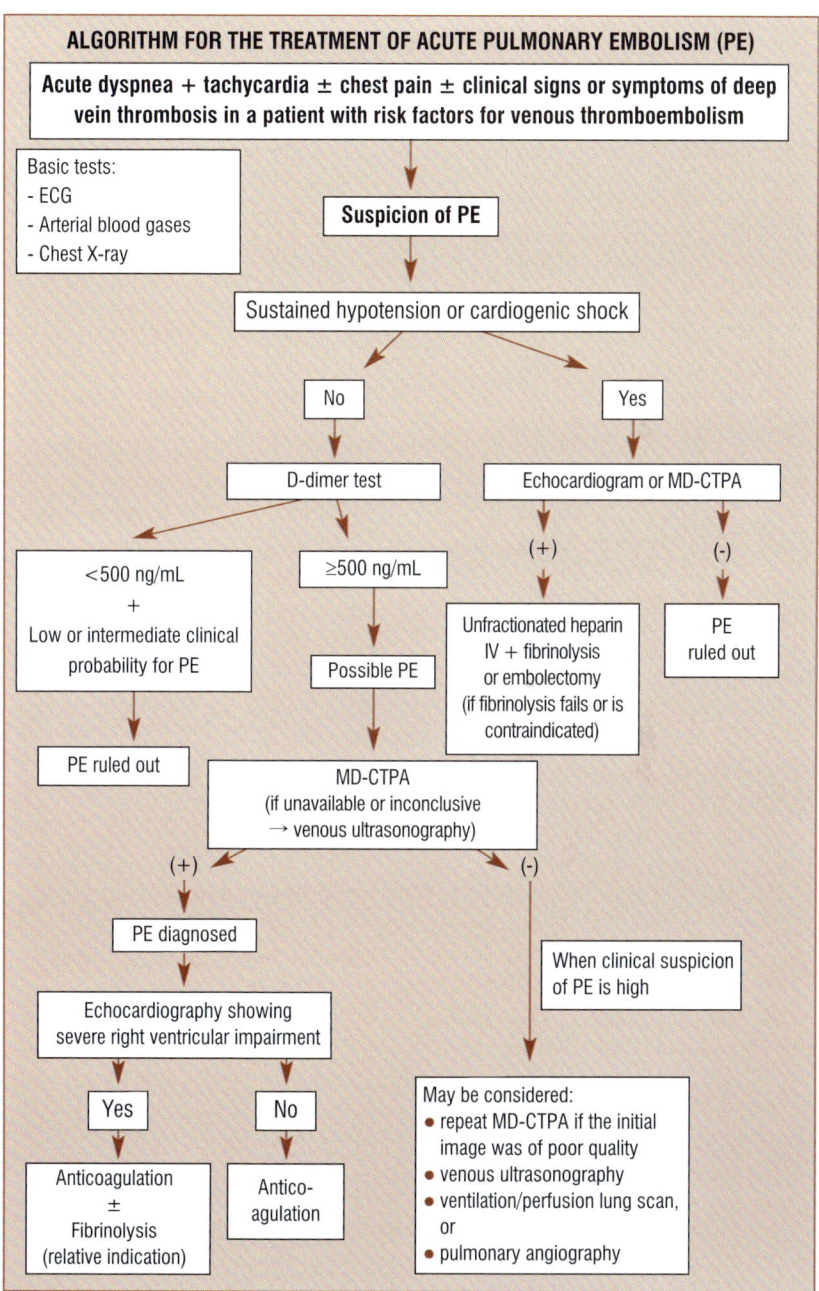

ALGORITHM FOR THE TREATMENT OF ACUTE PULMONARY EMBOLISM (PE)

Acute dyspnea + tachycardia ± chest pain ± clinical signs or symptoms of deep vein thrombosis in a patient with risk factors for venous thromboembolism

Basic tests:
- ECG
- Arterial blood gases
- Chest X-ray

Suspicion of PE

Sustained hypotension or cardiogenic shock

No

Yes

D-dimer test

Echocardiogram or MD-CTPA

(+)

(-)

<500 ng/mL
+
Low or intermediate clinical probability for PE

≥500 ng/mL

Unfractionated heparin IV + fibrinolysis or embolectomy (if fibrinolysis fails or is contraindicated)

PE ruled out

PE ruled out

Possible PE

MD-CTPA
(if unavailable or inconclusive → venous ultrasonography)

(+)

(-)

PE diagnosed

When clinical suspicion of PE is high

Echocardiography showing severe right ventricular impairment

Yes

No

May be considered:
- repeat MD-CTPA if the initial image was of poor quality
- venous ultrasonography
- ventilation/perfusion lung scan, or
- pulmonary angiography

Anticoagulation
±
Fibrinolysis
(relative indication)

Anticoagulation

MD-CTPA: multi-detector computed tomographic pulmonary angiography

5

Acute pulmonary edema (cardiogenic)

Cardiogenic **acute pulmonary edema** is characterized by acute severe dyspnea that is usually caused by an abrupt worsening of left ventricular systolic function (mostly due to heart failure decompensation) with adequate right ventricular function. This leads to a sudden increase in hydrostatic pressure in the lung capillaries, fluid transudation into the alveoli, impeded gas diffusion, and finally hypoxemia.

An acute pulmonary edema may also be noncardiogenic (acute respiratory distress syndrome, ARDS), caused primarily by an increase in alveolocapillary membrane permeability with no increase in pulmonary capillary pressure (pulmonary capillary wedge pressure [PCWP] <18 mmHg). The causes of cardiogenic and noncardiogenic acute pulmonary edema are listed in Table 5.1.

Most cases of cardiogenic acute pulmonary edema develop on a background of chronic compensated heart failure caused by preexisting organic heart disease (e.g. coronary artery disease, cardiomyopathy, etc.), which is decompensated acutely because of a triggering factor (Table 5.2). As Tables 5.1 and 5.2 show, certain conditions can act as both causative agents and triggering factors for acute pulmonary edema; examples are acute myocardial ischemia, arrhythmias and others. For example, an extensive acute myocardial infarction (AMI) may manifest with acute pulmonary edema (causative agent), while a small degree of acute myocardial ischemia in a patient with preexisting ischemic cardiomyopathy can also set off acute pulmonary edema (triggering factor).

We shall also mention that the above term of cardiogenic acute pulmonary edema does not cover all cases of acute cardiogenic dyspnea. A significant proportion, particularly among elderly and hypertensive patients, develop acute pulmonary edema in the setting of diastolic dysfunction and preserved left ventricular ejection fraction (>50%). In these cases the triggering factor may be: hypertensive crisis, onset of atrial fibrillation with rapid ventricular response, etc.

TABLE 5.1	Causes of cardiogenic and noncardiogenic acute pulmonary edema

1) Cardiogenic acute pulmonary edema
- Acute myocardial ischemia (usually acute myocardial infarction ± mechanical complications, i.e. ventricular septal rupture or acute mitral valve regurgitation)
- Hypertensive crisis (usually diastolic arterial blood pressure >120-130 mmHg and/or systolic blood pressure >200 mmHg)
- Rhythm disorders (e.g. atrial fibrillation with rapid ventricular response [>150 beats/min], ventricular tachycardia, severe bradycardia)
- Fluid overload (usually iatrogenic in postoperative elderly patients)
- Fluid retention in cases of renal failure (usually dialysis patients after intake of large amounts of fluids)
- Severe aortic or mitral valve stenosis (usually when complicated by atrial fibrillation)
- Acute aortic or mitral valve regurgitation (e.g. complication of infectious endocarditis)
- Dilated cardiomyopathy (e.g. when complicated by atrial fibrillation, respiratory tract infection, etc.)
- Acute thrombosis of mechanical heart valves (most commonly of the mitral valve)
- Acute myocarditis

2) Noncardiogenic acute pulmonary edema (ARDS)
- Pneumonia
- Aspiration of gastric contents
- Sepsis
- Acute pancreatitis
- Fat embolism
- Disseminated intravascular coagulation
- Smoke inhalation
- Near drowning
- Pulmonary contusion

Finally hypoalbuminemia (as in severe liver disease, nephrotic syndrome, etc.) lowers the threshold for acute pulmonary edema, which can develop with smaller increases of hydrostatic pressure in the lung capillaries.

Symptoms
- Severe dyspnea. The patient is usually sitting down with dangling legs, pallid, sweating and possibly cyanotic.
- Cough, nonproductive at the early stages, or with frothy red sputum in severe cases.
- Chest pain in cases of concomitant myocardial ischemia.

TABLE 5.2	Triggering factors for acute pulmonary edema

1) Acute myocardial ischemia

2) Hypertensive crisis

3) Arrhythmia with rapid ventricular response

4) Acute valvular regurgitation

5) Infection (usually of the respiratory tract)

6) Medication causing fluid retention (e.g. nonsteroidal antiinflammatory drugs)

7) Medication with negative inotropic effect or with cardiotoxic effect (e.g. anthracycline)

8) Patient noncompliance with treatment, e.g. discontinuation of diuretics or angiotensin-converting enzyme inhibitors, consumption of salt, etc.

9) Anemia

10) Thyrotoxicosis

Clinical signs

- Tachypnea (>20 breaths/min). A good indicator of response to treatment is the monitoring of the number of breaths/min.
- The systolic arterial blood pressure (BP) may be normal, elevated or lowered. Low BP is found in <10% of cases and is an unfavorable prognostic sign.

Warning! The BP is often elevated as a result of peripheral vasoconstriction and the acute pulmonary edema should not be attributed to an increased BP except when greatly elevated (for example, usually a systolic BP >200 mmHg).

- Jugular venous distention may be present (assessment at 45° incline).
- Heart auscultation: usually difficult. A galloping rhythm (usually a summation gallop due to coincident 3rd and 4th heart sounds because of the tachycardia) or a murmur due to underlying valvular heart disease may be noted.
- Lung auscultation: crackles in both lung bases, extending to the middle and upper lung fields in severe conditions ± wheezes (sibilant rhonchi due to precipitation of bronchospasm ± sonorous rhonchi due to the presence of secretions in the airways).

Warning! In the early phases of an acute pulmonary edema, crackles might be absent and only sibilant rhonchi might be heard (interstitial edema phase, where fluid effuses only into the interstitial tissue causing edema of the bronchiolar mucosa with subsequent narrowing). This clinical picture is called "cardiac asthma" and must be distinguished from a bronchial asthma attack.

Basic tests

1) **ECG:** primarily to rule out acute myocardial ischemia, recent onset atrial fibrillation, severe bradycardia or ventricular tachycardia.
2) **Blood tests:** complete blood count (to detect anemia or leukocytosis), cardiac troponin I or T, urea, creatinine, glucose, C-reactive protein (detection of inflammation/infection) and electrolytes. If a differential diagnosis for bronchial asthma attack is required, then measurement of natriuretic peptides, such as B-type natriuretic peptide (BNP) or N-terminal-proBNP (NT-proBNP), may be useful. These molecules are produced from myocardial cells, especially in the ventricles, in response to conditions that increase the ventricular wall stress. BNP consists of 32 amino acids, has a half-life of ~20 min and is cleared through the kidneys, as well as by cell-surface clearance receptors and by the widely expressed (kidneys, lungs, endothelial cells, etc.) enzyme neutral endopeptidase. NT-proBNP is an inactive molecule made of 76 amino acids, with a half-life of ~2 h, which is cleared mainly through the kidneys. BNP values >400 pg/mL or NT-proBNP values >1800 pg/mL* are highly suggestive of cardiogenic acute pulmonary edema, whereas BNP values <100 pg/mL or NT-proBNP values <300 pg/mL almost certainly rule out cardiogenic causes for the acute dyspnea. Table 5.3 lists the most important causes affecting BNP and NT-proBNP levels.
3) **Arterial blood sample** for blood gases and pH measurement. Hypoxemia and, in the early stages, hypocapnia will be found. If the clinical picture does not improve within 20-30 min after initial treatment, then the tests should be repeated. Pulse oximetry is not reliable when peripheral perfusion is poor.
4) **Chest X-ray:** characterized by a rapid change in findings. It may show:
   - Cardiomegaly ± pleural effusions.
   - Vascular redistribution (early stages): intensified perfusion in the upper pulmonary fields due to constriction of basilar vessels and direction of blood flow upwards.

This limit applies to people over 75 years of age. For people aged <50 and 50-75, the limits are >450 pg/mL and >900 pg/mL, respectively.

TABLE 5.3	Conditions affecting the levels of B-type natriuretic peptide (BNP) and N-terminal-proBNP (NT-proBNP)

1) Conditions associated with increased levels
- Acute or chronic heart failure
- Renal impairment (NT-proBNP levels are affected more than BNP levels)
- Acute coronary syndrome
- Acute pulmonary embolism
- High cardiac output conditions (sepsis, hyperthyroidism, cirrhosis)
- Advanced age
- Atrial fibrillation

2) Conditions associated with levels lower than expected
- Obesity
- Flash pulmonary edema, i.e. sudden onset pulmonary edema
- Decompensated end-stage heart failure
- Acute mitral valve regurgitation
- Mitral valve stenosis, left atrial myxoma
- Cardiac tamponade
- Constrictive pericarditis

- Interstitial edema due to extravasation of fluid into the interstitium:
  - Kerley B lines: horizontal, linear opacities, 1-2 cm long and 1 mm thick, at the costophrenic angles in contact with the pleura due to expansion of interlobular septa
  - Peribronchial cuffing: haziness around the bronchioles due to thickening of the bronchial walls.
- In the typical (alveolar) acute pulmonary edema, there are patchy infiltrates (haziness) with perihilar prominence (butterfly or bat's wing appearance).

Warning! In acute pulmonary edema, lung infiltrates do not extend to the peripheries. If this is observed, then ARDS should be suspected.

5) **Echocardiography**, primarily for:
- Assessment of left ventricular function (systolic and diastolic). Elderly people who develop acute pulmonary edema resulting from a hypertensive crisis often have a preserved ejection fraction (>50%), with only diastolic left ventricular dysfunction being observed.
- Ruling out mechanical complications of an AMI.
- Ruling out a large pericardial effusion (cardiac tamponade).
- Right ventricular function assessment for possible pulmonary embolism.
- Heart valve examination.

TABLE 5.4	Differential diagnosis of acute pulmonary edema

1) Bronchial asthma exacerbation (history, BNP <100 pg/mL or NT-proBNP <300 pg/mL)

2) Acute pulmonary embolism (D-dimers >500 ng/mL, MD-CTPA showing a filling defect, echocardiogram showing distension ± right ventricular impairment)

3) Cardiac tamponade (echocardiogram showing large pericardial effusion and diastolic collapse of the right ventricle)

4) Spontaneous pneumothorax (chest X-ray during expiration with a clear/avascular lung region)

5) Pneumonia (fever, productive cough, chest X-ray with consolidation)

6) Noncardiogenic acute pulmonary edema (concomitant severe noncardiac disease, diffuse infiltrates on the chest X-ray)

BNP: B-type natriuretic peptide, N-terminal-proBNP (NT-proBNP)
MD-CTPA: multi-detector computed tomographic pulmonary angiography

6) **Lung ultrasound examination:** a useful tool for discriminating between cardiogenic acute pulmonary edema and noncardiogenic dyspnea. The lung ultrasound examination can be performed within 2-3 min using any commercially available 2-D scanner, with the patient in a near-supine or supine position. The probe is positioned over the chest, usually the anterior and lateral wall. The differential diagnosis between cardiogenic and noncardiogenic dyspnea is based on the detection of the **comet-tail artifacts** or **B-lines** (ultrasonic equivalent of Kerley B lines). A B-line is a discrete, vertical, hyperechoic image that arises from the pleural line and extends to the bottom of the screen. These lines are reverberation artifacts produced by the reflection of the ultrasound beam off interlobular septa that have been thickened by edema. The detection of multiple, diffuse, bilateral B-lines with a homogeneous distribution in a patient with acute dyspnea is very sensitive for the diagnosis of cardiogenic acute pulmonary edema while the absence of these findings excludes cardiogenic dyspnea. Note that B-lines can also be found in pulmonary fibrosis, ARDS, etc.

Table 5.4 presents the most important diseases involved in the differential diagnosis of acute pulmonary edema.

Therapeutic manipulations

1) The patient is placed in a seated position, with dangling legs in order to reduce venous return to the lungs.

2) **Oxygen** (O_2) is administered at high concentrations (>40%) [usually with a Venturi mask]. If the hypoxemia persists (O_2 saturation <90%

	TABLE 5.5	Oxygen delivery systems

Device	Oxygen flow (L/min)	Oxygen concentration in the inhaled mixture, % (FiO$_2$)
• Nasal cannula	1	21-24
	2	24-28
	3	28-34
	4	34-38
	5	38-42
	6	42-46
• Simple face mask	5-10	30-50
• Mask with partial rebreather reservoir bag	5-10	35-80
• Mask with nonrebreather reservoir bag	10-15	60-90
• Venturi mask	4-12	24, 28, 31, 35, 40, 50, 60

measured using a pulse oximeter), O_2 is administered with a nonre-breather mask (Table 5.5) that can achieve inhaled O_2 concentrations up to 90% (target O_2 saturation ≥95% and partial pressure of O_2 [PaO$_2$] in arterial blood >60 mmHg).* If hypoxemia does not resolve, then nonin-vasive ventilation with a continuous positive airway pressure (CPAP) mask is applied to improve the symptoms. CPAP might lower the BP and therefore it should be avoided when the systolic BP is <85 mmHg.

Warning! If there is concomitant chronic obstructive pulmonary disease, O_2 is administered using a Venturi mask at initial concentrations of 24-28% because of the risk of CO_2 retention (target O_2 saturation >90%).

3) A peripheral venous line is placed for IV administration of drugs.
4) Administration of **furosemide** IV at a dose of 40-80 mg over 1-2 min (Lasix, Diuresal). It is prudent to avoid initial bolus injections >1 mg/kg because they can cause reflex vasoconstriction. Furosemide shows a biphasic action: venodilation at ~10 min, at which time the first signs of dyspnea improvement are expected, and diuresis at ~30 min. If dyspnea persists after 15-30 min then furosemide may be repeated (20-40 mg IV bolus). For an accurate assessment of diuresis in noncooperative pa-tients or in cases of severe acute pulmonary edema, a urinary catheter should be placed.

*PaO_2 in arterial blood (mmHg) can be roughly calculated using the formula: $100 - 0.3 \times age$ (years).

Remarks on furosemide administration

- If the systolic BP is <90 mmHg, furosemide is ineffective owing to reduced renal perfusion. The BP should be increased pharmaceutically for
  furosemide administration to be meaningful.
- After the initial bolus administration of furosemide and after patient's admission, furosemide can be administered either by continuous infusion or by
  intermittent bolus injections. Although continuous infusion results in greater
  diuresis it is unclear whether this is translated into an improved clinical outcome. The dose that the patient will receive in the first 24 h depends on the
  degree of congestion (jugular vein distention, lower limb edema, etc.), the
  patient's previous oral dose of furosemide, the response (diuresis) to the
  initial administration, and the patient's renal function. In patients with acute
  pulmonary edema due to acute decompensation of chronic heart failure
  and normal renal function, furosemide is administered IV in a dosage at
  least equal to the patient's previous oral dose of furosemide (Mebazaa A, et
  al. Eur J Heart Fail 2015;17:544-58). For example, if the patient was taking
  80 mg of furosemide po twice daily, then a total dose of ~160 mg IV should
  be given within the first 24 h, either by continuous infusion or by bolus injections every 8 or 12 h. In general, the dose of diuretic should be limited to
  the smallest amount necessary to provide clinical benefit and is subject to
  modification according to patient's response (diuresis).
- In new-onset heart failure or no previous maintenance diuretic therapy
  (diuretic-naive patients), a low initial bolus dose i.e. 40 mg furosemide IV,
  may result in significant clinical relief.
5) If the systolic BP is >100 mmHg, **nitrates** should be considered:
    - If no IV line is available, a sublingual nitrate is given, e.g. as a 5 mg
      isosorbide dinitrate tablet or 1-2 puffs (400-800 μg) of a nitroglycerin
      spray, which can be repeated after 5-10 min.
    - If an IV line is available: continuous infusion of a nitroglycerin solution.
      The initial rate is 5-10 μg/min, which is gradually increased by 5-10
      μg/min every 5-10 min as long as the systolic BP does not fall to <90
      mmHg. The beneficial effect of nitrates is mostly due to the decreased
      preload because of venodilation and to the decreased afterload because
      of arterial vasodilation. For the preparation of the nitrate solution, see
      Chapter 23.
    - Generally, in cases of acute pulmonary edema resulting from a hyperten-
      sive crisis, the mainstay of medical treatment is BP reduction by IV ad-
      ministration of nitrates. IV administration of furosemide is less important
      and initial doses >1 mg/kg should be avoided, as previously mentioned.
6) **Morphine** used to be one of the main treatments for acute pulmonary edema. However, good evidence supporting a beneficial hemodynamic effect
   is lacking and recent data suggest that morphine is associated with higher
   rates of mechanical ventilation, intensive care unit (ICU) admission, and

death. According to the latest European Guidelines (Ponikowski P, et al. Eur Heart J 2016;37:2129-200) the routine use of morphine is not recommended. Morphine may only be considered (class IIb recommendation) in selected cases, i.e. in particularly anxious, restless, or distressed patients, or patients with angina. It should be avoided in patients with a history of bronchial asthma and in cases of hypercapnia, lethargy or hypotension (systolic BP <90 mmHg). Morphine is administered diluted (1 mg/mL) slowly IV, at an initial dose of 3-5 mg. It has a triple effect as it causes mild venodilation (reduced preload), anxiolysis and reduced breathing work. Its beneficial hemodynamic effect is probably due to the anxiolysis, with a resulting decrease in catecholamine production and a decrease in systemic vascular resistance. Morphine should be coadministered with an antiemetic (e.g. metoclopramide 10 mg IV) to prevent nausea and vomiting, common side effects caused by morphine. Other side effects are hypotension, bradycardia and respiratory depression. Respiratory depression may be treated with administration of naloxone (Narcan) IV at a dose of 0.4 mg, repeated after 4 min to a maximum dose of 1.2 mg.

7) In cases of persistent hypertension despite administration of maximum nitrate doses (200 µg/min), **nitroprusside** is given. The starting dose is 0.25 µg/kg/min and the dosage is gradually increased every 5 min until the BP is controlled (see Chapter 23).

8) **Low-molecular-weight heparin** is given (e.g. 40 mg enoxaparin daily, subcutaneously) to reduce the risk of deep vein thrombosis and pulmonary embolism.

9) **Correction of triggering factors:**
   - Electrical cardioversion in the setting of ventricular tachycardia.
   - Electrical cardioversion in the setting of recent-onset atrial fibrillation and:
     – low systolic BP or
     – no clinical improvement despite initial treatment.
   - In cases of AMI, primary angioplasty is performed as soon as possible. If not available fibrinolysis is administered.
   - In cases of acute obstructive thrombosis of a mechanical mitral or aortic valve, the following are recommended (Vahanian A, et al. Eur Heart J 2012;33:2451-96):
     – Urgent or emergent valve replacement as long as the operative risk due to serious comorbidity is not prohibitive
     – Fibrinolysis (alteplase [rtPA] at doses 10 mg bolus + 90 mg IV over 90 min) if the operative risk is considered particularly high, or surgery is not immediately available.
   - In cases of severe renal failure and fluid retention resulting from oliguria or anuria, emergency dialysis is undertaken.
   - In cases of concomitant respiratory tract infection, appropriate antibiotic therapy is administered.

10) In cases of concomitant bronchospasm: β_2 agonists by nebulizer, e.g. 2.5-5 mg **salbutamol** (albuterol in the USA) [Ventolin, Airomir], or anti-cholinergics, e.g. **ipratropium** (Atrovent), or a combination of salbuta-mol and ipratropium (Combivent). The major side effects of bron-chodilators are arrhythmogenesis and tachycardia.
11) Administration (IV) of inotropes/vasopressors should be considered:
    - In cases of "mild" hypotension (systolic BP 80-90 mmHg): **dobuta-mine** (Dobutrex, Dobutamine Hydrochloride) starting at a dose of 2.5 µg/kg/min. The dose gradually increases depending on the response (improved cardiac output) and usually ranges between 2.5 and 20 µg/kg/min (see Chapter 23).
    - In cases of "severe" hypotension (systolic BP <80 or <70 mmHg):
        - **dopamine** (Intropin, Dopmin) at vasoconstrictive doses (>10 µg/kg/min) [see Chapter 23].
        - **noradrenaline** (Levophed) at a dose of 0.02-1 µg/kg/min, depend-ing on the response.
    - In case of satisfactory BP but low urine output (<30 mL/h for 2 con-secutive hours): dopamine at diuretic doses (<3 µg/kg/min).

    The general rule for the administration of inotropes/vasopressors is to give **the smallest effective dose for the shortest time necessary,** because they cause an "adverse" increase in myocardial oxygen de-mands. Consequently, they are given as a bridge to the main therapy, e.g. primary angioplasty in AMI. In the case of persistent severe hy-potension, as an alternative or complementary treatment to inotropes/va-sopressors, an intra-aortic balloon pump may be inserted.
12) Administration of **digoxin** (Lanoxin, Digoxin) only in cases of atrial fibril-lation with rapid ventricular response (0.5 mg IV slowly, and then 0.25 mg IV at 12 and at 24 h if rapid digitalization is required).
13) Intubation and **mechanical ventilation** if the dyspnea deteriorates de-spite initial treatment (Table 5.6). Mechanical ventilation improves oxy-genation and pH (since acidosis is often present), but usually at the price of a small decrease in cardiac output due to increased intratho-racic pressure.

TABLE 5.6	Indications for intubation and mechanical ventilation in acute pul-monary edema (after unsuccessful noninvasive ventilation)

1) Clinical signs and symptoms:
   - Respiration rate >40 breaths/min or respiratory arrest
   - Confusion or generally low level of consciousness in a patient with tachypnea

2) Hypoxemia (PaO_2 <60 mmHg)

3) Hypercapnia ($PaCO_2$ >50 mmHg) with concomitant acidosis (pH <7.35) [the hypercap-nia threshold for mechanical support is higher in patients with chronic respiratory disease]

14) Transfer to the ICU for further treatment. There, the patient is placed under hourly urinary recording and, if the clinical picture deteriorates or shock is established, then right-heart catheterization is performed with placement of a Swan-Ganz catheter (typically in alveolar acute pulmonary edema PCWP is >25 mmHg).

Differential diagnosis of cardiogenic and noncardiogenic acute pulmonary edema (Table 5.7)

The following are indicative of noncardiogenic acute pulmonary edema: absence of a 3rd heart sound; absence of cardiomegaly and presence of

TABLE 5.7	Differences between cardiogenic and noncardiogenic acute pulmonary edema	
	Cardiogenic acute pulmonary edema	**Noncardiogenic acute pulmonary edema**
Mechanism	Increased hydrostatic pressure in the pulmonary capillaries resulting from acute left heart failure	Increased alveolocapillary membrane permeability
Previous history of heart disease (previous MI, etc.)	Usually yes	Usually no
Concomitant noncardiac disease (sepsis, pneumonia, etc.)	Usually no	Yes
3rd heart sound or summation gallop	Yes	No
Jugular distension	Usually yes	No
ECG	Pathological	Usually normal
Chest X-ray	• Usually cardiomegaly • Bilateral perihilar shadowing • Patchy infiltrates with perihilar prominence	• Normal heart size • Diffuse infiltrates with peripheral prominence
Echocardiography	Pathological	Usually normal
BNP	Usually >400 pg/mL	Usually <100 pg/mL
Pulmonary capillary wedge pressure	≥18 mmHg	<18 mmHg

MI: myocardial infarction, BNP: B-type natriuretic peptide

TABLE 5.8	Causes of pulmonary edema of unknown etiology

1) High altitude (rapid ascent to >2500 meters)

2) Neurogenic (stroke, seizures, traumatic brain injury)

3) Following electric cardioversion (<0.5% of cases)

4) Acute pulmonary embolism

5) Following anesthesia

6) Following coronary artery bypass graft surgery

7) Large doses of heroin

diffuse infiltrates in the lungs with peripheral prominence on the chest X-ray; normal ECG; PCWP <18 mmHg; and presence of triggering agents such as sepsis, pneumonia, aspiration of gastric contents, etc.

It should be noted that in rare cases (~2%) the acute pulmonary edema (cardiogenic) is unilateral (most commonly in the right lung) and usually complicates severe acute mitral valve regurgitation. The reason why the right lung is most frequently affected might be the fact that prolapse of the posterior leaflet is the most common manifestation of myxomatous mitral valve disease and directs the eccentric regurgitant jet towards the right pulmonary veins.

Lastly, there is also a type of acute pulmonary edema with unknown pathogenesis (Table 5.8).

Key points

- The three prongs of initial pharmaceutical treatment for acute (cardiogenic) pulmonary edema are O_2 (concentration >40%), furosemide and if systolic BP >100 mmHg nitrates IV. Morphine may be given in selected cases (particularly anxious, restless, or distressed patients or patients with angina). In parallel, the causative agent is corrected.

- If, despite the initial treatment, the patient does not improve, then noninvasive ventilation must be applied. If the patient continues to present tachypnea (>40 breaths/min) and becomes confused, they should be intubated quickly and placed under mechanical ventilation.

- Do not forget the administration of low-molecular-weight heparin to reduce the risk of deep vein thrombosis and pulmonary embolism in patients with acute pulmonary edema.

- Acute pulmonary edema with a low systolic BP has a poor prognosis. Inotropes ± vasopressors are administered and the patient should be treated etiologically as soon as possible, e.g. with primary angioplasty in case of AMI.

- When noncardiogenic acute pulmonary edema is suspected (presence of severe extracardiac disease, normal ECG, chest X-ray with diffuse infiltrates, etc.), the patient should be transferred promptly to the ICU.

- A patient with known heart disease, who presents to the Emergency Room with the clinical picture of "acute bronchial asthma" but no previous history of asthma, probably has acute pulmonary edema (early stage with only interstitial edema).

- IV solutions in acute pulmonary edema are always administered in the form of isotonic glucose solution (D/W 5%), whereas normal saline solutions (NaCl 0.9%) are avoided.

ALGORITHM FOR THE TREATMENT OF CARDIOGENIC ACUTE PULMONARY EDEMA

Patient with dyspnea, sweating, sitting, possibly cyanotic and usually with a history of heart disease (lung auscultation: crackles on both sides ± wheezes, but in very early stages there might only be auscultatory findings of bronchospasm)

ACUTE PULMONARY EDEMA

Differential diagnosis
1) Bronchial asthma exacerbation (history, BNP <100 pg/mL)
2) Pulmonary embolism (D-dimers >500 ng/mL, MD-CTPA showing filling defect)
3) Cardiac tamponade (echocardiogram with pericardial fluid and right ventricular collapse)
4) Spontaneous pneumothorax (chest X-ray with avascular region)
5) Pneumonia (fever, chest X-ray with consolidation)
6) Noncardiogenic acute pulmonary edema (severe extracardiac disease, diffuse infiltrates on the chest X-ray, BNP <100 pg/mL)

Basic tests
1) ECG (to exclude myocardial ischemia, arrhythmias, etc.)
2) Complete blood count, cardiac troponin, BNP, urea, creatinine, glucose and Na, K
3) Arterial blood gases (hypoxemia)
4) Chest X-ray: perihilar shadowing (butterfly pattern)

Therapeutic manipulations

First actions
1) Seated position
2) O_2 administration at concentrations >40% (in cases of chronic obstructive pulmonary disease: concentration 24-28%)
3) IV line placement

General manipulations
1) Furosemide (40-80 mg IV)
2) If SBP >100 mmHg: IV nitroglycerin (start at 5-10 μg/min)
3) Morphine (3-5 mg IV slowly) in selected cases (cautiously)
4) In case of bronchospasm: salbutamol ± ipratropium inhalation solution
5) Low-molecular-weight heparin
6) If SBP <90 mmHg: consider inotropes/vasopressors

Special manipulations
1) In case of AMI: primary angioplasty (preferable) or fibrinolysis
2) In case of recent-onset atrial fibrillation or ventricular tachycardia: electrical cardioversion
3) In case of fluid retention in kidney patients: dialysis

MD-CTPA: multi-detector computed tomographic pulmonary angiography
BNP: B-type natriuretic peptide, SBP: systolic blood pressure, AMI: acute myocardial infarction

6

Acute pericarditis

Acute pericarditis is an inflammation of the pericardium with ("wet") or without ("dry") the presence of pericardial fluid (normally, the pericardial fluid volume is <50 mL). The fluid may be serous, hemorrhagic or, in rare cases, purulent. The most common cause of pericarditis is idiopathic (Table 6.1). In fact, most cases of idiopathic pericarditis are due to viral infection of the pericardium and constitute 80-90% of all pericarditis cases in developed countries.

The prognosis of acute pericarditis depends on the underlying cause. Idiopathic/viral pericarditis has the best prognosis while neoplastic and purulent pericarditis have the worst.

Symptoms
- Retrosternal or precordial pain (in >90% of cases), usually with sudden onset, sharp, lasting several hours or days, that may radiate to the trapezius muscle ridge (especially the left) due to irritation of the phrenic nerve (highly specific sign). Radiation to the left arm is not unusual and can lead to confusion with acute myocardial ischemia; in other cases, pain is localized in the epigastrium, raising the problem of differential diagnosis from acute abdomen. Pericarditis is more likely when there is aggravation of pain in the supine position or on swallowing, cough or deep inspiration. The latter two signs indicate pleural involvement due to the inflammation spreading to the adjacent pleura.
- Dyspnea, as a result of either shallow breathing due to inspiratory chest pain or a large pericardial effusion.
- May be preceded or accompanied by fever (or symptoms of upper respiratory tract infection) if it caused by a viral illness, as opposed to pericarditis complicating acute myocardial infarction (AMI), in which case pain precedes the fever.

TABLE 6.1	Most common causes of pericarditis*

1) Idiopathic (the most common cause of all)

2) Viral (mostly due to Coxsackie B and echovirus)

3) Bacterial (purulent, tuberculous [~4%]** etc.)

4) Postinfarct
- Early (1-5 days >AMI)
- Late or Dressler syndrome (1 week to several months >AMI) [<1%]

5) Advanced renal failure (uremic)

6) Autoimmune diseases (rheumatoid arthritis, lupus erythematosus, scleroderma, etc.) [~7%]

7) Neoplasms (~5%)
- Primary: rare, e.g. pericardial mesothelioma
- Secondary: metastatic or by direct extension due to lung or breast malignancies, Hodgkin's lymphoma, etc.

8) Traumatic

9) Hypothyroidism

10) Use of certain drugs (procainamide, isoniazid, hydralazine, etc.)

11) Radiation (particularly for Hodgkin's lymphoma, breast or lung neoplasms)

12) Postpericardiotomy syndrome (1-12 weeks after heart surgery)

Mnemonic for the causes of pericarditis (other than idiopathic): TUMOR, where T=trauma, U=uremia, M=myocardial infarction or medication, O=other infections: bacterial, fungal, tuberculosis, R=rheumatoid arthritis or radiation.
** *The rates in the table apply to developed countries.*
AMI: acute myocardial infarction

Clinical signs

1) Upon heart auscultation, the pathognomonic finding is a **pericardial friction rub** (~35% of cases) that:
- Classically it is triphasic (~50%): the 3 phases correspond to ventricular contraction (the loudest component), early diastolic ventricular filling, and atrial contraction (presystolic component). It is described as a scratchy, grating, high-pitched sound similar to the sound of new leather rubbing on leather. In ~30% it is biphasic and in the remainder monophasic (only a systolic component, in which case it needs to be differentiated from a systolic murmur).
- It is heard more clearly in a seated position with the body leaning forward, in the left parasternal area at the 3rd-4th intercostal space.

- It is often dynamic (may disappear and reappear during the course of the disease) and thus patients should be examined repeatedly.
2) Tachycardia and low-grade fever (fever >38° is rare in idiopathic pericarditis).

Diagnostic tests

1) **ECG:** in the acute phase shows:
   - Concave upward (saddle-shaped) ST-segment elevation in all leads (except for aVR and V_1, where the ST-segment may be depressed).
   - PR-segment depression in all leads except for aVR and V_1 (highly specific but relatively rare).
   - Sinus tachycardia.

   The acute phase is followed by a return of the ST-segment to the isoelectric line, with T-wave flattening and then reversal that might persist for several weeks or months. This needs to be differentiated from AMI (Table 6.2).
2) **Chest X-ray:** of little diagnostic value, as cardiomegaly will be noted only when the pericardial fluid exceeds 250 mL. A pleural effusion on the left is noted in ~25% of cases.
3) **Echocardiography:** permits
   - Detection (requires minimal time) and quantification of pericardial fluid (present in ~60% of cases). If the pericardial fluid is uniformly distributed around the heart, then its quantity can be roughly estimated by measur-

TABLE 6.2	Differential diagnosis for acute myocardial infarction (AMI) and acute pericarditis based on the ECG	
	AMI	**Acute pericarditis**
ST-segment elevation	Convex upward	Concave upward
PR-segment depression	No	Yes
Involved leads	ST-segment elevation in some leads (adjacent)	ST-segment elevation in almost all leads (at least 8)
Reciprocal changes	Usual	Absent (except for ST-segment depression in leads aVR and V_1)
Course of changes	T waves reversed before the ST-segment returns to the isoelectric line	T waves reversed after the ST-segment returns to the isoelectric line

ing, on diastole, the distance between the visceral and the parietal laminae of the pericardium (Table 6.3). The measurements can be made in
the parasternal long axis, apical 4-chamber or subxiphoid view.

- Assessment of left ventricular function for potential myopericarditis (in
  few cases a mild global or segmental left ventricular dysfunction can be
  detected) or AMI (regional abnormalities in systolic thickening) complicated by pericardial effusion. Note that significant left ventricular dysfunction (in the absence of AMI) denotes a substantial myocardial inflammatory involvement, and a predominant myocarditic syndrome
  (perimyocarditis).
- Assessment of any impairment of the right heart chambers, and examination of transmitral and transtricuspid flow in order to identify signs
  of cardiac tamponade (see page 115).
- Assessment of inferior vena cava size and its respiratory variations.
  Distension and lack of respiratory variations may suggest cardiac tamponade or less commonly constrictive pericarditis.

Warning! The absence of pericardial fluid does not exclude the diagnosis
of acute pericarditis, as this is often dry. Therefore, the diagnosis of acute
pericarditis is mainly clinical.

4) **Blood tests**
   a) *Basic*
   - Complete blood count (usually leukocytosis), creatinine (to exclude
     uremic pericarditis), electrolytes.
   - Cardiac troponin I or T in order to detect myocardial necrosis in
     case of acute myopericarditis or AMI. In acute myopericarditis the
     increase in cardiac troponins is usually mild (seen in 15-30% of a-
     cute pericarditis patients) and typically resolves within 1-2 weeks. It
     suggests a minor extension of the inflammatory process to the
     subepicardial myocardium and in most cases left ventricular func-

TABLE 6.3	Approximate quantification of the pericardial fluid by measuring the distance between the two pericardial laminae (echo-free space) on diastole using a 2D echocardiogram.

- <5 mm → minimal effusion (50-100 mL)
- 5-10 mm → small effusion (100-250 mL)
- 10-20 mm → moderate effusion (250-500 mL)
- >20 mm → large effusion (>500 mL)

tion is normal and prognosis is good. Therefore, the term myoperi-carditis indicates a primarily pericarditic syndrome.
- Inflammatory markers: C-reactive protein (CRP), erythrocyte sedimentation rate.
- Serology testing for viruses is of limited clinical usefulness.

b) Additional tests, depending on clinical suspicion
- T3, T4, TSH to exclude hypothyroidism.
- Tuberculin skin test (Mantoux test) when tuberculosis is suspected. However, it should be noted that it has a low diagnostic accuracy.
- Rheumatology testing (antinuclear antibodies, rheumatoid factor, etc.).
- Blood cultures x 3 if the patient is septic.
- Tumor associated markers if a metastatic process is suspected.

Treatment

1) Patients with acute pericarditis and with at least one high-risk feature (Table 6.4) should be admitted to a hospital. If symptoms are mild and no high-risk features are present, the patient may remain at home after undergoing basic laboratory testing (complete blood count, cardiac troponin, echocardiogram, chest X-ray) and treatment is administered.
2) Nonspecific treatment:
   - **Exercise restriction** is recommended until resolution of symptoms, and normalization of CRP, ECG and echocardiogram.
   - **Nonsteroidal antiinflammatory drugs (NSAIDs):** ibuprofen is preferable to indomethacin because it causes less gastrointestinal irritation. It is administered at a dose of 400-800 mg x 3 daily. Indomethacin

TABLE 6.4	High-risk features in acute pericarditis, dictating the patient's hospitalization and full etiologic research *(European Guidelines for Pericardial Diseases, Adler Y, et al. Eur Heart J 2015;36:2921-64)*

1) Fever >38°C
2) Subacute onset (symptoms developing over several days or weeks)
3) Cardiac tamponade
4) Large pericardial effusion
5) Lack of response to nonsteroidal antiinflammatory drugs after at least 1 week of therapy
6) Myopericarditis (increased cardiac troponin ± mild left ventricular dysfunction on the echocardiogram)
7) Immunosuppression
8) Traumatic pericarditis
9) Oral anticoagulant therapy

is administered at a dose of 25-50 mg x 3 daily. The medication of choice in postinfarct pericarditis is acetylsalicylic acid (aspirin), at a dose of 750-1000 mg x 3 daily. NSAIDs are used at lower doses for a-cute myopericarditis. They are always coadministered with proton pump inhibitors to reduce gastrointestinal irritation.

- **Colchicine:** administered in case of nonresponse to NSAIDs or recurrence (relapse) of pericarditis in combination with NSAIDs. The combination of colchicine and NSAIDs is also recommended as initial treatment for acute pericarditis. Colchicine is administered at a dose of 0.5 mg x 2 daily (with or without a loading dose of 2 mg on the first day). For people aged >70 years, weighing <70 kg, and in cases of moderate chronic renal failure (creatinine clearance 30-60 mL/min), the dosage is halved. In severe renal impairment (creatinine clearance 10-30 mL/min) the dose is 0.5 mg every 2 to 3 days. Colchicine's major side effects involve the gastrointestinal system (nausea, vomiting, diarrhea) and occur in 10-15% of cases. More rarely (<1%), it can cause bone marrow suppression, increased transaminase levels or myotoxicity, so a complete blood count with transaminase, creatine kinase (CK) and creatinine measurement is recommended after one month of treatment. Colchicine is metabolized by cytochrome P450 3A4 and great caution is required when it is coadministered with similarly metabolized drugs (cyclosporine, macrolides, certain statins, etc.).
- **Corticosteroids:** their use is becoming ever more rare today because they are associated with an increased rate of pericarditis relapse after discontinuation. As a result, corticosteroids are only given when an infectious cause has been excluded and:
  a) pericarditis does not respond* or relapses after coadministration of NSAIDs and colchicine. In these cases they are usually coadministered with colchicine and NSAIDs.
  b) pericarditis complicates an autoimmune disease, or
  c) NSAIDs and colchicine are contraindicated, e.g. when acute pericarditis appears in a pregnant woman after gestational week 20 (NSAIDs can cause constriction of the ductus arteriosus).

  Nowadays, the recommended dose of corticosteroids is 0.2-0.5 mg/kg/day of prednisone (instead of 1 mg/kg/day given in the past) or equivalent dose of other corticosteroids [Table 6.5]. The lower prednisone dosage reduces the complications without any loss of effectiveness.

In our clinical practice, when acute pericarditis is associated with a large pericardial effusion (without clinical signs of cardiac tamponade) and there is no response to the coadministration of NSAIDs and colchicine within few days, we proceed to pericardiocentesis and continue the coadministration of NSAIDs and colchicine.

TABLE 6.5	A comparison of major corticosteroids		
Corticosteroid	**Antiinflammatory action**	**Mineralocorticoid action**	**Dosage equivalence (mg)**
Cortisol (or hydrocortisone)	1	1	20
Prednisone	4	0.8	5
Prednisolone	4	0.8	5
Methylprednisolone	5	0.5	4

Remarks on medication duration and discontinuation (tapering)

- The duration of administration of antiinflammatory treatment is individualized. It is administered until symptoms have fully receded and CRP levels have returned to normal; CRP levels should be tested weekly. The usual duration of NSAID administration is 2-3 weeks, whereas for colchicine it is 3 months in acute and 6-12 months in recurrent pericarditis. The NSAID dose should be gradually tapered after the first 1-2 weeks provided that the symptoms have resolved.
- Regarding corticosteroids, low to moderate dose (i.e. 0.2-0.5 mg/kg/day of prednisone) is administered for 2-4 weeks, and thereafter **very slow tapering** over 6-12 months. According to the European Guidelines for Pericardial Diseases (Adler Y, et al. Eur Heart J 2015;36:2921-64) the tapering schedule is as follows:
  - >50 mg: 10 mg/day every 1-2 weeks
  - 50-25 mg: 5-10 mg/day every 1-2 weeks
  - 25-15 mg: 2.5 mg/day every 2-4 weeks
  - <15 mg: 1.25-2.5 mg/day every 2-6 weeks.

Note that the critical threshold for pericarditis recurrence is the reduction of the prednisone dose to 10-15 mg/day. Every decrease in prednisone dose should be done only if the patient is asymptomatic and has normal CRP levels.

When the corticosteroid dose tapering begins, NSAIDs or colchicine (usually at 0.5 mg daily) must be coadministered in order to reduce the risk of recurrence. In addition, with prolonged (>3 months) corticosteroid use, osteoporosis prevention should be considered (i.e. prescription of calcium 1200-1500 mg daily and vitamin D 800-1000 IU daily). In addition, bisphosphonates are recommended in men ≥50 years and postmenopausal women.

Warning! Concomitant use of oral anticoagulants in the setting of acute pericarditis was traditionally considered as a possible risk factor for the worsening of pericardial effusion and was contraindicated. However, recent data showed that the continuation of oral anticoagulants is not associated with an increased risk of cardiac tamponade.

3) Specific treatment depending on the cause: for uremic pericarditis in a patient under dialysis, for example, the dialysis regimen is intensified.

Complications of idiopathic-viral pericarditis
- Recurrent pericarditis (15-30%) defined as recurrence of pericarditis after a symptom-free interval of 4-6 weeks or longer
- Cardiac tamponade (<5%)
- Constrictive pericarditis (<1%).

The complication rates vary depending on the underlying cause of the pericarditis: the risk of cardiac tamponade is greater in cases of metastatic involvement of the pericardium, whereas the risk of constrictive pericarditis is greater in purulent (~30%) and tuberculous pericarditis (20-50%).

With regard to the etiology of constrictive pericarditis, the most common cause is idiopathic, followed by cardiovascular surgery and mediastinal irradiation (usually a late complication).

Key points

- Acute pericarditis is diagnosed when at least two of the following criteria are present: pericarditic chest pain (>90% of cases), pericardial friction rub (~35% of cases), new widespread ST-segment elevation or PR-segment depression on ECG (up to 60% of cases), and pericardial effusion (~60% of cases).

- A patient with acute pericarditis and with at least one high-risk feature (fever >38°C, subacute onset, cardiac tamponade, large pericardial effusion, lack of response to NSAIDs after at least 1 week of therapy, myopericarditis, immunosuppression, traumatic pericarditis, oral anticoagulant therapy) requires hospital admission and etiology research.

- An ECG must be recorded, cardiac troponin must be requested in order to exclude myopericarditis and/or AMI, and an echocardiographic examination must be performed to assess the amount of pericardial fluid (for wet pericarditis) and to exclude signs of cardiac tamponade, as well as to evaluate left ventricular function.

- First line treatment for idiopathic acute pericarditis is NSAIDs (ibuprofen is preferred) given for 2-3 weeks.

- Colchicine is given
  - as first line treatment for acute pericarditis (x 3 months) in combination with NSAIDs
  - in recurrent pericarditis (x 6-12 months) usually in combination with NSAIDs.

- For postinfarction pericarditis, the drug of choice is acetylsalicylic acid (aspirin).

- Corticosteroids are given in cases of pericarditis, at low to moderate doses (i.e. prednisone 0.2–0.5 mg/kg/day or equivalent dose of other corticosteroids), only if:
  a) Pericarditis does not respond or relapses after coadministration of NSAIDs and colchicine.
  b) Pericarditis complicates an autoimmune disease
  c) NSAIDs and colchicine are contraindicated.

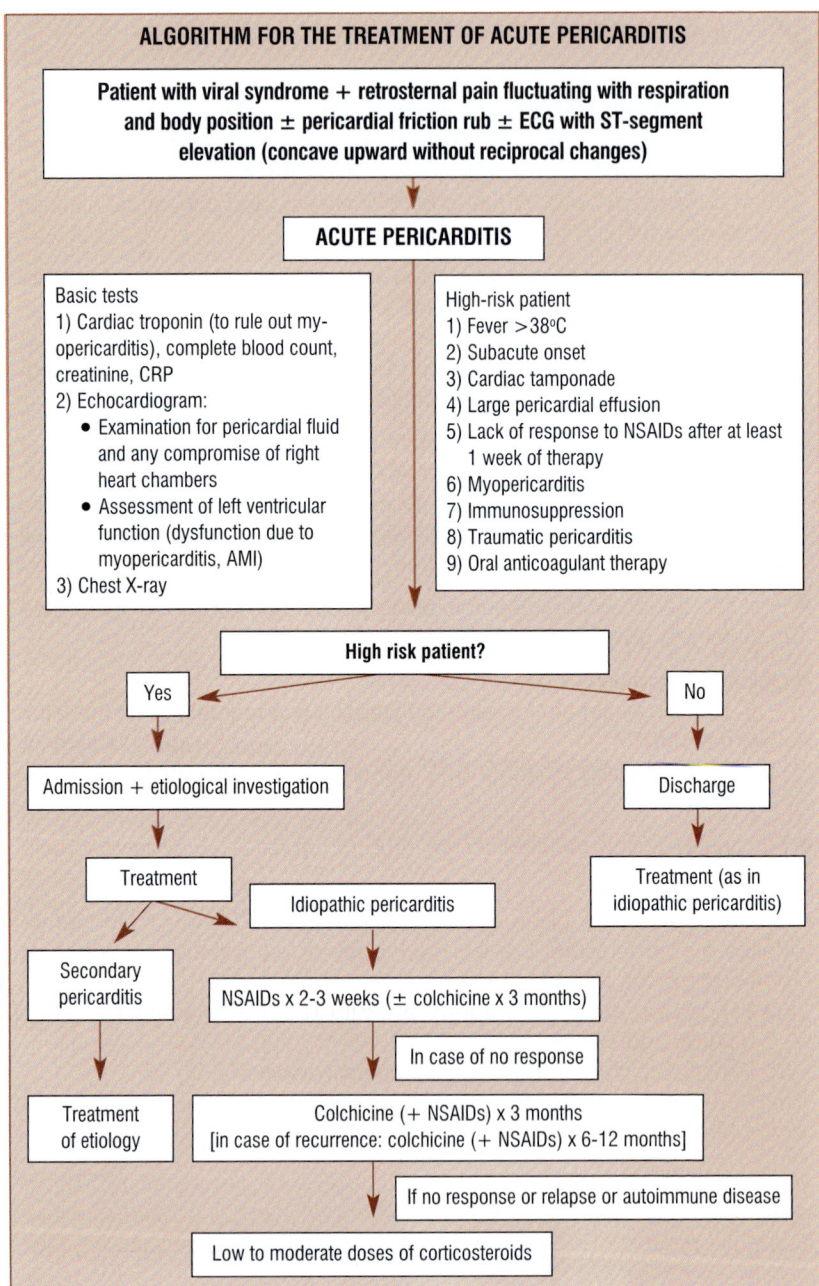

ALGORITHM FOR THE TREATMENT OF ACUTE PERICARDITIS

Patient with viral syndrome + retrosternal pain fluctuating with respiration and body position ± pericardial friction rub ± ECG with ST-segment elevation (concave upward without reciprocal changes)

ACUTE PERICARDITIS

Basic tests
1) Cardiac troponin (to rule out my-opericarditis), complete blood count, creatinine, CRP
2) Echocardiogram:
 • Examination for pericardial fluid and any compromise of right heart chambers
 • Assessment of left ventricular function (dysfunction due to myopericarditis, AMI)
3) Chest X-ray

High-risk patient
1) Fever >38ºC
2) Subacute onset
3) Cardiac tamponade
4) Large pericardial effusion
5) Lack of response to NSAIDs after at least 1 week of therapy
6) Myopericarditis
7) Immunosuppression
8) Traumatic pericarditis
9) Oral anticoagulant therapy

High risk patient?

Yes   No

Admission + etiological investigation   Discharge

Treatment   Treatment (as in idiopathic pericarditis)

Idiopathic pericarditis

Secondary pericarditis

NSAIDs x 2-3 weeks (± colchicine x 3 months)

In case of no response

Treatment of etiology

Colchicine (+ NSAIDs) x 3 months
[in case of recurrence: colchicine (+ NSAIDs) x 6-12 months]

If no response or relapse or autoimmune disease

Low to moderate doses of corticosteroids

CRP: C-reactive protein, NSAIDs: nonsteroidal antiinflammatory drugs, AMI: acute myocardial infarction

7

Cardiac tamponade

Cardiac tamponade is caused by the accumulation of a large amount of pericardial fluid, or of a small amount (150-200 mL) increasing rapidly (e.g. due to acute dissection of the aorta) and causing elevated intrapericardial pressure up to 15-30 mmHg (which is normally zero or negative) and decreased diastolic ventricular filling. In the early stages, cardiac output is maintained through sympathetic activation, leading to tachycardia and systemic vasoconstriction. After decompensation, cardiac output is reduced.

Cardiac tamponade is an emergency cardiological condition. Its most common causes are presented in Table 7.1. Note that ~50% of pericardial

TABLE 7.1	Causes of cardiac tamponade

1) Metastatic pericardial involvement (especially due to lung or breast malignancy, lymphoma, etc.) [~35%]
2) Idiopathic pericarditis (~30%)
3) Uremia
4) Acute aortic dissection (type A)
5) Chest trauma, e.g. traffic accident
6) Iatrogenic, e.g. myocardial wall puncture by a catheter
7) Chest irradiation
8) Use of anticoagulants (rare)
9) After heart surgery

Warning! When clinical signs of cardiac tamponade develop after cardiac surgery, exclude pericardial hematoma located behind the right or left atrium (regional tamponade), usually visible only by transesophageal echocardiogram.

effusions in cancer patients are not caused by metastasis, in which case the prognosis is poor, but by other, more "benign" causes (e.g. idiopathic, radiation, tuberculosis, etc.).

Clinical signs

- Tachypnea with "clear lungs".
- Tachycardia (usually >100 beats/min), but it can be absent in the setting of hypothyroidism, conduction system defects, or when a preterminal bradycardic reflex has supervened.
- Distended jugular veins (loss of the y descent and preservation of the x descent, since venous return occurs only during ventricular systole).
- Muffled heart sounds ± pericardial friction rub. If the cardiac tamponade is severe, the peripheral pulse might weaken or even disappear on inspiration.
- Signs of low cardiac output (low blood pressure [BP], oliguria, etc.).
- Large pericardial effusion may be associated with **Ewart's sign**: dullness to percussion, bronchial breath sounds, and egophony below the angle of left scapula secondary to compression of the left lower lobe of the lung.
- **Pulsus paradoxus,** defined as an inspiratory drop in the systolic BP >10 mmHg during normal breathing. This constitutes an exaggeration of a normal phenomenon, since the systolic BP normally drops <10 mmHg on inspiration. The pulsus paradoxus is caused by the increased venous blood return to the right ventricle on inspiration. The increased intrapericardial pressure restricts the diastolic expansion of the ventricles (particularly the right), and causes the interventricular septum to protrude into the left ventricle. Combined with the reduced venous blood return from the lungs, this results in reduced filling of the left ventricle, which leads to a reduced stroke volume and a drop in systolic BP on inspiration. The measurement technique for pulsus paradoxus is presented in Table 7.2.

Warning! Pulsus paradoxus is not pathognomonic for cardiac tamponade because it is also observed in severe obstructive pulmonary disease, hypovolemic shock, acute massive pulmonary embolism, right ventricular infarction, and constrictive pericarditis, whereas is it absent in cases of right ventricular hypertrophy, regional cardiac tamponade, severe aortic regurgitation, and atrial septal defect.

Diagnostic tests

1) **ECG:** findings of acute pericarditis (see page 105), low-voltage QRS complexes (nonspecific finding) and electrical alternans (beat-to-beat

TABLE 7.2	**Technique for measuring a pulsus paradoxus by manual sphygmomanometer**

1. Increase the pressure in the sphygmomanometer cuff above the patient's systolic blood pressure (BP)
2. Slowly deflate the sphygmomanometer cuff and follow the patient's breathing. Record the systolic BP when the first Korotkoff sound is heard. The first Korotkoff sound will only be heard during exhalation, because in this phase the systolic BP is higher than during inhalation. Therefore, the first Korotkoff sounds will be heard intermittently and only during exhalation
3. Continue deflating the cuff and record the systolic BP when the Korotkoff sounds also start to be heard during inhalation, i.e. when they are heard "rhythmically" throughout the respiratory cycle
4. The difference in the levels of systolic BP (mmHg) between the first Korotkoff sound and the multiple "rhythmic" Korotkoff sounds is the measure of the pulsus paradoxus

variation in both the amplitude and the axis of the QRS complexes) caused by swinging of the heart in the pericardial sac.

2) **Chest X-ray:** in cases of large pericardial effusion, the heart assumes a rounded, flask-like appearance with an acute right cardiophrenic angle. Signs of pulmonary congestion are generally absent.

3) **Echocardiogram:** the most useful modality for the assessment of the amount of pericardial fluid and the degree to which the right cardiac chambers are affected. The most common echocardiographic signs in cases of tamponade are:

- Early diastolic collapse of the free wall of the right ventricle (highly specific with good sensitivity sign) [Figure 7.1]. It is not present in cases of right ventricular hypertrophy. The longer the duration of collapse, the more severe tamponade physiology is.
- Late diastolic collapse of the wall of the right atrium, extending into the systolic period (more sensitive but less specific than the previous sign).
- Inferior vena cava distension (its diameter is normally ≤21 mm) and absence of respiratory variations of its diameter (its diameter should decrease by >50% on inspiration).
- Doppler: inspiratory reduction of the transmitral flow E wave >30%, and inspiratory increase of the transtricuspid flow E wave >40%.

Warning! The diagnosis of cardiac tamponade is mainly clinical. The presence of echocardiographic signs of cardiac tamponade is not always synonymous with clinical tamponade.

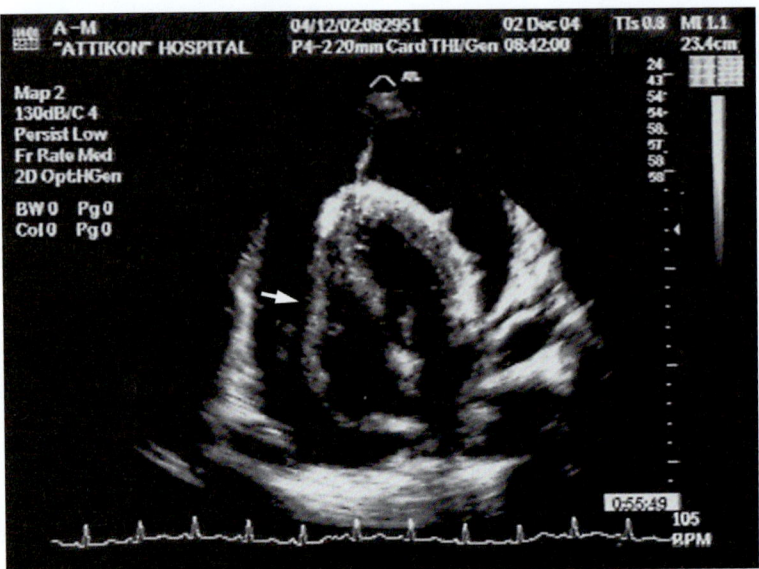

Figure 7.1. Echocardiogram with a large pericardial effusion and early diastolic compression (arrow) of the lateral wall of the right ventricle (4-chamber apical view).

Treatment

Emergency percutaneous **pericardial paracentesis** to drain the fluid and send samples for laboratory diagnostic investigation. For fuller drainage, a pigtail catheter is introduced and usually kept in place until fluid drainage is <25 mL/day (see Chapter 22). While waiting for the paracentesis, IV normal saline is administered (e.g. 500 mL over one hour).

> **Warning!** For cardiac tamponade, it is contraindicated to administer drugs that cause bradycardia (tachycardia is a compensation mechanism), diuretics (which lower the preload and further reduce the cardiac output) or vasodilators.

In cases of frequent relapse of pericardial effusion (as in the case of metastases), a pericardial window may need to be opened (surgically or percutaneously). In cases of traumatic hemopericardium and purulent pericarditis, surgical drainage is required. If cardiac tamponade is a complication of acute aortic dissection, then emergency surgical treatment of the acute dissection, instead of pericardiocentesis, is required (see also page 127).

Key points

- Suspicion of cardiac tamponade is raised in dyspneic patients with low cardiac output (hypotension, oliguria), distended jugulars, and absence of auscultatory findings from the lungs, with no improvement after inotrope administration.

- Cardiac tamponade is caused by the accumulation of a large amount of pericardial fluid, or of a small amount (150-200 mL) increasing rapidly (e.g. acute dissection of the aorta or trauma).

- The diagnosis of cardiac tamponade is mainly clinical and is confirmed by echocardiography. Echocardiographic detection of pericardial fluid (usually large) + diastolic collapse of right ventricle confirm the diagnosis of tamponade only if associated with clinical signs of cardiac tamponade.

- The presence of echocardiographic signs of cardiac tamponade in a patient without hemodynamic compromise is not an indication for emergency pericardiocentesis.

- A "normal" chest X-ray in a patient with dyspnea does not exclude the diagnosis of cardiac tamponade.

- Treatment of cardiac tamponade requires emergency percutaneous pericardiocentesis for fluid drainage.

- ~50% of cases of pericardial effusion in cancer patients are not caused by metastasis but by other, more "benign" causes (idiopathic, radiation, tuberculosis, etc.).

ALGORITHM FOR THE TREATMENT OF CARDIAC TAMPONADE

Acute dyspnea + distended jugulars + hypotension + pulsus paradoxus + "clear lungs" on auscultation
+
history of malignancy (lungs, breasts, etc.), chronic renal failure, chest trauma, or presence of stabbing chest pain (acute aortic dissection)

↓

Suspicion of CARDIAC TAMPONADE

Placement of IV line and urinary catheter

Basic tests:
1) ECG: exclusion of acute myocardial infarction
2) Chest X-ray: detection of cardiomegaly, widened mediastinum (suspected aortic dissection), lung infiltrations, etc.

↓

Emergency echocardiographic assessment

↓

Pericardial fluid (usually large effusion) + diastolic collapse of right ventricle

Yes   No

Rapid loading with 500 mL of normal saline while waiting for pericardiocentesis

Emergency palliative and diagnostic pericardiocentesis

Avoid paracentesis and perform immediate heart surgery for treatment of acute aortic dissection

Exclude other causes of dyspnea, e.g. acute pulmonary embolism

Introduce a pigtail catheter for fuller drainage (left in place until fluid drainage is <25 mL/day) and send fluid for testing

8

Acute aortic dissection

Acute aortic dissection is a relatively rare (2 to 3.5 cases per 100.000 person-years) condition with high early mortality. Without surgical treatment, 40-50% of patients with acute aortic dissection (proximal) will die within the first 48 h (~1% mortality per hour for the first 48 h), whereas mortality is 10-20% if the condition is treated surgically. The diagnosis of aortic dissection is often delayed or missed. Almost 30% of patients with acute aortic dissection are treated initially for acute coronary syndrome, congestive heart failure, pulmonary embolism or pericarditis.

Acute aortic dissection is classically caused by a rupture of the aortic intima, allowing blood to enter the media, which is usually abnormal, e.g. due to cystic medial degeneration. The site which most commonly ruptures is the proximal segment of the ascending aorta (65% of intimal tears occur within 10 cm of the aortic root). Less commonly, rupture of the vasa vasorum within the aortic wall may separate the intima from the media and lead to intimal disruption and aortic dissection. Table 8.1 presents the most important predisposing factors for the development of an acute aortic dissection. The inflow of blood tears and splits the wall of the aorta in two. The detached part of the wall that projects into the aortic lumen is called the **intimal flap.** The new lumen that forms between the flap and the remainder of the media is the **false lumen.** The dissection then extends, usually anterogradely (in the direction of blood flow), and ischemia develops, depending on which arteries are blocked along the course of the false lumen. In addition, the weakened aortic wall of the false lumen can rupture into the pericardium (hemopericardium) or into the pleura (hemothorax), usually leading

TABLE 8.1	Predisposing factors for the development of acute aortic dissection

1) Hypertension (70% of cases have a history of hypertension)
2) Advanced age (>60 years old)
3) Aneurysm of the thoracic aorta
4) Bicuspid aortic valve (due to the common occurrence of cystic medial degeneration of aorta)
5) Marfan and Ehlers–Danlos syndromes (due to cystic medial degeneration of aorta)
6) Coarctation of the aorta
7) Pregnancy (usually in the 3rd trimester)
8) Iatrogenic (underlying aortic disease is usually present) [e.g. during placement of an intra-aortic balloon pump]
9) Previous cardiac surgery (usually after aortic valve replacement for a bicuspid valve)

to death. If the dissection extends into the aortic root, severe aortic valve insufficiency usually develops.

Table 8.2 lists the various classification systems and Figure 8.1 gives a schematic representation of the various types of aortic dissection, based on its anatomical location.

TABLE 8.2	Aortic dissection classification
Type	**Description of location**
DeBakey	
Type I	Origin in the ascending aorta, extending to the aortic arch and in many cases even more distally ("walking stick" distribution)
Type II	Limited to the ascending aorta
Type III	Origin in the descending aorta (distal to the left subclavian artery) extending distally (usually) or proximally (rarely)
Stanford	
Type A	Any dissection involving the ascending aorta, regardless of origin (includes 2/3 of all dissections)
Type B	Any dissection not involving the ascending aorta
Descriptive	
Proximal	Includes: DeBakey types I and II and Stanford type A
Distal	Includes: DeBakey type III and Stanford type B

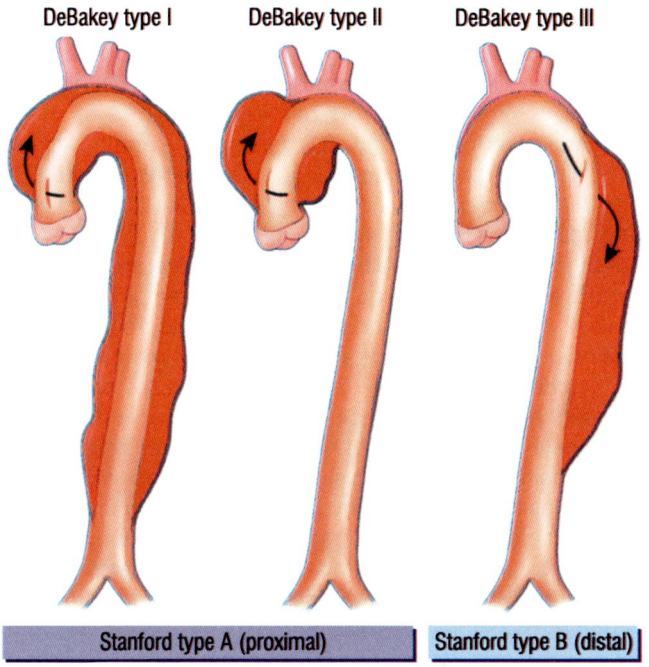

Figure 8.1. Schematic representation of the various types of aortic dissection. (Modified from Braunwald's Heart Disease by Zipes, Libby, Bonow and Braunwald, 7th edition, p 1416).

In addition, and according to chronicity, dissections are classified as:
- Acute: occurs <14 days after onset of pain (high mortality period).
- Subacute: occurs between 15-90 days after onset of pain.
- Chronic: occurs >90 days after onset of pain.

Atypical forms of aortic dissection
- **Aortic intramural hematoma (IMH)*:** approximately 10-15% of patients presenting with a clinical picture of aortic dissection have an IMH. This is caused by bleeding into the aortic media after rupture of the wall vessels (vasa vasorum), without tearing of the intima. It may progress to classic aortic dissection (30-50%), regress (~10%), or rupture (~30%). IMH has a

---

*Acute aortic dissection, aortic intramural hematoma and penetrating aortic ulcer are collectively described by the term "acute aortic syndrome".

higher rate of rupture compared to aortic dissection due to its closer re-
lationship to the adventitia. The clinical picture and treatment are similar
to those of a classic dissection. Diagnosis is made by transesophageal
echocardiogram (TEE) [localized echolucent aortic wall thickness cres-
cent-shaped or circumferential >7 mm in the absence of an intimal flap
or tear], computed tomography (CT) [area in the aortic wall with higher
tissue density than unenhanced blood], contrast-enhanced CT (area in
the aortic wall without enhancement after contrast administration), or by
magnetic resonance imaging (MRI).

- **Penetrating aortic ulcer (PAU):** is defined as ulceration of an aortic ath-
erosclerotic plaque penetrating through the internal elastic lamina into
the media. It is often associated with a variable degree of IMH formation.
Such lesions represent ~5% of all acute aortic syndromes and they are
usually located (~90%) in the descending aorta. Its clinical manifestations are sudden pain in the back or on the anterior surface of the chest.
A pseudoaneurysm forms in ~25% of cases, whereas rupture of the aorta or progression to a typical dissection occurs less frequently. A PAU
can be diagnosed by aortography, TEE, contrast-enhanced CT (imaging
modality of choice) or magnetic resonance angiography (MRA, i.e. MRI
enhanced with IV gadolinium). Initial treatment includes pain relief and
blood pressure (BP) control. Surgical treatment is required in cases of
aortic rupture, continued or recurrent pain, signs of contained rupture
(rapidly growing aortic ulcer, associated periaortic hematoma, or pleural
effusions), expanding pseudoaneurysm or PAUs located in ascending
aorta (i.e. type A). For complicated type B PAUs thoracic endovascular
aortic repair (TEVAR) should be considered.

Symptoms

- Pain (>90%): sudden (like "gunshot"), very intense (peak intensity at onset, as opposed to an acute myocardial infarction [AMI] where pain intensity increases gradually), stabbing, located in the anterior thorax
(proximal dissection) and/or in the interscapular or lumbar area (distal
dissection), occasionally (~15%) migrating along the course of the dissection.

Warning! Painless aortic dissection occurs in ~5% of patients.

- Dyspnea due to left heart failure caused by severe aortic insufficiency, or
to hemopericardium caused by rupture of the aorta within the pericardium.
- Symptoms due to obstruction of aortic branches along the dissection:
  – coronary artery (right >left) → AMI (usually inferior) [1-5%]
  – anonymous or left common carotid artery → hemiplegia (3-6%)
  – intercostal arteries → paraplegia (<5%) [spinal cord ischemia]

- mesenteric artery → abdominal pain, bloody diarrhea (<5%)
- renal artery → hematuria, anuria, refractory hypertension (5-8%)
- iliac artery → acute lower limb ischemia (<10%).
- Syncope (~10%).
- Cardiac arrest.

Warning! In cases of inferior AMI, the small possibility that it is caused by an acute proximal aortic dissection should always be investigated. Administration of fibrinolytics in such cases will have devastating results (mortality >70%, usually by cardiac tamponade). The administration of antiplatelet agents or heparin is also contraindicated.

Clinical signs

- The BP in acute aortic dissection may be:
  - elevated (usually)
  - normal
  - truly low (~25% of proximal aortic dissection): unfavorable sign since it usually indicates acute aortic valve insufficiency, cardiac tamponade (rupture in the pericardium) or rupture of aortic wall in other cavities (intrapleural or intraperitoneal)
  - falsely low (pseudohypotension) due to an obstruction of the anonymous or left subclavian artery while central arterial pressure is normal or high
  - unequal in upper limbs (systolic BP difference >20 mmHg): may indicate an obstruction of the anonymous or left subclavian artery.
- Pulse deficit: weak or absent peripheral pulses (in 20-30% of proximal and 15% of distal aortic dissection). Pulse deficit may be transient.
- New murmur of aortic insufficiency (in ~50% of proximal aortic dissections) of fluctuating intensity depending on the BP.
- Neurological focal signs: persistent or transient ischemic stroke (~5%), ischemic neuropathy (limb pain with sensory or motor deficit), etc., from hypotension, cerebral malperfusion, distal thromboembolism, or nerve compression.

Warning! In cases of suspected aortic dissection, BP should be measured in both arms, all peripheral arteries should be palpated and a gross neurological assessment should be performed.

Diagnostic tests

1) **Blood tests:** complete blood count, urea, creatinine, myocardial necrosis markers (preferably cardiac troponin I or T), D-dimers, blood typing

and cross-matching. Elevated levels of D-dimers (>500 ng/mL) are high-ly sensitive (>90%) for the diagnosis of acute aortic dissection, whereas low levels (<500 ng/mL) almost exclude the diagnosis, especially in pa-tients with low risk for the condition. However, because of the devastat-ing consequences of misdiagnosing this condition, **a low D-dimer level should in no case be the only examination excluding aortic dissec-tion.**

Warning! Normal D-dimer levels have been reported in aortic dissection with thrombosed false lumen and in cases of aortic IMH or PAU.

2) **ECG:** nonspecific findings. This is most useful for excluding the possi-bility of acute myocardial ischemia in patients presenting with acute chest pain. Thirty percent of cases will have left ventricular hypertrophy, while rarely (1-5% of cases) there may be a picture of inferior AMI caused by the dissection extending up to the origin of the right coro-nary artery.
3) **Chest X-ray:** this test can only raise suspicions, but not confirm the diag-nosis of aortic dissection. It is normal in ~10% of cases, or it may show:
   ● Widened mediastinum (~85%).
   ● In cases of calcified intima in the aortic arch, the "calcium sign" may be observed: there will be a distance of >10 mm between the external border of the aortic arch and the (calcified) intima.
   ● Left-side pleural effusion (~20%) [may be reactive, not indicating rup-ture of the aorta].
4) **Echocardiogram:** a transthoracic echo is useful for assessing aortic in-sufficiency and the presence of pericardial fluid, but has low sensitivity (~70%) in diagnosing acute aortic dissection. TEE is highly sensitive (~98%) and specific (~95%) for diagnosing a dissection, and has the added important advantage that it can be performed at the patient's bedside within 10-15 min. It is preferable to a CT scan in hemodynami-cally unstable patients. The study needs to be conducted after the pa-tient is sedated, in order to reduce the risk of a BP spike from the pa-tient's distressed reaction to the test. Usually, midazolam [Dormicum] (a short-acting benzodiazepine) is given at a dose of 2-5 mg IV. After the study, flumazenil is administered at a dose of 0.2-1 mg IV to reverse the effect of midazolam. A TEE can image:
   ● The detached part of the aortic wall (intimal flap). It appears as a linear mobile structure and should be differentiated from linear artifacts usu-ally due to reverberations.

Warning! Features that favor the diagnosis of intimal flap are: motion independent of the surrounding structures i.e. aortic wall (not parallel), never extends beyond the aortic wall and there is different color Doppler flow on either side of the flap.

- The site of blood entry (entry point) into the false lumen and the site of blood exit (exit point) from the false into the true lumen.
- The false and the true lumen (the false is usually larger and the blood flows more slowly through it while the smaller true lumen shows systolic expansion).
- Any involvement of the origins of the coronary arteries.

A TEE cannot image the distal ascending aorta and the proximal segment of the aortic arch because of the interposition of the trachea and left bronchus (blind spot).

5) **Contrast-enhanced CT:** a helical (spiral) CT scan can produce a three-dimensional reconstruction of the aorta and its branches, and has sensitivity and specificity of ~98%. It is the most commonly used test in cases of suspected aortic dissection, with TEE being the second most common.

6) **MRI:** has a sensitivity and specificity of nearly 100% in diagnosing an acute aortic dissection, and does not involve administering contrast medium or exposing the patient to ionizing radiation. However, it is time-consuming and only available in a few institutions, and therefore it has no place as a diagnostic test in the emergency diagnosis of acute aortic dissection. It is however the test of first choice for monitoring patients with chronic aortic dissection. It is contraindicated for patients with a pacemaker, implantable cardioverter defibrillator or older-generation mechanical heart valves.

7) **Aortography:** rarely used today because of the availability of alternative diagnostic tests.

What is the role of preoperative coronary angiography?

Usually, the patient is transferred to the operating room without undergoing coronary angiography to reveal any concurrent coronary artery disease (which is present in ~25% of patients), because of the delay this involves and the associated increase in mortality.

Treatment

1) A peripheral venous line is placed (blood sampling for laboratory testing and IV drug administration).

2) Pain suppression with IV **morphine**. Four to 8 mg are administered by slow intravenous infusion and 2 mg are readministered after an interval

of 5-15 min depending on the intensity of the pain. An antiemetic is also administered (10 mg of metoclopramide IV).

3) The patient is transferred to an intensive monitoring unit until the surgical team takes over, if there is an indication for surgical treatment.

4) BP monitoring by arterial route and hourly urine measurement.

5) Immediate therapeutic measures:

- Reduce the myocardial contraction intensity and hence the rate of BP increase (dP/dt) in order to limit the extension of the dissection. This is achieved by IV administration of short-acting beta-blockers. The target is to maintain a systolic BP between 100-120 mmHg and a heart rate ≤60 beats/min. It should be noted that beta-blockers are also administered in cases of "normal" BP. There is a preference nowadays (especially in hemodynamically unstable patients) for the ultra-short-acting cardioselective beta1-blocker esmolol. **Esmolol** (Brevibloc) is given at a loading dose of 0.5 mg/kg over 1 min, followed by continuous infusion of a maintenance dose of 50 µg/kg/min over 4 min. If the desired result is still not achieved, the loading dose is repeated and the maintenance dose is increased to 100 µg/kg/min for another 4 min. If the desired result is still not achieved, the same titration procedure is repeated up to 4 times (maximum maintenance dose 300 µg/kg/min). A ready-made esmolol solution is available for continuous IV administration, in a 100 or 250 mL bag of 0.9% NaCl. Alternatively, the noncardioselective beta-blocker **propranolol** (Inderal) can be administered at a dose of 1 mg IV every 5 min (the maximum initial dosage is 10 mg). For maintenance, 4 mg IV are administered every 4-6 h. A reduction in dP/dt and in BP can also be achieved with administration of **labetalol** (Trandate), which has the combined effects of an alpha- and a beta-blocker. Labetalol may be given as repeated IV injections, i.e. 20 mg IV over 2 min and then at a dose of 40-80 mg every 15 min until the desired response is achieved. Alternatively, it may be administered by continuous IV infusion at an initial rate of 1-2 mg/min (titrated up to 10 mg/min if required). Note that with both methods of administration the maximum cumulative or daily dose is 300 mg. In case of a contraindication for beta-blockers (e.g. bronchospasm, signs of heart failure, etc.), IV **diltiazem** or **verapamil** is administered. Diltiazem (Cardizem) is administered at a dose of 0.25 mg/kg (usually 15-20 mg) over 2 min, followed by a continuous infusion of 5-15 mg/h. For continuous infusion, 100 mg of diltiazem are dissolved in 250 mL of 5% D/W and administered at a rate between 12-37 mL/h.
- In cases of elevated BP, the target is a systolic BP between 100-120 mmHg. If this is not achieved with beta-blockers, **nitroprusside** is given at an initial dose of 0.25 µg/kg/min, which is gradually increased depending on the response (maximum dose 10 µg/kg/min) [see Chapter 23]. Alternatively, **nicardipine, nitroglycerin** or **fenoldopam** IV can be used.

Warning! Vasodilators always follow the administration of beta-blockers provided that a systolic BP <120 mmHg has not been achieved. Vasodilator therapy without prior beta blockade may cause reflex tachycardia and an increased force of ventricular contraction (dP/dt), leading to greater aortic wall stress and potentially causing extension of the aortic dissection.

- In cases of refractory hypertension, it is necessary to exclude the possibility of ischemia in one or both kidneys due to an extension of the dissection up to the renal arteries (overproduction of renin). In this case, the antihypertensive of first choice is **enalaprilat** IV (Vasotec). It is administered initially at a dose of 0.625-1.25 mg IV/6 h, and thereafter the dose might need to be increased up to 5 mg/6 h.
- If the BP is decreased (poor prognostic sign), then large fluid volumes are administered IV while waiting for emergency surgery and, if a vasopressor is required, then **noradrenaline** (Levophed) is used because it does not increase the dP/dt. Adrenaline and dopamine should be avoided.
- If cardiac tamponade is present (rupture of the aorta into the pericardial space):
  - in relatively stable patients pericardiocentesis must be avoided (contraindicated) because it will lead to exsanguination; surgical treatment should be expedited.
  - in unstable patients who will not survive until surgery, controlled pericardiocentesis with aspiration of only enough fluid (usually 20-40 mL) to temporarily stabilize the patient before surgery may be attempted.
- Emergency surgical treatment or TEVAR. The indications are listed in Table 8.3.

TABLE 8.3	**Indications for emergency surgical treatment or thoracic endovascular aortic repair (TEVAR) of acute aortic dissection** *(Erbel R, et al. Eur Heart J 2014;35:2873-926)*

a) Acute type A aortic dissection (surgical treatment)

b) Complicated acute type B aortic dissection (TEVAR is preferred in most cases), i.e. associated with:
  - Signs of rupture (hemothorax, increasing periaortic and mediastinal hematoma)
  - Malperfusion syndrome i.e. visceral ischemia
  - Early aortic expansion
  - Persistent or recurrent pain
  - Retrograde extension of dissection to the ascending aorta
  - Uncontrolled hypertension despite full medication

Key points

■ Acute aortic dissection is a relatively rare condition associated with very high mortality.

■ In cases of acute aortic dissection (proximal or type A), mortality increases dramatically over time and therefore surgery should be performed as soon as possible. Surgical treatment should not be postponed to allow time for coronary angiography.

■ In elderly hypertensive patients or patients with a known aneurysm of the thoracic aorta or with features of Marfan syndrome who develop intense sudden chest and/or interscapular pain with a nonischemic ECG, acute aortic dissection should be suspected until proven otherwise.

■ If acute aortic dissection is suspected, measure BP in both arms, palpate all peripheral arteries and perform a gross neurological examination.

■ In patients with risk factors for aortic dissection and an ECG picture of inferior AMI, consider the possibility of aortic dissection before the administration of antithrombotics or fibrinolysis.

■ True hypotension is an ominous sign, usually from acute aortic insufficiency, cardiac tamponade or aortic wall rupture (intrapleural or intraperitoneal) and requires immediate operation. In the meantime aggressive volume replacement should be initiated and noradrenaline is the preferred vasopressor.

■ While waiting for surgery, the patient should be given analgesics, betablockers (to maintain the heart rate at ≤60 beats/min), and nitroprusside if the systolic BP is >120 mmHg.

■ The diagnosis of acute aortic dissection can be established with a TEE or contrast CT, which have approximately equal levels of sensitivity and specificity. TEE should be preferred in hemodynamically unstable patients.

■ A normal chest X-ray or normal transthoracic echocardiogram does not rule out acute aortic dissection.

■ Around 15-20% of patients who present in the Emergency Room with a clinical picture of acute aortic dissection have aortic IMH, or more rarely PAU, conditions "invisible" to transthoracic echocardiography (absence of intimal flap). In addition, these conditions have fewer clinical signs, i.e. usually lack of pulse deficit, etc., than classical aortic dissection due to their more localized distribution.

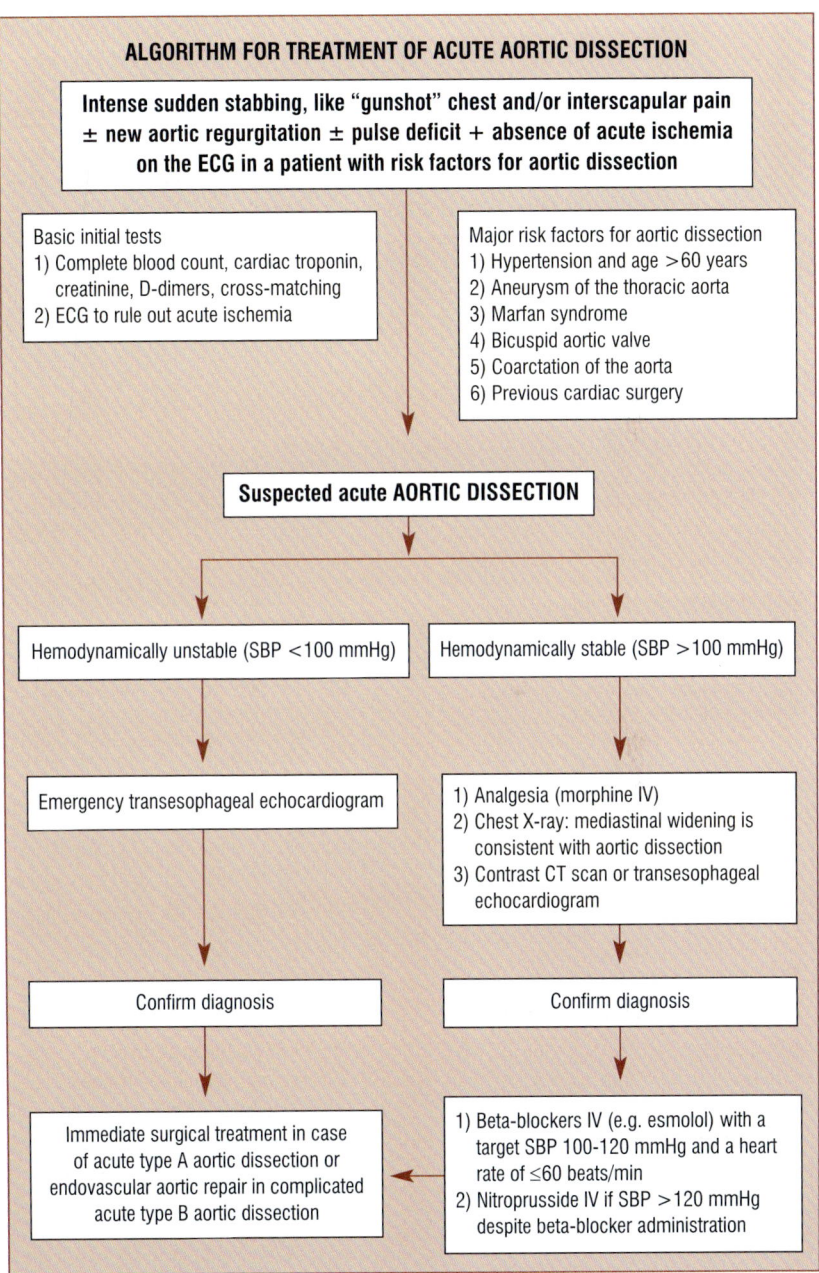

ALGORITHM FOR TREATMENT OF ACUTE AORTIC DISSECTION

Intense sudden stabbing, like "gunshot" chest and/or interscapular pain ± new aortic regurgitation ± pulse deficit + absence of acute ischemia on the ECG in a patient with risk factors for aortic dissection

Basic initial tests
1) Complete blood count, cardiac troponin, creatinine, D-dimers, cross-matching
2) ECG to rule out acute ischemia

Major risk factors for aortic dissection
1) Hypertension and age >60 years
2) Aneurysm of the thoracic aorta
3) Marfan syndrome
4) Bicuspid aortic valve
5) Coarctation of the aorta
6) Previous cardiac surgery

Suspected acute AORTIC DISSECTION

Hemodynamically unstable (SBP <100 mmHg)

Hemodynamically stable (SBP >100 mmHg)

Emergency transesophageal echocardiogram

1) Analgesia (morphine IV)
2) Chest X-ray: mediastinal widening is consistent with aortic dissection
3) Contrast CT scan or transesophageal echocardiogram

Confirm diagnosis

Confirm diagnosis

Immediate surgical treatment in case of acute type A aortic dissection or endovascular aortic repair in complicated acute type B aortic dissection

1) Beta-blockers IV (e.g. esmolol) with a target SBP 100-120 mmHg and a heart rate of ≤60 beats/min
2) Nitroprusside IV if SBP >120 mmHg despite beta-blocker administration

SBP: systolic blood pressure, CT: computed tomography

9   *Syncope*

Syncope is a sudden, brief and transient loss of consciousness with simultaneous loss of postural muscle tone due to global cerebral hypoperfusion. It is characterized by rapid and complete spontaneous recovery. It is usually triggered by an abrupt fall in systolic blood pressure (BP) to ≤60 mmHg, which interrupts the blood flow to the brain for ≥6-8 s. The term **presyncope** refers to a condition characterized by relatively nonspecific and always self-limiting symptoms, similar to those appearing in the prodromal phase of syncope, such as dizziness, lightheadedness, weakness, blurred vision, sweating and nausea. The main differentiating characteristic of presyncope is that it does not cause loss of consciousness.

Syncope accounts for ~3% of all visits to an Emergency Room. It may be the cause of injury or accident, and in some cases it is a harbinger of sudden death. It is recurrent in one third of all cases. The prognosis depends on the cause; when the etiology is cardiac, the annual mortality is up to 30%.

Table 9.1 lists the major causes of syncope or conditions that resemble syncope but do not meet its definition. These conditions include situations with loss of consciousness but absence of generalized cerebral hypoperfusion (e.g. epilepsy, metabolic causes, transient cerebrovascular accidents due to ischemia of the vertebrobasilar system) or situations with no true loss of consciousness (e.g. psychiatric causes). With regard to metabolic causes, hypoglycemia usually presents with confusion and/or weakness, and very rarely as syncope. Lastly, transient cerebrovascular accidents originating from the carotid arteries do not cause syncope.

When diagnosing the cause of syncope, particular importance should be given to the history, the clinical examination and the ECG; these allow a diagnosis to be made in 40-50% of cases.

TABLE 9.1	Major causes of syncope or syncope-like conditions

A) Syncope
  1) Cardiovascular (10-20% of syncopal episodes)
   a) Anatomical
     a1) Severe aortic valve stenosis
     a2) Hypertrophic cardiomyopathy
     a3) Acute myocardial infarction (usually inferior wall) / myocardial ischemia
     a4) Mitral valve stenosis
     a5) Atrial myxoma (usually in left atrium)
     a6) Acute pulmonary embolism / pulmonary hypertension
     a7) Cardiac tamponade
     a8) Acute aortic dissection
   b) Arrhythmological
     b1) Bradyarrhythmias
       • Sick sinus syndrome (marked sinus bradycardia, pauses, sinoatrial block)
       • Second or third degree atrioventricular block (i.e. Stokes-Adams attacks)
       • Pacemaker or implantable cardioverter defibrillator malfunction
     b2) Tachyarrhythmias
       • Ventricular tachycardia (monomorphic or polymorphic)
       • Supraventricular tachycardia (rare cause of syncope)
  2) Reflex (neurally-mediated) syncope
   a) Vasovagal or common faint (~35% of cases)
   b) Carotid sinus syndrome
   c) Situational (during or immediately after coughing, defecation, micturition, laughing, etc.)
  3) Syncope due to orthostatic hypotension (10-15% of syncopal episodes)
   a) Primary autonomic failure (Parkinson's disease, pure autonomic failure, etc.)
   b) Secondary autonomic failure (diabetes mellitus, amyloidosis, etc.)
   c) Drug-induced (antihypertensives, tricyclic antidepressants, etc.)
   d) Volume depletion (bleeding, diarrhea, vomiting, etc.)

B) Syncope-like conditions
  1) Neurological causes (epilepsy, migraine, transient cerebrovascular episodes due to vertebrobasilar ischemia)
  2) Subclavian steal syndrome
  3) Metabolic causes (hypoglycemia, hypoxia, hyperventilation with hypocapnia)
  4) Psychiatric causes (panic attacks, hysteria)

C) Syncope of unknown etiology (20-30% of cases)

TABLE 9.2	Features from the clinical history suggesting specific causes of syncope
Clinical history	**Causes of syncope**
Syncope after strong fear, intense pain, unpleasant sight, emotional stress or prolonged standing. Preceded by a brief prodromal period	Vasovagal syncope or common faint
Syncope during or immediately after coughing, defecation, micturition, laughing, sneezing or within 30-60 min after meals	Situational syncope
Syncope when turning the head or applying pressure to the carotid sinus (e.g. shaving)	Carotid sinus syndrome
Syncope associated with vertigo, dysarthria or diplopia	Ischemia of the vertebrobasilar system
Syncope within a few seconds or minutes of standing up	Orthostatic hypotension
Syncope on intense exercise of the arm	Subclavian steal syndrome
Syncope during exercise	Severe aortic valve stenosis, hypertrophic cardiomyopathy or myocardial ischemia
Syncope immediately after exercise	Neurally-mediated syncope
Palpitations immediately prior to syncope	Arrhythmological cause
Syncope when changing body position (e.g. from seated to supine, bending over, etc.)	Atrial myxoma
Sudden loss of consciousness (lasting usually >3 min) with tonic-clonic seizures, cyanosis, urinary incontinence (usually), confusion and drowsiness after recovery	Epilepsy (tonic-clonic or grand mal seizures)

History (Table 9.2)

- **Vasovagal syncope or common faint:** this is the most frequent cause of syncope (~35% of all cases). It is most commonly observed in young women and it is triggered by intense fear, strong pain, a warm environment, an unpleasant sight (e.g. blood), emotional stress or prolonged standing. It never occurs in reclining individuals. It is characterized by gradual onset and gradual offset. The duration is usually <20 s. It is almost always preceded by a precursor (prodromal) period of a few seconds or minutes, which may include weakness, nausea, epigastric discomfort, sweating or vision disturbances. Pallor (but never cyanosis) and usually bradycardia occur during the faint.

The common faint is caused by "inappropriate" and excessive stimulation of the parasympathetic system after an initial stimulation and subsequent withdrawal of the sympathetic system. Specifically, people susceptible to this type of syncope after certain stimuli or in certain situations, such as prolonged standing that causes blood to pool in the lower limbs and reduces its return to the heart, initially present the expected compensatory sympathetic stimulation aimed at maintaining a normal BP. However, this initial sympathetic activation, through vigorous contraction of the volume-depleted ventricles and activation of mechanoreceptors located in the inferior and posterior wall of the left ventricle, inappropriately triggers the Bezold–Jarisch parasympathetic reflex. This reflex is responsible for causing peripheral vasodilation and bradycardia, which lead to loss of consciousness.

- **Syncope by orthostatic hypotension:** syncope within a few seconds or minutes after standing up. This can also occur after prolonged standing and thus raises the issue of differential diagnosis from vasovagal syncope. It is most commonly observed in elderly people, and is extremely rare in persons younger than 40 years. Its causes may include:
  a) Autonomic failure:
    – Primary: Parkinson's disease, pure autonomic failure, etc.
    – Secondary: diabetic neuropathy, amyloidosis, etc.
  b) Drugs: antihypertensives, tricyclic antidepressants, alpha-blockers for prostatic hyperplasia, etc., including alcohol consumption.
  c) Volume depletion: bleeding, diarrhea, vomiting, etc.
  Therefore, it is important to look for "suspect" drugs and to rule out bleeding or dehydration when taking the patient's history.
- **Carotid sinus syndrome:** syncope when turning the head or otherwise applying pressure on the carotid sinus (e.g. tight collar, shaving, etc.), which causes parasympathetic stimulation.
- **Situational syncope:** occurs during or immediately after coughing, defecation, micturition, laughing, sneezing, etc. It can also occur within 30-60 min after meals (postprandial syncope) or immediately after exercise (postexercise).
- **Stokes–Adams attacks:** these are episodes of syncope observed in elderly people. They are usually caused by transient ventricular asystole due to a delay in establishing a ventricular escape rhythm following complete atrioventricular (AV) block. These episodes are sudden, unexpected, often recurrent, without warning signs, and they occur regardless of body position (even supine). A patient who is standing will fall quickly to the ground (injuries are frequent), become pulseless and pallid, and when cardiac function resumes (usually within 15-30 s), they will recover quickly without neurological symptoms. The quick return of facial color is characteristic.

- **Epilepsy (tonic-clonic or grand mal seizures):** sudden loss of consciousness (lasting usually >3 min) accompanied by generalized tonic-clonic seizures (tonic phase lasting <1 min/clonic phase usually ~1-3 min) and cyanosis. During seizures urinary incontinence (not pathognomonic since it can rarely be observed in syncope), and tongue-biting (if lateral, it is highly specific) may occur. The clonic phase of the seizures is characterized by coarse and rhythmic contractions. After recovering, the patient is confused, somnolent and without memory of the incident (postictal state). The epileptic seizure may be preceded by an aura (perception of unusual unpleasant smell, visual or auditory hallucinations, etc.). Loss of consciousness is characterized by abrupt onset and gradual offset.

Warning! Brief (<15 s) clonic movements (myoclonic jerks) of the limbs (usually small and arrhythmic) may occur in cases of prolonged syncope. It should, however, be noted that the seizures in this case occur a few seconds (usually >15 s) after syncope and not concurrently with the loss of consciousness, as in the case of epilepsy.

- **Vertebrobasilar system ischemia:** in rare cases this can manifest with syncope, which may be associated with vertigo, dysarthria or diplopia. Most commonly, however, it manifests with a sudden fall to the ground (drop attacks), without associated loss of consciousness but with a sudden loss of muscle tone in the lower limbs. Ischemia of the vertebrobasilar system is also caused by the subclavian steal syndrome, which is due to proximal to the origin of the vertebral artery significant stenosis or obstruction of the subclavian artery (usually on the left). During exercise of the ipsilateral arm, the vertebrobasilar system becomes ischemic, because of blood being "stolen" (reversed flow to the arm) through the vertebral artery originating distally to the lesion of the subclavian artery.
- **Syncope due to tachyarrhythmia:** preceded by palpitations.
- **Aortic valve stenosis, hypertrophic cardiomyopathy or myocardial ischemia:** syncope usually occurs during exercise, due to reduced cardiac output (impeded ejection in the case of aortic valve stenosis or hypertrophic obstructive cardiomyopathy or ischemia with subsequent left ventricular dysfunction) in combination with reduced systemic resistance. May also be caused by tachyarrhythmias.

Warning! Syncope during exercise should raise serious concern about cardiac disease, while syncope immediately after exercise is most commonly neurally-mediated and therefore benign.

- **Subclavian steal syndrome:** syncope (rarely) occurs during exercise of the arm ipsilateral to the affected subclavian artery.

Clinical examination

- Systolic murmur on auscultation in the aortic valve region: consider aortic valve stenosis.
- Left parasternal systolic murmur: consider hypertrophic obstructive cardiomyopathy (arrhythmogenic background).
- 3rd heart sound in individuals >30 years old: consider dilated cardiomyopathy (arrhythmogenic substrate).
- Carotid sinus hypersensitivity: gentle carotid sinus massage for 5 s is consistent with carotid sinus hypersensitivity if it causes a ventricular pause of >3 s (cardioinhibitory response in ~70% of cases), a fall in systolic BP by >50 mmHg (vasodepressive response in ~20% of cases) or both (mixed response). Carotid sinus syndrome is defined as a pathological response to carotid sinus massage associated with reproduction of spontaneous symptoms. Massaging of the carotid sinus must be avoided if a bruit is heard over the carotid arteries (unless a Doppler study excludes significant stenosis) or if there is a history of cerebrovascular accident within the last three months. It is performed under continuous ECG monitoring and periodic measurement of BP with the patient supine. If no abnormal response is elicited, it should be repeated with the patient sitting upright, since 30% of patients show a pathological response only in the upright position. Carotid sinus syndrome is exceptional in patients <40 years old while a positive response to carotid sinus massage is relatively common, even in asymptomatic, elderly patients.

Warning! A positive response to carotid sinus massage is considered diagnostic of the causes of syncope if it reproduces the symptoms and after excluding other potential causes of syncope.

- Orthostatic hypotension: a fall of ≥20 mmHg in systolic BP or ≥10 mmHg in diastolic BP compared to baseline, or a decrease in systolic BP to <90 mmHg within 3 min (measured at 1 and 3 min) of standing up after 5 min in a supine position, regardless of symptoms.
- Bruit in the subclavian region, a difference in systolic BP of >20 mmHg (usually >40 mmHg) between the arms, and weakened pulse in the ipsilateral arm: consider subclavian steal syndrome.

Diagnostic investigation

1) Blood tests

Depend on the clinical suspicion:

- If the patient is pale: complete blood count
- If electrolyte disturbances are possible: creatinine, Na, K, Mg
- If acute pulmonary embolism or acute aortic dissection is suspected: D-dimers.

2) ECG

May show:

- Signs of acute myocardial ischemia. In 5-10% of cases, an inferior acute myocardial infarction manifests with syncope caused by parasympathetic stimulation (Bezold–Jarisch reflex).
- Signs of a previous myocardial infarction, i.e. abnormal Q waves (arrhythmogenic substrate).
- Sustained or nonsustained ventricular tachycardia.
- Long QT interval (>500 ms). Since this interval depends on the heart rate, it is preferable to calculate the corrected QT interval (QTc) using Bazett's formula.* The QTc is considered prolonged if >440 ms in men and >460 ms in women. The prolongation may be due to medications, electrolyte disturbances, etc., or may be congenital, in which case it is called long-QT syndrome (LQTS). The prevalence of the syndrome is 1:2000. More than 12 related mutations have been identified, of which 3, which are responsible for LQT_1, LQT_2, and LQT_3, make up ~80% of cases. The probability that somebody suffers from LQTS is high when they have a prolonged QT (especially QTc >460 ms) + a history of syncope or polymorphic ventricular tachycardia (torsades de pointes), or a family member with definite LQTS. The recent European Guidelines (Priori SG, et al. Eur Heart J 2015;36:2793-867) set the threshold for the diagnosis of LQTS as a QTc ≥480 ms in repeated ECGs. A QTc >500 ms poses a high risk for cardiac events. Episodes of syncope are caused by self-terminating episodes of torsades de pointes.
- Short QT interval (QTc <330 ms). May be acquired (hyperkalemia, hypercalcemia or acidosis) or may very rarely be due to a hereditary disorder (short-QT syndrome). This syndrome may be manifested by episodes of atrial fibrillation, syncope, or cardiac arrest.

---

*Corrected QT interval $= QTc = \dfrac{QT_{max}\ (ms)}{\sqrt{R\text{-}R\ (s)}}$

Warning! In syncopal episodes the QTc should always be measured. Unfortunately, the majority of physicians overlook the QT-interval pathology while reading the ECG.

- Delta wave + short PR interval (<120 ms) + wide QRS complex (>120 ms) + ST-segment/T wave changes (directed opposite to the major delta wave and QRS complex), indicative of Wolff–Parkinson–White (WPW) syndrome. Syncope may occur due to the development of supraventricular tachycardia with a very rapid ventricular response due to stimuli descending via an accessory pathway (regular tachycardia with wide QRS complexes) or due to development of atrial fibrillation with rapid ventricular response.
- AV conduction disturbances:
  - AV block: Mobitz type II or 3rd degree AV block
  - bifascicular block:
    left bundle branch block (LBBB)
    right bundle branch block (RBBB) + left anterior hemiblock or
    RBBB + left posterior hemiblock
  - trifascicular block: bifascicular block + prolonged PR interval.
- Other intraventricular conduction abnormalities (QRS duration ≥120 ms).
- Sinus bradycardia (<50 beats/min) or sinus pauses (typically >3 s).
- Ventricular extrasystoles: frequent, multifocal, couplets, R-on-T phenomenon (arrhythmogenic substrate).
- Negative T waves in leads V_1–V_3 (in those aged >14 years and in the absence of complete RBBB) + epsilon wave (notching in the terminal segment of the QRS complex) in leads V_1–V_3 + prolonged QRS complex (>110 ms) in leads V_1–V_3, indicative of arrhythmogenic right ventricular cardiomyopathy (Figure 9.1). In addition, ventricular tachycardia with LBBB morphology should raise suspicion for this condition.
- ST-segment elevation in at least two right precordial leads (V_1–V_3) ± negative T waves indicative of Brugada syndrome (arrhythmogenic substrate). This is a rare hereditary disorder (1:5000) of the heart's electrical system that may be manifested as a syncopal episode (self-terminating polymorphic ventricular tachycardia) or sudden death (at rest or during sleep). There are three types of ECG changes:
  - type 1 (diagnostic of Brugada syndrome): a coved ST-segment elevation ≥2 mm in more than one right precordial lead (V_1-V_3) followed by negative T waves (Figure 9.2). The recent European Guidelines

(Priori SG, at al. Eur Heart J 2015;36:2793-867) suggest that the diagnosis of Brugada syndrome can be made even if ST-segment elevation with type 1 morphology is present in leads V_1 and/or V_2.

- type 2 (suggestive of Brugada syndrome): ST-segment elevation ≥2 mm in more than one precordial lead (V_1-V_3) followed by positive or biphasic T waves, resulting in a saddleback appearance, and

- type 3 (suggestive of Brugada syndrome): defined as any of the 2 previous types if ST-segment elevation is ≤1 mm.

Note that the ECG is dynamic and patients with Brugada syndrome may have a normal ECG. In addition, the 3 aforementioned patterns may coexist in the same patient at different times. If there is suspicion of Brugada syndrome and the ECG is not diagnostic, the administration of sodium channel inhibitors (procainamide, flecainide, or ajmaline) can unmask the typical diagnostic ECG.

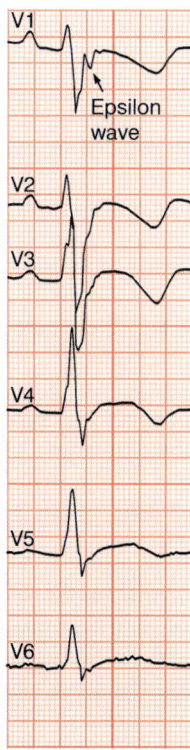

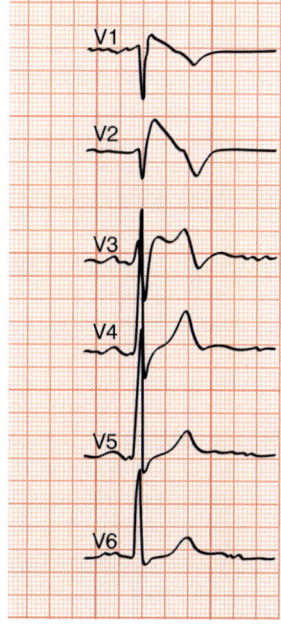

◄ **Figure 9.1.** ECG of a patient with arrhythmogenic right ventricular cardiomyopathy, showing negative T waves in leads V_1–V_4, epsilon wave in lead V_1, and a widened QRS complex >110 ms. Recording speed 50 mm/s, sensitivity 20 mm/mV.

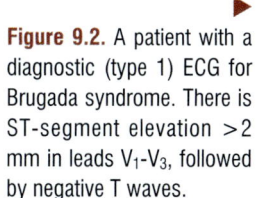

► **Figure 9.2.** A patient with a diagnostic (type 1) ECG for Brugada syndrome. There is ST-segment elevation >2 mm in leads V_1-V_3, followed by negative T waves.

Warning! When the diagnosis of Brugada syndrome is suspected but the standard ECG is uncertain, repeat the ECG with placement of leads V_1 and V_2 in the 2nd or 3rd intercostal space (instead of the 4th, where they are normally placed). This may bring out the typical Brugada ECG pattern.

3) Echocardiogram

Although this examination contributes little when the clinical examination and the ECG are normal, there is a tendency to perform it routinely when investigating syncope. The only exception is the investigation of syncopal episodes in young persons (<30 years old) with features of common faint, in which the clinical examination and ECG are normal. An echocardiogram can:

- Assess left ventricular function (important in risk stratification):
  - in ischemic cardiomyopathy it usually shows segmental disturbances of left ventricular systolic wall thickening
  - in dilated cardiomyopathy it usually shows diffuse wall hypokinesia of left ± right ventricle.
- Assess right ventricular function:
  - in arrhythmogenic right ventricular cardiomyopathy it will show ventricular dilation and regional akinetic or aneurysmal regions in the wall of right ventricle
  - in pulmonary embolism may show dilation ± right ventricular impairment, etc.
- Diagnose valvular diseases, such as aortic valve stenosis.
- Diagnose hypertrophic cardiomyopathy.
- Rule out a myxoma in the cardiac cavities (usually in the left atrium), etc.

4) 24-48-h ECG recording (Holter monitoring)

The diagnostic yield of Holter monitoring in unselected patients with syncope is low (<5%). It is more useful in patients with frequent episodes of syncope or presyncope or in whom there is high suspicion of an arrhythmic cause.

5) Tilt testing

Useful in the diagnosis of reflex syncope (sensitivity 60-70%, specificity ~90%). For this test, the patient is strapped to a special bed (tilt table) and placed at an angle of 60-70° for 30-45 min (isoproterenol IV or nitroglycerin sublingually may also be administered to increase the sensitivity of the test). The test examines whether the patient will become symptomatic (onset of syncope) because of bradycardia (cardioinhibitory response) or hypotension (vasodepressive response) or a combination of the two (mixed response). It should be emphasized that a negative tilt testing response does not exclude the diagnosis of reflex syncope.

The tilt testing is primarily indicated for:

- Unexplained single syncope associated with injury or in people whose occupation places their own or others' lives at risk (aircraft pilots, etc.).
- Recurrent episodes of syncope in the absence of organic heart disease, or if there is organic heart disease but cardiac causes have been excluded.

6) Carotid sinus massage

Indicated for patients >40 years old who present episodes of syncope with negative initial investigation, or patients presenting syncope when pressure is applied to the area of the carotid sinus, e.g. when turning their head, shaving, etc. Note that ~10% of elderly people in the general population show a positive response to carotid sinus massage, so a positive test result should always be interpreted based on the patient's history.

7) Exercise stress testing

This is considered necessary when active myocardial ischemia is suspected to be the cause of syncope. In addition, exercise stress testing is indicated for those presenting syncope during or shortly after exercise (provided there is no severe valvular disease).

8) Electrophysiological study

If an arrhythmic cause for the syncope is suspected and other tests have failed to make the diagnosis, then an electrophysiological study should be considered, primarily:

- In order to induce monomorphic ventricular tachycardia, which is diagnostic for syncope causes in patients with previous myocardial infarction or to induce rapid symptomatic supraventricular tachycardia.
- In order to study AV conduction by measuring the HV interval. An HV interval ≥100 ms in a patient with bundle branch block is consistent with syncope due to a disturbance of AV conduction. Additionally, development of AV block (2nd or 3rd degree) in patients with bundle branch block during atrial pacing or by pharmaceutical challenge is indicative of increased future risk for developing AV block.
- In order to measure the corrected sinus node recovery time (CSNRT). A sinus bradycardia and a prolonged CSNRT (>525 ms) are consistent with syncope due to sinus node dysfunction.

9) Implantable continuous ECG recording devices (implantable loop recorders)

These devices are implanted subcutaneously under local anesthesia and their battery lasts up to 36 months. Their placement is recommended primarily:

- For the investigation of patients with recurrent syncope of unknown etiology, who do not have the characteristics of high-risk patients (Table 9.3), and have a high likelihood of syncope recurrence while the device is in place.
- For high-risk patients in whom other investigations have not revealed the cause of syncope.

Finally, Table 9.3 presents the characteristics of high-risk syncope patients who should be admitted to a hospital for diagnostic investigation and treatment and Table 9.4 the clinical features that suggest cardiovascular syncope in patients evaluated in the Emergency Department.

TABLE 9.3	**Characteristics of high-risk patients who should be admitted for diagnostic investigation and treatment of syncope** *(modified from the European Guidelines for the Diagnosis and Management of Syncope. Moya A, et al. Eur Heart J 2009;30:2631-71)*

1) Clinical characteristics
  - Known or suspected underlying severe cardiac disease
  - Palpitations immediately prior to syncope
  - Syncope during exercise or in supine position
  - Syncope causing severe injury
  - Family history of sudden cardiac death
  - Presence of neurological signs
  - Presence of severe anemia or electrolyte disorders
2) ECG findings
  - Sustained or nonsustained ventricular tachycardia
  - Signs of acute myocardial ischemia or previous myocardial infarction
  - Bifascicular or trifascicular block or other intraventricular conduction abnormalities (QRS ≥120 ms)
  - Delta wave + short PR interval + wide QRS complex + ST-segment repolarization disorders (WPW syndrome)
  - Negative T waves + epsilon wave + wide QRS complex (>110 ms) in leads V_1–V_3 (arrhythmogenic right ventricular cardiomyopathy)
  - ST-segment elevation in at least two right precordial leads (V_1-V_3) ± negative T waves (indicative of Brugada syndrome)
  - Prolonged or short QT interval
  - Second or third degree atrioventricular block
  - Sinus bradycardia (<50 beats/min) or sinus pause ≥3 s without the use of bradycardic drugs or physical training

Treatment
- **Vasovagal syncope:**
  - *Nonpharmacological treatment:* is the first line treatment. This includes reassurance to the patient that the condition is benign, instructions to avoid possible triggering factors (e.g. dehydration, hot environment, prolonged standing) and education for early recognition of prodromal symptoms and performing maneuvers to abort syncope i.e. leg crossing combined with tensing of muscles may prevent syncope by increasing venous return. If dizziness or fainting occurs, the patient should be placed in a horizontal position with the lower limbs elevated.
  - *Pharmacological treatment:* if lifestyle measures fail, midodrine may be considered (class IIb recommendation, Moya A, et al. Eur Heart J 2009;30:2631-71). Midodrine (Gutron) stimulates α_1-receptors and is a strong vasoconstrictor of both arteries and veins. It is given in dose of 5 mg x 3/day.

  Other drugs that have been used for the treatment of vasovagal syncope, such as beta-blockers, fludrocortisone and selective serotonin reuptake inhibitors, failed to show effectiveness in clinical trials and their use cannot be recommended.
  - *Cardiac pacing:* dual-chamber pacing may play a role in selected cases. It should be considered in patients with frequent recurrent vasovagal syncope, age >40 years and documented spontaneous bradycardia or asystole during monitoring.
- **Orthostatic hypotension:**
  - *Nonpharmacological treatment:* avoidance of triggering factors (e.g. reduce or discontinue antihypertensive medication), patient education (the patient should stand up from a reclining position slowly and after remaining seated for a while) and increased fluid intake (2-3 L/day) and salt (10 g/day).

TABLE 9.4	Features that suggest cardiovascular syncope in patients evaluated in the Emergency Department

1) Known severe cardiac disease
2) Sudden onset of palpitations immediately followed by syncope
3) Syncope during exercise or in supine position
4) Family history of sudden death or channelopathy
5) Auscultatory findings suggestive of heart disease i.e. murmur of severe aortic stenosis
6) Abnormal ECG (see Table 9.3)

– **Pharmacological treatment:** if nonpharmaceutical measures fail, the following may be administered:

- **Midodrine** (Gutron, tablets of 2.5, 5 and 10 mg): 2.5-20 mg x 3 daily (class IIa recommendation, Moya A, et al. Eur Heart J 2009;30:2631-71). Midodrine has a short duration of action (2-3 h). Its major side effect is the development of supine hypertension. Last daily dose should be taken 3 to 4 h before bedtime to minimize nighttime supine hypertension.
- **Fludrocortisone** (Florinef, tablet of 0.1 mg): initial dose 0.1-0.2 mg daily up to 0.4-0.6 mg daily (class IIa recommendation, Moya A, et al. Eur Heart J 2009;30:2631-71). It is preferred in normotensive patients. Its major side effects are hypokalemia and supine hypertension.
- **Pyridostigmine** (Mestinon, tablet of 60 mg): initial dose 30 mg x 2 or x 3 daily up to 60 mg x 3 daily. It is a cholinesterase inhibitor, has a relatively weak action, and is given in mild forms of orthostatic hypotension. It has the advantage of not affecting the supine BP.
- **Droxidopa** (Northera, capsules of 100, 200, 300 mg): initial dose 100 mg x 3 daily up to 600 mg x 3 daily. It is a prodrug that is directly metabolized in the body to noradrenaline. In 2014 the US Food and Drug Administration approved droxidopa for the treatment of neurogenic orthostatic hypotension caused by primary autonomic failure (Parkinson's disease, multiple-system atrophy, and pure autonomic failure). To reduce the potential for supine hypertension during sleep, elevate the head of the bed and give the last dose at least 3 h prior to bedtime.

- **Situational syncope:** urination in a seated position, avoidance of constipation through administration of laxatives, etc.
- **WPW syndrome:** accessory pathway ablation.
- **Carotid sinus syndrome:** avoidance of tight collars or neckties, dual-chamber pacing for patients with a predominantly cardioinhibitory response. The European Guidelines (Brignole M, et al. Eur Heart J 2013;34:2281-329) recommend dual-chamber pacing when carotid massage performed in supine and erect position causes asystole >6 s and reproduces the syncope.
- **Sick sinus syndrome or AV block (second or third degree):** cardiac pacing.
- **Brugada syndrome:** an implantable cardioverter defibrillator (ICD) should be considered in patients with a spontaneous diagnostic type 1 ECG who have a history of syncope judged to be likely caused by ventricular arrhythmias (class IIa recommendation, Priori SG, et al. Eur Heart J 2015;36:2793-867).

- **Long-QT syndrome:** an ICD should be considered in patients who experienced syncope while receiving adequate dose of a beta-blocker (class IIa recommendation, Priori SG, et al. Eur Heart J 2015;36:2793-867).
- **Arrhythmogenic right ventricular cardiomyopathy:** ICD.
- **Ventricular tachycardia:** an ICD may be required, depending on the underlying condition and the left ventricular ejection fraction.
- **Severe aortic valve stenosis, atrial myxoma:** surgical treatment.
- **Myocardial ischemia:** revascularization.

Key points

- Syncope due to cardiac causes is a severe and recurrent condition, with an annual mortality up to 30%.

- Almost 50% of cases are diagnosed through their history, the clinical examination and the ECG.

- Vasovagal syncope or common faint accounts for one third of cases and is usually observed in young people, with no signs of organic heart disease.

- The primary concern of an on-duty doctor treating a patient with syncope in the Emergency Room should be to determine whether this is a high-risk patient (pathological ECG, syncope on exercise or in the supine position, family history of sudden death, palpitations immediately prior to syncope, etc.), who needs to be admitted to the hospital.

- For every "unexplained" syncopal episode D-dimers should be determined, since their normal levels almost rule out the diagnosis of acute pulmonary embolism or acute aortic dissection. However, this only holds provided that the clinical probability of those diseases is low.

- Prolonged syncope may be accompanied by clonic seizures of very short duration (<15 s) because of cerebral ischemia. If such seizures occur concurrently with loss of consciousness, however, this indicates an epileptic attack.

- If the history is typical of vasovagal syncope, then a tilt testing is unnecessary. It is, however, indicated in cases of:
  a) Unexplained single syncope accompanied by injury or in those whose profession entails a high risk of injury
  b) Recurrent syncope in the absence of heart disease, or when heart disease is present but cardiac causes of syncope have been ruled out.

- In the treatment of vasovagal syncope, the most important measure is to reassure the patient that the condition is benign and to educate him how to prevent syncope. If this fails, midodrine may be administered.

- Syncope during exercise is more ominous than that occurring in the postexertion period.

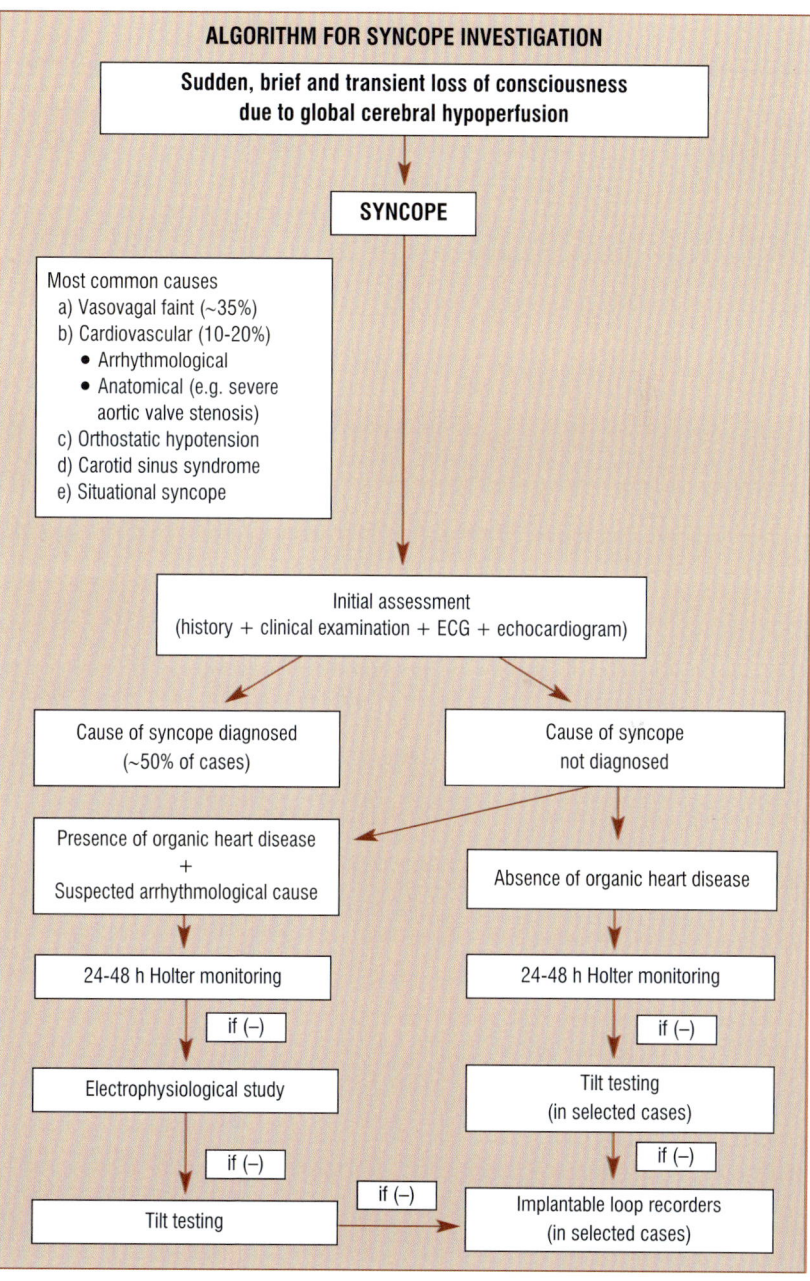

ALGORITHM FOR SYNCOPE INVESTIGATION

**Sudden, brief and transient loss of consciousness
due to global cerebral hypoperfusion**

SYNCOPE

Most common causes
a) Vasovagal faint (~35%)
b) Cardiovascular (10-20%)
  • Arrhythmological
  • Anatomical (e.g. severe
    aortic valve stenosis)
c) Orthostatic hypotension
d) Carotid sinus syndrome
e) Situational syncope

Initial assessment
(history + clinical examination + ECG + echocardiogram)

Cause of syncope diagnosed
(~50% of cases)

Cause of syncope
not diagnosed

Presence of organic heart disease
+
Suspected arrhythmological cause

Absence of organic heart disease

24-48 h Holter monitoring

if (−)

24-48 h Holter monitoring

if (−)

Electrophysiological study

Tilt testing
(in selected cases)

if (−)

if (−)

Tilt testing

if (−)

Implantable loop recorders
(in selected cases)

10

Cardiac arrest

Cardiac arrest is the abrupt cessation of effective mechanical activity in the heart, which may be reversible or may lead to cardiac death if not treated promptly and successfully. It is recognized by the absence of carotid pulsation for ≥5 s (the examination should not exceed 10 s by trained medical professionals) in an unconscious (unresponsive) person with no respiratory motions or with occasional (agonal) gasps. However, it should be noted that checking the carotid pulse is a relatively inaccurate method for confirming the presence or absence of circulation. Therefore, cardiopulmonary resuscitation (CPR) should be considered in an unconscious person with no breathing or with agonal gasps without the need for carotid artery palpation. Note that ~75% of cardiac arrests occur at home.

Cardiac arrest may be due to:

- **Ventricular fibrillation (VF) or pulseless ventricular tachycardia (VT).** This is the first monitored rhythm in ~25% of cardiac arrests. The first priority in this case is immediate defibrillation. During CPR, any potentially reversible causes should be checked for (Table 10.1) and attempts should be made to correct them. The most common causes are: acute myocardial infarction (AMI), previous myocardial infarction, dilated cardiomyopathy and hypertrophic cardiomyopathy.

- **Asystole or pulseless electrical activity.** Asystole (i.e. lack of cardiac electrical activity) or pulseless electrical activity (i.e. presence of organized cardiac electrical activity in the absence of effective mechanical function, formerly called electromechanical dissociation), has a worse prognosis than VF. Asystole or pulseless electrical activity is not treated by defibrillation; the first priority is to look for potentially reversible causes of cardiac arrest during CPR. Only if the underlying cause is treated can the patient be resuscitated successfully (Table 10.2). If the reversible causes are not treated, the survival rate is discouraging (1-2% in cases of asystole).

TABLE 10.1	Potentially reversible causes of cardiac arrest (these are listed as "4H's" and "4T's", as a mnemonic device)
• 4H's:	Hypoxia Hypovolemia Hypo-/hyperkalemia/metabolic Hypothermia
• 4T's:	Thrombosis (acute myocardial infarction or massive pulmonary embolism) Tamponade, cardiac Toxins Tension pneumothorax

The role of the precordial thump

If defibrillation is delayed in a person with cardiac arrest, then the sternum may be thumped (hit sharply with closed fist) once, from a height of 20 cm. Such a thump is equivalent to ~5-15 Joules (J) of energy. According to the European Guidelines for Resuscitation, a precordial thump may be applied only to patients in arrest who are under ECG monitoring indicating VF, when immediate defibrillation is not possible (Nolan JP, et al. Resuscitation 2010;81:1219-76). However, many experts feel that the precordial thump may be used in cases of arrest in heart patients where immediate ECG monitoring and defibrillation are not possible; the reasoning is that, if the underlying rhythm is pulseless VT, then the worst possible effect of an "asynchronous" precordial thump would be a conversion to VF, which is of course treated by defibrillation, the same as pulseless VT. If the precordial thump is delivered within 10 s after the arrest is established, there is a very small possibility that the VT, or more rarely the VF, will revert to sinus rhythm.

Performing CPR

The first act when starting CPR would be to open the airway by tilting the head and lifting the chin. Until the patient is intubated (if this is not done immediately), an oropharyngeal tube is placed and the patient is ventilated with a self-inflating bag (ambu bag) connected to an oxygen supply. This will achieve ventilation with an oxygen concentration of ~45% in the inhaled air. If a reservoir bag is used, it is possible to achieve ventilation with 85% inhaled oxygen (oxygen flow at 10-15 L/min). At the same time, defibrillator paddles or self-adhesive pads (which allow ECG monitoring) are put in place in order to allow immediate defibrillation if indicated. If defibrillation is delayed, and as long as signs of circulation are still absent, chest compressions and artificial

TABLE 10.2	Conditions that cause pulseless electrical activity, asystole or refractory ventricular fibrillation and their treatment		
Condition	**Diagnostic evidence**	**Treatment**	
Massive pulmonary embolism	History (postoperative immobilization, hip fracture, etc.)	Fibrinolysis, anticoagulation, embolectomy	
Acute myocardial infarction	History, ECG, cardiac troponin	Intra-aortic balloon pump and primary angioplasty	
Cardiac tamponade	History (malignancy, chest trauma, chronic renal failure, etc.), distended jugular veins	Pericardiocentesis	
Hypovolemia	History (severe bleeding from trauma, rupture of aortic aneurysm, etc.), empty jugular veins	Restore fluid volume, urgent surgery to stop the bleeding	
Hypoxia	History of respiratory disease, arterial blood gases	Ventilation (probably with mechanical support)	
Hyperkalemia	History (chronic renal failure, use of potassium-increasing drugs, etc.)	• Calcium (chloride or gluconate) • Glucose + insulin solution • Sodium bicarbonate	
Hypothermia	Exposure to cold, low central body temperature	Warming	
Tension pneumothorax	History (asthma, chest trauma), distended jugular veins	Needle decompression	
Attempted poisoning with tricyclic anti-depressants, digoxin, beta-blockers, calcium antagonists, etc.	Bradycardia, empty vials of drugs next to the patient, psychiatric history	Gastric lavage, activated charcoal, specific antidotes	

ventilation using an ambu bag (or mouth-to-mouth ventilation) are applied at a ratio of 30 compressions to 2 rescue breaths (30:2 ratio). The frequency of compressions should be 100-120/min; however, the actual number of chest compressions in the nonintubated patient is lower (80-90/min) because of the interruption for ~5 s to deliver rescue breaths every 30 compressions. During CPR, the patient is intubated: this is the best way to preserve airway patency and achieve good ventilation. The aspiration of gastric fluid is also avoided. The intubation attempt should not exceed 10 s, so it should be undertaken by a physician with experience in intubation (usually an anesthesiologist). Ideally, waveform capnography should be used to confirm and monitor the position of the endotracheal tube. Once the patient is intubated, CPR continues at a rate of 100-120 chest compressions/min and 10 ventilations/min performed a-synchronously, meaning that the compressions are continuous, without pause for ventilation.

On compression, the sternum should be depressed by 5-6 cm allowing the chest to recoil completely after each compression and the carotid pulse should be palpable. Note that a successful compression will cause a systolic pressure spike of ~60-80 mmHg, whereas cardiac output will not exceed 30% of the normal cardiac output.

Warning! If there is no airway/ventilation equipment (usually out-of-hospital cardiac arrest) and the rescuer is unwilling to perform mouth–to-mouth ventilation, then compression-only CPR (continuous chest compressions or cardiocerebral resuscitation [CCR] at a rate of 100-120/min) should be performed. CCR performed by bystanders in out-of-hospital cardiac arrest victims is associated with higher survival rates compared to standard CPR.

Defibrillation during CPR

1) One paddle or self-adhesive pad of the defibrillator is placed below the right clavicle and the other (apical) is placed to the left of the left nipple.
2) Any nitrate transdermal patches are removed, the paddles are placed at least 8 cm away from the generator of the pacemaker or implantable cardioverter defibrillator, if the patient has such a device, and the oxygen supply is disconnected (this does not apply to intubated patients connected to a contactless ventilator circuit). Pressure is applied and bystanders are warned to stay clear of the patient and the bed during the shock.
3) In case of **ventricular fibrillation** or **pulseless ventricular tachycardia (shockable rhythms):**
   • A shock is delivered immediately (360 J monophasic or 150-200 J biphasic). For every minute of delay in applying defibrillation, survival is reduced by 10-12%. After the **first shock** the heart rhythm is not checked; instead, CPR is performed immediately for 2 min (compression:ventilation ratio of 30:2 in nonintubated patient) starting with chest compressions. This is done because, even if a perfusing rhythm has been restored, only rarely can the pulse be palpated immediately after defibrillation. If CPR is interrupted for the palpation attempt, the myocardium will be further burdened if the rhythm has not been restored. Even if it has, compressions will not produce any adverse effects (for example, there is no increased risk of VF recurrence).

- After CPR has been performed for 2 min, it is interrupted briefly in order to check the rhythm on the monitor. If VF or VT persists, a **second shock** (360 J monophasic or 150-360 J biphasic) is delivered, followed by 2 min CPR.
- After CPR has been performed for 2 min, it is interrupted briefly in order to check the rhythm on the monitor. If VF or VT persists, a **third shock** (360 J monophasic or 150-360 J biphasic) is delivered, and again CPR continues for another 2 min. If an IV or intraosseous route has been found, 1 mg adrenaline (epinephrine) and 300 mg amiodarone are administered rapidly (bolus) once compressions have restarted. The dose of adrenaline is repeated every 3-5 min throughout CPR (alternate cycles) and until the return of spontaneous circulation (ROSC), i.e. purposeful movement, breathing (more than occasional gasp), or coughing.
- After CRP has been performed for 2 min, it is briefly interrupted to check the rhythm on the monitor. If VF or VT persists, another shock is delivered and the algorithm described above is repeated.
- If an organized rhythm is found (regular and/or narrow QRS complexes), then an attempt is made to quickly palpate the pulse. If there is doubt as to the presence of pulses, CPR is continued. If an organized rhythm appears during the 2-min CPR, the compressions are not interrupted in order to check the pulse unless the patient shows signs of recovery (ROSC).

Warning! If VF or pulseless VT occurs during cardiac catheterization or during the immediate postoperative period after heart surgery, up to three successive (stacked) shocks are delivered instead of only one, before chest compressions begin.

4) In case of **asystole** or **pulseless electrical activity (nonshockable rhythms)**:
- CPR is started immediately (30 compressions : 2 ventilations) and 1 mg of adrenaline is administered IV (or via intraosseous route) as soon as a vascular access is found. After CPR has been performed for 2 min, it is briefly interrupted for a rhythm check on the monitor. If asystole is present, CRP is resumed immediately. If an organized rhythm is present, an attempt is made to palpate a pulse. If there is no pulse or if there is any doubt about the presence of a pulse, CPR is continued.

Warning! If asystole is displayed on the monitor make sure that this is the correct diagnosis. Check the gain settings and the position of the leads.

- Defibrillation is not indicated in cases of asystole or pulseless electrical activity. Even if it is unclear whether the cause is asystole or fine VF, it is preferable to continue CPR rather than to defibrillate. Continued CPR will increase the likelihood of fine VF converting to coarse, as well as the chances of successful defibrillation.
- If the heart rhythm converts to VF during CPR, the algorithm for VF or pulseless VT is followed.

Warning! Shock is always applied asynchronously in cases of cardiac arrest even if the underlying rhythm is VT (pulseless), in order to avoid any delay.

The role of ultrasound imaging

Ultrasound imaging during CPR can demonstrate, particularly if there is ongoing cardiac activity during imaging, certain potentially reversible causes of cardiac arrest (cardiac tamponade, acute massive pulmonary embolism, complicated proximal acute aortic dissection, AMI [i.e. mechanical complications], hypovolemia, pneumothorax, etc.). Note that AMI and massive pulmonary embolism are the most common causes of cardiac arrest (~50-70% of out-of-hospital cases). Prerequisites for performing an ultrasound examination are:
- The examiner performing the study must be experienced, so that diagnostic images can be obtained within 10 s.
- The transducer must be placed at a subxiphoid site so that CPR is not impeded.
- Imaging should begin at the end of the 2-min CPR and the interruption should be utilized for a planned rhythm check.

Routes for drug administration

1) It is preferable to locate a peripheral rather than a central vein, because the procedure is faster and safer. Each time a drug is administered, the line should be flushed with at least 20 mL of normal saline and the limb should be elevated for at least 10 s.
2) Intraosseous administration is proposed as an alternative route if IV access is difficult or impossible. Infusion through the intraosseous route (usually at the tibial tuberosity) produces satisfactory plasma levels of the drug within a timeframe comparable to that achieved by infusion through a central venous line.
3) Endotracheal administration is no longer recommended, because it produces unpredictable drug concentrations and the optimal dose for most drugs is unknown. However, if IV or intraosseous access cannot be es-

tablished, adrenaline and lidocaine may be administered by the endotracheal route (diluted in 5 to 10 mL of sterile water or normal saline). The endotracheal dose is 2 to 2.5 times the recommended IV dose.
4) Intracardiac drug administration is contraindicated. Hazards of intracardiac drug administration are:
   - Interruption of chest compressions.
   - Coronary artery or myocardial laceration.
   - Intramyocardial infusion and provocation of intractable VF.
   - Pneumothorax.
   - Cardiac tamponade.

Drugs
1) **Adrenaline (epinephrine):**
   - In cases of VF or pulseless VT, it is administered immediately after the third shock and only if CPR compressions have begun. It is then repeated every 3-5 min throughout CPR until the ROSC.
   - In cases of asystole or pulseless electrical activity, it is administered as soon as vascular access is established, and then repeated every 3-5 min throughout CPR until the ROSC.

   Adrenaline stimulates β_1, β_2 and, at higher doses (such as the doses administered for cardiac arrest), α-adrenergic receptors ($\beta_1=\beta_2>\alpha$). It has a half-life of ~2 min. The dose at each IV infusion is 1 mg; it is available in ampoules containing 1 mg in 1 mL (a dilution of 1:1000). Before administration, it should be further diluted to 1:10,000 (by drawing up the ampoule in a syringe containing sterile water to a final volume of 10 mL). Table 10.3 describes the effects of adrenaline.
2) **Amiodarone:** administered in cases of VF or pulseless VT, at a dose of 300 mg IV bolus immediately after the third shock (similar to the first dose of adrenaline). If the arrhythmia recurs or persists, an additional

TABLE 10.3	Effects of adrenaline on cardiac arrest

1) Increased myocardial contractility
2) Increased likelihood of successful defibrillation
3) Increased systemic resistances and therefore arterial blood pressure on systole (chest compression) leading to better brain perfusion, and on diastole (chest release) leading to better myocardial perfusion
4) Increased probability of conversion of electromechanical dissociation to electromechanical coupling

150 mg may be administered, followed by an infusion of 900 mg over 24 h. As an alternative to amiodarone (if unavailable), lidocaine may be administered at a dose of ~100 mg (1-1.5 mg/kg IV), but should not be given if amiodarone has been administered previously. If VF or pulseless VT persists, additional doses of 0.5 to 0.75 mg/kg IV may be administered at 5 to10-min intervals to a maximum dose of 3 mg/kg.

Amiodarone is available as Cordarone ampoules containing 150 mg/3 mL, and lidocaine as 50 mL Xylocaine solution for injection at a concentration of 2%, i.e. 1 mL contains 20 mg of lidocaine.

3) **Atropine:** its routine use for asystole or pulseless electrical activity is no longer recommended, because there is no evidence of benefit. In any case, asystole is mostly due to myocardial damage, not to excessive parasympathetic stimulation.

4) **Sodium bicarbonate (NaHCO$_3$):** routine use is not recommended. It may be used in:

- Arrest due to hyperkalemia.
- Arrest due to poisoning by tricyclic antidepressants or phenobarbital.
- Prolonged cardiac arrest (>20 min) [relative indication].
- Metabolic acidosis, i.e. pH <7.1 despite good ventilation (there are conflicting data).

It should be noted that the best way to treat acidosis is to maintain the circulation by chest compressions, and to ensure good lung ventilation. Sodium bicarbonate is given at a dose of 1 mEq (mmol)/kg IV or usually 50 mEq, i.e. 50 mL of 8.4% solution, which contains 50 mEq HCO$_3$, over 2-3 min. Side effects of the administration of sodium bicarbonate include:

- Decreased release of oxygen from oxyhemoglobin, due to a leftward shift of the oxyhemoglobin saturation curve as a result of extracellular alkalosis caused by the drug.
- Reduction of systemic vascular resistance.
- Hypernatremia and hyperosmolarity.
- Contribution to intracellular acidosis by the production of excess CO_2 (liberated from NaHCO$_3$), which freely diffuses into myocardial (suppressive effect) and cerebral cells.

Sodium bicarbonate is available in solutions of 4.2% (provides 0.5 mEq/mL of HCO$_3$), 8.4% (provides 1 mEq/mL of HCO$_3$), etc.

5) **Calcium (chloride or gluconate):** administered only in cases of cardiac arrest with severe hyperkalemia, severe hypocalcemia, or overdose of calcium channel blockers. The initial dose is 10 mL of 10% calcium chloride IV over 2-3 min (or an equivalent dose of calcium gluconate).

A 10 mL ampoule of 10% calcium chloride contains 13.6 mEq of calcium, and a 10 mL ampoule of 10% calcium gluconate contains 4.6 mEq of calcium. This means that 1 ampoule of 10% calcium chloride is equivalent to ~3 ampoules of 10% calcium gluconate with regard to calcium ion content.

6) **Magnesium sulfate:** administered in cases of refractory VF if hypomagnesemia is suspected or if the arrest is due to torsades de pointes or to digitalis toxicity. A 2 g dose of magnesium sulfate is administered IV over 1-2 min and the same dose may be repeated >10-15 min.

Magnesium sulfate for IV administration is available in various concentrations, i.e. 25% in 10 mL ampoules (provides 2 mEq/mL of Mg), 50% in 10 mL ampoules (provides 4 mEq/mL of Mg), etc.

7) **Fibrinolysis:** consider it when cardiac arrest is caused by proven or suspected acute massive pulmonary embolism.

Warning! When drugs are administered during CPR, it is very important not to interrupt CPR.

When is CPR terminated?

There is no generally accepted rule dictating the time at which CPR should be terminated when a person does not recover. The current trend is to discontinue if the underlying rhythm is asystole or pulseless electrical activity, provided:

- The person is normothermic with no indication of toxic drug effects, and
- Asystole or pulseless electrical activity continues after 20 min of CPR, provided there are no potentially reversible causes.

However, if the rhythm persisting after 20 min of CPR is **VF** then CPR should be continued for a longer period. Furthermore, CPR should be continued in cases of arrest due to **hypothermia** (body temperature reduced to <35°C), because hypothermia protects the vital organs and such individuals may make a full neurological recovery despite prolonged CPR. Finally, if fibrinolysis has been administered because of proven or suspected **massive pulmonary embolism,** then CPR should be continued for at least 60-90 min.

Warning! The presence of mydriasis should not be used as a criterion for discontinuing CPR as an indication of irreversible brain damage, because it may also be due to the drugs administered (e.g. adrenaline). Furthermore, mydriasis occurs within 60-90 s from establishment of cardiac arrest and therefore develops before brain death.

Early actions after successful CPR

- Check vital signs, perform ECG and continuous ECG monitoring.

- Send blood for complete blood count, urea, creatinine, glucose, electrolytes and markers of myocardial necrosis (preferably cardiac troponin).
- Check arterial blood gases and pH.
- Ensure good ventilation to maintain an oxygen saturation in the range of 94-98%. Oxygen saturation should be monitored using a pulse oximeter (less reliable in case of severe peripheral vasoconstriction). The patient will require mechanical ventilation if they are in a coma or have severe hypoxemia or hypercapnia, despite receiving 100% oxygen.
- Insert a urinary catheter and measure hourly urinary output.
- Administer IV antiarrhythmics (preferably amiodarone) for 24-48 h; these are usually discontinued after that, as long as the arrhythmia does not recur.
- Restore myocardial perfusion in cases of acute ischemia. In cases of AMI with ST-segment elevation, primary percutaneous coronary intervention (PCI) is the preferred treatment. If there are no facilities for PCI, fibrinolytic treatment will be administered. Note that in survivors of out-of-hospital cardiac arrest, early coronary angiography and PCI, if appropriate, should be performed irrespective of the ECG pattern if no obvious noncardiac cause is present.
- Potassium serum levels should be maintained at >4 mEq/L and magnesium at >2 mEq/L.
- Administer insulin if blood glucose levels are >180 mg/dL and with great care to avoid hypoglycemia.
- Perform neurological assessment (Glasgow Coma Scale).
- Examine the patient to ensure that there is no other medical or surgical condition requiring specific treatment
- Obtain a chest X-ray using a portable scanner, primarily to exclude the possibility of rib fractures and pneumothorax and to check the position of the tracheal tube.
- Perform right heart catheterization to measure pulmonary capillary wedge pressure and to guide the administration of fluids and inotropes/vasopressors in cases of hemodynamic instability despite the restoration of the heart rhythm. Also consider placing an intra-aortic balloon pump in cases of persisting hypotension. Note that significant myocardial dysfunction after ROSC (component of the postcardiac arrest syndrome) is common and usually recovers by 2-3 days.
- Control of seizures with benzodiazepines, phenytoin, sodium valproate, propofol, or a barbiturate. Note that seizures increase cerebral metabolism and may cause cerebral injury.
- Apply therapeutic hypothermia to comatose patients, as there is evidence that this can improve their neurological outcome.
- Safely transfer the patient to an intensive care unit.

Key points

■ In cases of cardiac arrest due to VF or pulseless VT, the only truly life-saving intervention is immediate defibrillation, while drugs play a minor role during CPR. It is also important, particularly in cases of refractory VF or pulseless VT, to identify and treat potentially reversible causes.

■ A single shock is delivered and is repeated every 2 min until ROSC in VF or pulseless VT. However, if VF or pulseless VT occurs during cardiac catheterization or during the immediate postoperative period after heart surgery, up to three successive shocks are delivered.

■ In cases of cardiac arrest due to asystole or pulseless electrical activity, the only life-saving intervention is the identification and treatment of potentially reversible causes. Otherwise, CPR will not be effective.

■ For ease of memory, the potentially reversible causes of cardiac arrest are divided into 4H's (hypoxia, hypovolemia, hypo-/hyperkalemia, hypothermia) and 4T's (thrombosis, tamponade [cardiac], toxins, tension pneumothorax).

■ In an intubated patient with cardiac arrest perform uninterrupted (except for shock delivery, rhythm assessment or pulse check when indicated) chest compressions at rate of 100-120/min and ventilations at approximately 10 breaths/min.

■ If IV or intraosseous access cannot be established, adrenaline and lidocaine may be administered by the endotracheal route.

■ In cases of VF or pulseless VT cardiac arrest, adrenaline is administered after the third shock once chest compressions have restarted, i.e. ~4 min after starting CPR, while in cases of asystole or pulseless electrical activity, it is administered immediately, provided that a vascular access site has been found.

■ During CPR, administration of adrenaline every 3-5 min until ROSC should not be overlooked.

■ Fibrinolysis should not be used routinely in cardiac arrest. However, if there is proven or suspected acute massive pulmonary embolism, then fibrinolysis should be used and the resuscitation team should be prepared to do prolonged CRP (for at least 60-90 min).

Key points - *continued*

- During CPR, pulse check should be undertaken only if an organized rhythm appears, either
  - a) at the end of each 2-min cycle (prior to shock delivery in VF or pulseless VT cardiac arrest), or
  - b) at any time that signs of recovery appear (normal breathing, coughing, or movements).

- By itself, mydriasis should not be taken as a sign of brain death and should not be the reason to discontinue CPR.

- In cases of cardiac arrest where the immediate commencement of CPR is not possible and the resuscitator is not willing to perform mouth-to-mouth ventilation, CCR, i.e. chest compressions alone at a rate of 100-120/min, should be applied immediately. This intervention can serve as a bridge to the application of CPR.

- Successful performance of CPR requires the coordinated efforts of a resuscitation team, which should include a cardiologist, an anesthesiologist and a nurse.

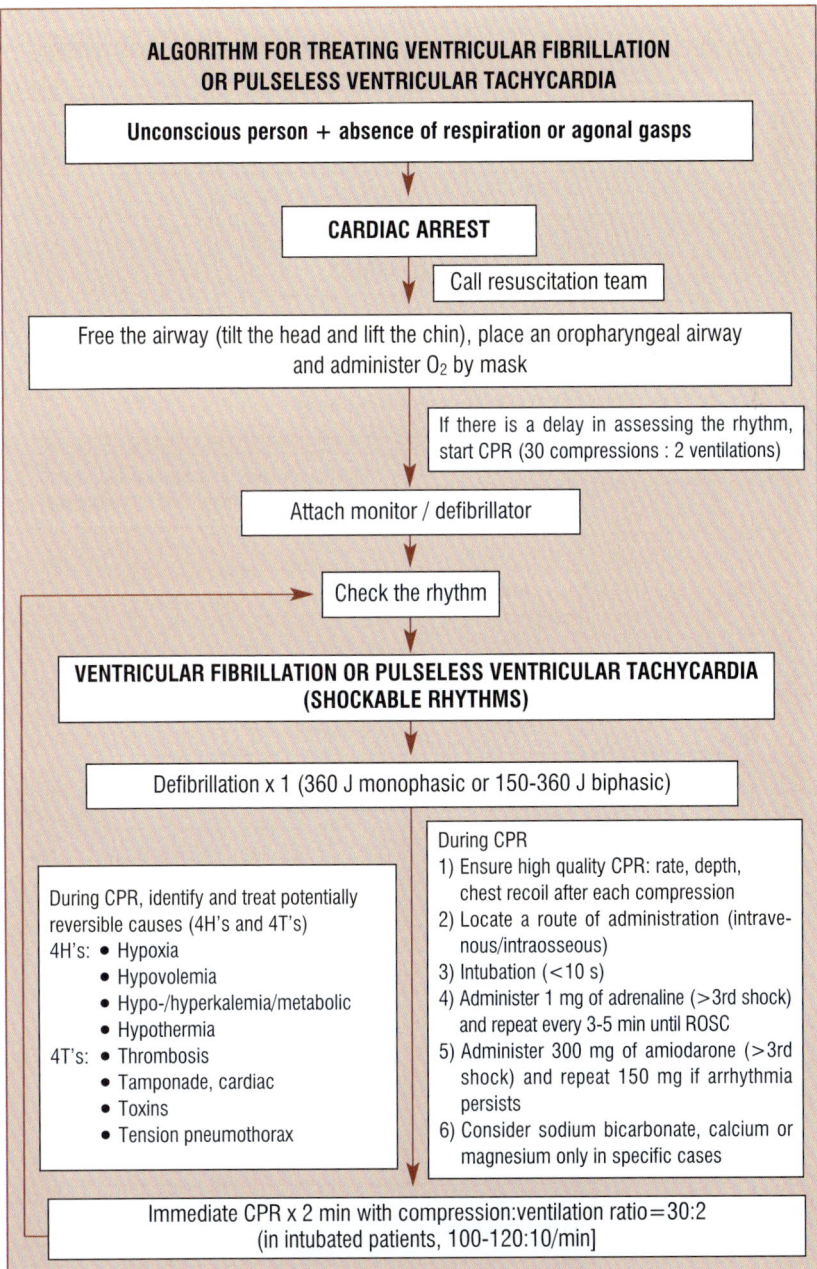

ALGORITHM FOR TREATING VENTRICULAR FIBRILLATION OR PULSELESS VENTRICULAR TACHYCARDIA

Unconscious person + absence of respiration or agonal gasps

CARDIAC ARREST

Call resuscitation team

Free the airway (tilt the head and lift the chin), place an oropharyngeal airway and administer O_2 by mask

If there is a delay in assessing the rhythm, start CPR (30 compressions : 2 ventilations)

Attach monitor / defibrillator

Check the rhythm

VENTRICULAR FIBRILLATION OR PULSELESS VENTRICULAR TACHYCARDIA (SHOCKABLE RHYTHMS)

Defibrillation x 1 (360 J monophasic or 150-360 J biphasic)

During CPR, identify and treat potentially reversible causes (4H's and 4T's)

4H's: • Hypoxia
• Hypovolemia
• Hypo-/hyperkalemia/metabolic
• Hypothermia

4T's: • Thrombosis
• Tamponade, cardiac
• Toxins
• Tension pneumothorax

During CPR
1) Ensure high quality CPR: rate, depth, chest recoil after each compression
2) Locate a route of administration (intravenous/intraosseous)
3) Intubation (<10 s)
4) Administer 1 mg of adrenaline (>3rd shock) and repeat every 3-5 min until ROSC
5) Administer 300 mg of amiodarone (>3rd shock) and repeat 150 mg if arrhythmia persists
6) Consider sodium bicarbonate, calcium or magnesium only in specific cases

Immediate CPR x 2 min with compression:ventilation ratio=30:2 (in intubated patients, 100-120:10/min]

CPR: cardiopulmonary resuscitation, ROSC: return of spontaneous circulation

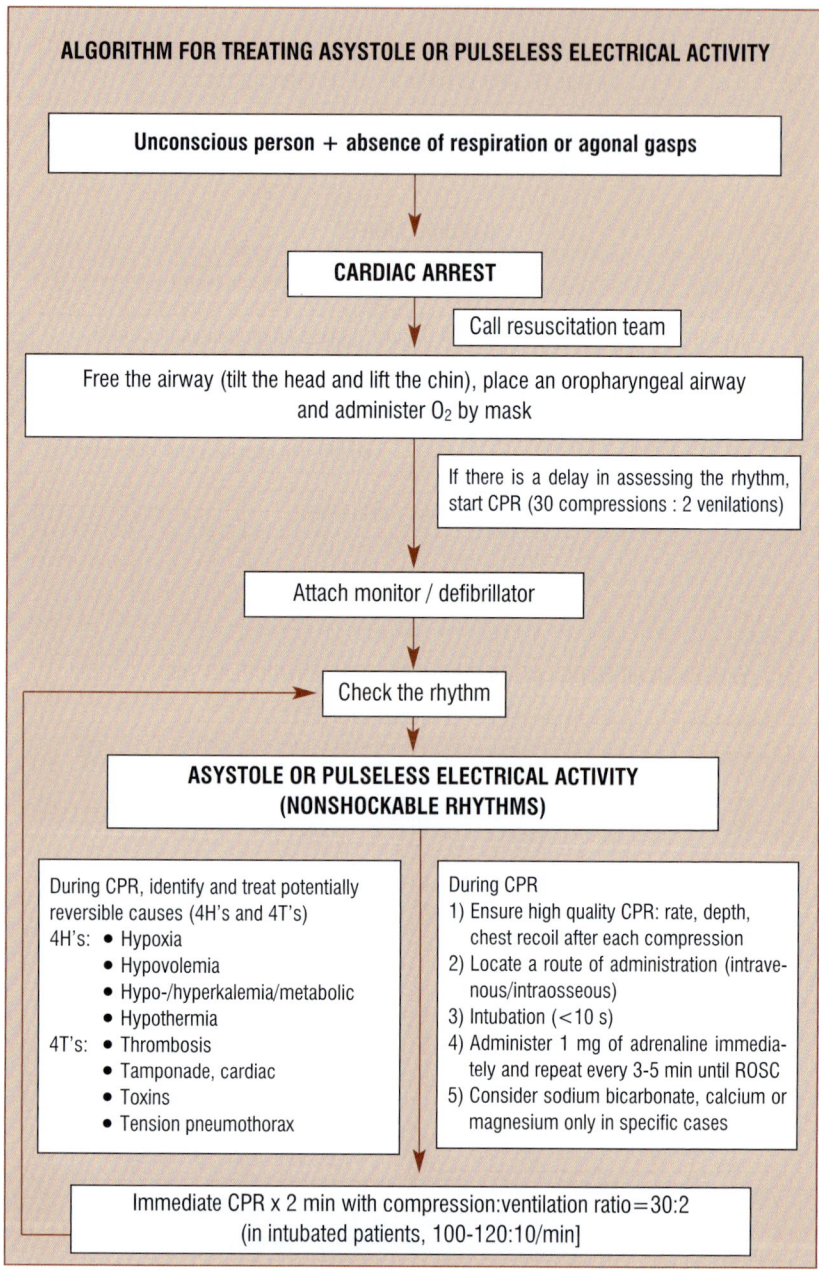

ALGORITHM FOR TREATING ASYSTOLE OR PULSELESS ELECTRICAL ACTIVITY

Unconscious person + absence of respiration or agonal gasps

CARDIAC ARREST

Call resuscitation team

Free the airway (tilt the head and lift the chin), place an oropharyngeal airway and administer O₂ by mask

If there is a delay in assessing the rhythm, start CPR (30 compressions : 2 venilations)

Attach monitor / defibrillator

Check the rhythm

ASYSTOLE OR PULSELESS ELECTRICAL ACTIVITY
(NONSHOCKABLE RHYTHMS)

During CPR, identify and treat potentially reversible causes (4H's and 4T's)
4H's: • Hypoxia
      • Hypovolemia
      • Hypo-/hyperkalemia/metabolic
      • Hypothermia
4T's: • Thrombosis
      • Tamponade, cardiac
      • Toxins
      • Tension pneumothorax

During CPR
1) Ensure high quality CPR: rate, depth, chest recoil after each compression
2) Locate a route of administration (intravenous/intraosseous)
3) Intubation (<10 s)
4) Administer 1 mg of adrenaline immediately and repeat every 3-5 min until ROSC
5) Consider sodium bicarbonate, calcium or magnesium only in specific cases

Immediate CPR x 2 min with compression:ventilation ratio=30:2
(in intubated patients, 100-120:10/min]

CPR: cardiopulmonary resuscitation, ROSC: return of spontaneous circulation

11

Acute elevations in blood pressure

In the international literature a number of different terms have been used for acute elevations of blood pressure (BP). Most authors use the general term **hypertensive crisis** to define both hypertensive emergencies and urgencies, i.e. acute and marked BP increase (systolic and/or diastolic), regardless of the presence of acute or rapidly progressive end-organ (target organ) damage. The latest European Guidelines (Mancia G, et al. Eur Heart J 2013;34:2159-219) define hypertensive emergencies as large elevations in systolic or diastolic BP (>180 mmHg or >120 mmHg, respectively) associated with impending or progressive organ damage. It is estimated that ~1% of hypertensive adults will present with hypertensive crisis. Most of them are the result of untreated or inadequately treated mild-to-moderate hypertension, or nonadherence to antihypertensive treatment.

In this chapter, for practical reasons, the cutoff values of BP threshold for hypertensive crisis have been slightly modified and the term hypertensive pseudocrisis has also been introduced. Therefore, an acute elevation in BP includes three entities:

1) **Hypertensive emergencies:** a sudden and marked increase in BP (usually diastolic BP >120-130 mmHg and/or systolic BP >200 mmHg) accompanied by acute or rapidly progressive end-organ damage (Table 11.1):
   - Eyes: fundoscopic findings such as hemorrhage, exudates, papilledema.
   - Brain: hypertensive encephalopathy (headache, nausea, vomiting, irritability, disturbances or loss of vision, confusion and convulsions), intracerebral hemorrhage (focal neurological deficits), subarachnoid hem-

TABLE 11.1	Hypertensive emergencies

1) Hypertensive encephalopathy
2) Acute aortic dissection
3) Acute pulmonary edema
4) Acute coronary syndrome
5) Eclampsia (preeclampsia + convulsions) or severe preeclampsia
6) Pheochromocytoma crisis
7) Subarachnoid or intracerebral hemorrhage
8) Acute ischemic stroke
9) Overdose of sympathomimetics (e.g. cocaine, LSD)
10) Rebound hypertension following abrupt withdrawal of certain antihypertensive agents (clonidine, methyldopa)
11) Cranial or cerebral injury
12) Postoperative hypertension

orrhage (sudden "explosive" headache, nausea, vomiting, loss of consciousness, stiff neck) or ischemic stroke (focal neurological deficits).
- Heart: dyspnea, orthopnea, acute pulmonary edema or acute coronary syndrome.
- Aorta: acute aortic dissection.
- Kidneys: acute renal failure.
- Arteries: microangiopathic hemolytic anemia (direct endothelial damage)

In hypertensive emergencies, the marked BP elevation is usually the direct cause of the acute end-organ damage, i.e. the heart may be affected in a hypertensive emergency presenting as acute pulmonary edema, etc. In other cases, as in ischemic stroke, the acute elevation in BP may exacerbate the existing damage to the affected organ, i.e. an acute elevation in BP is more likely to cause intracerebral hemorrhage, but if marked BP elevation is present in an ischemic stroke (usually caused by *in situ* occlusion of a cerebral artery or by embolization of carotid plaque material to distal cerebral arteries) it may adversely affect the progression of the disease. In hypertensive emergencies, BP reduction is critically urgent and needs to be achieved within 30-60 min. Hypertensive emergencies make up only a small percentage of all acute elevations in BP that are encountered in the Emergency Room. It is important to note, however, that very high BP levels are not always a prerequisite when an acute BP elevation is judged to be a hypertensive emergency. The definitive criterion is the presence of acute or rapidly progressive end-organ damage, which may be associated with BP levels lower than those referred to above, namely diastolic BP <120-130 mmHg or systolic BP <200 mmHg.

2) **Hypertensive urgencies:** a sudden and marked increase in BP (usually diastolic BP >120-130 mmHg and/or systolic BP >200 mmHg) that is not accompanied by acute or rapidly progressive end-organ damage.

In a hypertensive urgency, BP reduction is urgent and needs to be achieved within a few hours, and no more than 24 h. The patient is usually asymptomatic or has mild symptoms, such as headache (~20%), chest pain (~10%), dyspnea (~10%), etc. For the treatment of a hypertensive urgency, oral antihypertensive medication (e.g. captopril) is usually given, and in general the treatment is the same as for hypertensive pseudocrisis, as described below.

Hypertensive urgency includes conditions such as preoperative hypertension, acute glomerulonephritis, as well as some of the cases in Table 11.1, such as pheochromocytoma crisis, use of sympathomimetic substances, and abrupt cessation of certain antihypertensive medications, provided that there is no acute target organ damage. Table 11.2 presents the main differences between hypertensive emergencies and hypertensive urgencies.

3) **Hypertensive pseudocrises:** asymptomatic (usually) increase in BP (systolic BP ~180-220 mmHg and/or diastolic BP ~100-120 mmHg) with no accompanying acute or rapidly progressive end-organ damage. Hypertensive pseudocrisis can be considered as a milder form of hypertensive urgency.

Warning! The greatest risk in hypertensive urgencies or hypertensive pseudocrises lies in the overtreatment of these conditions and inciting a hypotensive crisis with subsequent cerebral or myocardial ischemia.

Pathophysiology of hypertensive encephalopathy

Also known as posterior reversible encephalopathy syndrome (PRES), this is a hypertensive emergency in which manifestations from the brain predominate and are reversible with a reduction in BP. It is characterized by headache, nausea, vomiting, irritability, confusion, convulsions, disturbances or loss of vision (cortical blindness) or stupor. Focal neurological signs are rare and when present they should raise the suspicion of an ischemic stroke or intracerebral hemorrhage. If the treatment of hypertensive encephalopathy is delayed it may progress to coma or death.

Hypertensive encephalopathy occurs when the autoregulation of blood

TABLE 11.2	Main differences between hypertensive emergencies and hypertensive urgencies	
	Hypertensive emergency	**Hypertensive urgency**
Rapidity of blood pressure reduction	Immediate reduction (within 30-60 min)	Gradual reduction (within 12-24 h)
Acute target organ damage	Present	Absent
Admission to hospital	Always required	Usually not required
Antihypertensive treatment	Intravenous infusion of titratable agents	Oral short-acting agents

flow to the brain is acutely compromised by a marked elevation of BP compared to the patient's baseline.

The brain is capable of maintaining a stable blood supply (autoregulation mechanism) within a wide range of BP values. In normotensive individuals this means that cerebral blood flow is relatively constant over a range of mean BP* between 50-150 mmHg (Figure 11.1). This is achieved by vasoconstriction of the arterioles when BP increases and vasodilation when BP decreases. When the BP increases beyond the limits of autoregulation, the compensatory mechanism breaks down, resulting in vasodilation of the previously constricted vessels, hyperemia, perivascular leakage of fluid (because of associated damage to the endothelium), and cerebral edema (papilledema is present).

In chronic hypertensives, because of adaptation of the brain vessels (mainly by thickening of the arterioles), the autoregulation curve is shifted to the right (autoregulation limits of mean BP between 110-180 mmHg) and the compensatory mechanism fails when mean BP exceeds 180 mmHg. This means that chronic hypertensives have better tolerance of large increases in BP compared to normotensives. Rapid correction of BP in chronic hypertensives to normotensive levels, because of the reduced capability for autoregulation at those levels, may cause cerebral ischemia. In contrast, in previously normotensive persons, severe encephalopathy can occur with relatively mild BP elevations, i.e. in pregnant women convulsions may occur (eclampsia) even at BP levels around 170/110 mmHg. In particular, the lower threshold for neurologic symptoms in pregnant women with eclampsia

---

$$* \ Mean \ BP \ = \ \frac{(systolic \ BP) \ + \ (diastolic \ BP \ x \ 2)}{3}$$

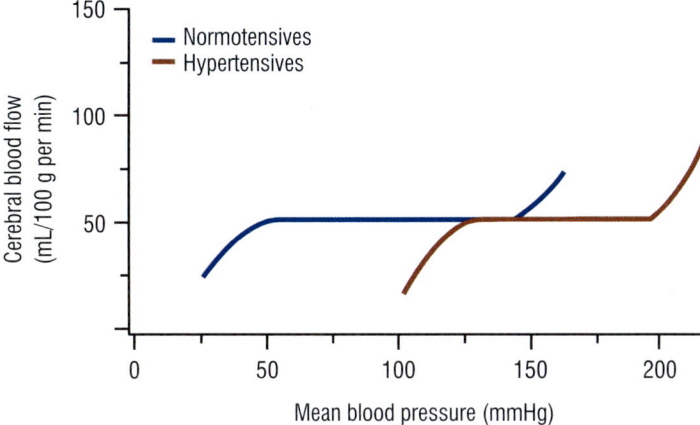

Figure 11.1. In normotensives the brain is able to maintain autoregulation of perfusion for mean blood pressure values ranging from 110-150 mmHg, while in chronic hypertensives (right-shifted curve) the equivalent values are 110-180 mmHg. (From Braunwald's Heart Disease by Zipes, Libby, Bonow and Braunwald, 7th edition, p 984, with permission).

may be due to impaired dynamic cerebral blood flow autoregulation, increased blood-brain barrier permeability, etc.

Warning! Apart from the brain, autoregulatory mechanisms that maintain blood flow despite fluctuations in BP are also found in the heart and kidneys. However, the brain is more vulnerable to variations in BP because it is encased in a finite space and because it maximally extracts oxygen at baseline.

Clinical evaluation of acute hypertensive episodes
The presence of the following symptoms makes treatment emergent:
- Acute dyspnea (orthopnea, acute pulmonary edema).
- Constrictive retrosternal pain (angina, acute coronary syndrome).
- Stabbing pain in the anterior thoracic or midscapular region, of migratory nature (acute aortic dissection).
- Headache, nausea, vomiting, irritability, disturbances or loss of vision, confusion, convulsions, stupor (hypertensive encephalopathy), focal neurological signs (intracerebral hemorrhage or ischemic stroke).
- Neck stiffness, sudden intense headache, vomiting, confusion (subarachnoid hemorrhage).

Clinical examination

- Measurement of BP in both arms: a difference in systolic BP >20 mmHg may be observed in proximal aortic dissection.
- Palpation of peripheral pulses: a weakening or absence of these may reflect acute aortic dissection.
- Check for a new aortic insufficiency murmur: observed in ~50% of proximal aortic dissections.
- Check for signs of heart failure: 3rd heart sound, crackles at the bases of the lungs, etc.
- Neurological examination: mental status and focal neurological signs.
- Fundoscopy: hemorrhages, exudates and papilledema.

Basic laboratory tests

- Complete blood count (check for hemolysis), urea, creatinine, glucose, electrolytes, markers of myocardial necrosis (in acute coronary syndrome) and D-dimers (on suspicion of acute aortic dissection).
- ECG.
- Chest X-ray.
- Urine analysis (check for red blood cells and protein when renal involvement is suspected).
- Brain computed tomography (CT) in the setting of possible cerebrovascular accident, magnetic resonance imaging (MRI) for hypertensive encephalopathy (edema localizes in posterior brain regions) or contrast chest CT on suspicion of acute aortic dissection.

Treatment of hypertensive emergencies

As stated above, emergency treatment is required. The decision to treat hypertensive emergencies is not determined only by the level of BP, but mainly by the underlying target organ damage. Thus, the BP threshold used for treatment is lower in acute pulmonary edema, acute coronary syndrome, acute aortic dissection, eclampsia, etc.

Remarks on the treatment of hypertensive emergencies

- The treatment requires admission to a hospital (preferably to the intensive care unit [ICU] or coronary care unit) and intra-arterial BP monitoring.
- Oral antihypertensive medications are avoided, since they often cause a sudden drop in BP, they are less effective, and they cannot be titrated.
- The treatment of hypertensive emergencies does not mean under any circumstances a swift restoration of BP to normal levels, because this may disturb the autoregulation mechanism and cause hypoperfusion of vital organs. This particularly applies to patients who present with hypertensive emergency and are unaware of their preexisting hypertension. For this reason the target is a BP reduction within 30-60 min to levels of

diastolic BP ~100 mmHg and systolic BP ~160 mmHg, or a reduction in mean BP by 25%. An exception is acute aortic dissection, where the aim is a rapid reduction (<10 min) in systolic BP to 100-120 mmHg.

- The need for a gradual reduction in BP is even greater in patients who have a history of chronic arterial hypertension, where the autoregulation mechanism for blood supply to the vital organs, such as the brain, kidneys, and heart, is shifted towards higher BP levels. This leads to hypoperfusion of these organs when BP is restored to normal levels within 30-60 min.
- In intracerebral hemorrhage the target is a reduction in systolic BP to levels of ~140 mmHg if systolic BP at presentation is between 150-220 mmHg.
- In ischemic stroke (acute phase) BP reduction is sought only when it is >220/120 mmHg, or >185/100 mmHg if fibrinolysis is to be administered. The target is a reduction in BP by 15-25% within the first 24 h.
- Severe preeclampsia is defined as preeclampsia (hypertension + proteinuria [≥300 mg/24 h] in a pregnant woman >20th week of gestation) that is complicated by any of the following (Obstet Gynecol 2013;122:1122-31):
  - severe hypertension (systolic BP ≥160 mmHg or diastolic BP ≥110 mmHg)
  - new onset cerebral (e.g. severe headache) or visual abnormalities
  - pulmonary edema
  - progressive renal failure
  - thrombocytopenia (platelets <100,000/mm³)
  - impaired liver function.

  If not treated promptly, it may lead to eclampsia, which nowadays is rarely encountered. In severe preeclampsia the patient should be immediately admitted to the obstetrics department and there should be close cooperation between the obstetrician and the cardiologist. For the treatment of hypertension labetalol is given IV (if it is contraindicated or fails to reduce BP hydralazine should be considered) targeting systolic BP ~140-150 mmHg and diastolic ~90-100 mmHg. For the prevention of convulsions magnesium sulfate is given IV in a dose of 4-6 g over 20 min, followed by a maintenance dose of 1-2 g/h. It should be noted that delivery is the definitive treatment for severe preeclampsia or eclampsia.

Warning! A pregnant woman with systolic BP ≥170 mmHg or diastolic BP ≥110 mmHg requires immediate hospital admission and emergency treatment (Regitz-Zagrosek V, et al. Eur Heart J 2011;32:3147-97)

- Postoperative hypertension with values of systolic BP ≥190 mmHg and/or diastolic BP ≥100 mmHg is usually treated as an emergency. This refers particularly to vascular surgical procedures because of the risk of bursting the sutures in the vessels, interventions for traumatic brain injuries, etc. Factors that contribute to the increase of BP postoperatively are excessive stimulation of the sympathetic nervous system re-

sulting from the stress of the procedure and the postoperative pain, interruption of antihypertensive medication the patient may have been taking before the procedure (e.g. beta-blockers), fluid overload during the
procedure or immediately postoperatively, etc.

Treatment of hypertensive pseudocrises

Hypertensive pseudocrisis is a "benign" deviation of BP (systolic BP ~180-
220 mmHg and/or diastolic BP ~100-120 mmHg) and should not be confused
with hypertensive crisis. In a hypertensive crisis, as has already been stated,
there is a large increase in BP with accompanying acute end-organ damage
(hypertensive emergency) or, if there is no acute damage, the risk of it remains
as long as BP levels are increased (hypertensive urgency). In contrast, a hypertensive pseudocrisis is characterized by milder increases in BP, there is no a-
cute end-organ damage or any immediate threat of it, and hyperstimulation of
the sympathetic nervous system predominates. In addition, specific risk factors
for end-organ damage, such as cardiovascular or chronic renal disease, are
usually absent. Hypertensive pseudocrisis is the most common type of acute
(but not marked) elevation in BP encountered in the Emergency Room. Individuals with hypertensive pseudocrisis are usually anxious, with or without a history
of arterial hypertension. They sometimes complain of headache, or a feeling of
"heat and pressure" in the head, but a more careful evaluation of the history
usually reveals that in most cases the symptoms occurred after the discovery or
announcement of the increase in BP.

The management of hypertensive pseudocrisis includes:
- Clinical evaluation of the individual and recording of an ECG (usually
  without pathological findings).
- Refraining from disclosing the initial high BP level, which can only rein-
  force the anxious reaction and is likely to result in a further increase in BP.
- Reassuring the patient.
- Reevaluation of BP after 15-30 min, assuming that the patient is in a
  calm environment.
- If, during the reevaluation, the systolic BP continues to be >180 mmHg
  or diastolic BP is >100 mmHg, medication is given. It must be stressed,
  however, that these **BP limits should not be taken as absolute criteria
  for the administration of antihypertensive medication** in the Emergency Room: the decision should rather be taken on an individual basis.
  Thus, in a slightly built individual whose usual systolic BP is around 100-
  110 mmHg, the possibility of drug administration should be considered
  when there is a smaller BP increase, e.g. systolic BP ≥170 mmHg.
- The drug of choice for the treatment (at least in the initial phase) of hypertensive pseudocrisis is captopril (Capoten), since it causes a mild
  drop in BP and does not entail the risk of cerebral or myocardial ischemia. It is given orally in a dose of 25 mg (swallowed or sublingual af-

ter chewing). Its action starts within 15-30 min and lasts for 4-6 h. Captopril is contraindicated in moderate or severe renal failure (creatinine >2.5 mg/dL) and in bilateral renal artery stenosis.

- As an alternative to captopril in a patient with coronary artery disease, sublingual nitrates may be given, e.g. isosorbide dinitrate 5 mg, or 1-2 puffs of nitroglycerin spray (i.e. Nitrolingual Pumpspray, one puff delivers 400 μg nitroglycerin).
- In very anxious individuals a supplementary anxiolytic may be given, e.g. diazepam po (2 or 5 mg).
- If the BP remains high despite the administration of captopril (e.g. systolic BP >180 mmHg and/or diastolic BP >100 mmHg) on reevaluation after 1-2 h, additional 25 mg of captopril po or 5 mg of amlodipine (Norvasc) po or 20 mg of furosemide (Lasix, Diuresal) usually IV can be given. The patient is reassessed after 2-3 h and the aim is to achieve a systolic BP ~150-180 mmHg and a diastolic BP <100 mmHg.

Warning! Immediate release nifedipine capsules (5 or 10 mg) should be avoided in the treatment of hypertensive pseudocrisis because they cause a sudden fall in BP, with a risk of cerebral or myocardial ischemia. They used to be given in a dose of 5-10 mg po (usually after breaking the capsule and allowing the contents to be absorbed by the oral mucosa). Their antihypertensive action begins after 5-15 min and lasts 3-5 h.

- Once BP has fallen to <180/100 mmHg and the patient is asymptomatic, they can be discharged, with a recommendation to adopt a salt free diet and to have their BP reevaluated on the following day and treated by the family doctor.

Table 11.3 summarizes the treatment of hypertensive pseudocrisis.

TABLE 11.3	Treatment of hypertensive pseudocrisis

1) Clinical evaluation of the patient and ECG recording
2) Refrain from disclosing the initial high blood pressure (BP) level, reassure the patient
3) Reevaluation of BP after 15-30 min
4) If BP continues to be >180/100 mmHg on reevaluation, captopril is administered in a dose of 25 mg per os (swallowed or sublingual after chewing)
5) As a supplement to captopril, particularly in individuals who are very anxious, an anxiolytic may be given
6) If, despite captopril administration, BP remains high (>180/100 mmHg) on reevaluation at 1-2 h, additional 25 mg of captopril po or 5 mg of amlodipine po or 20 mg of furosemide IV may be given and the patient is reassessed after 2-3 h
7) Once BP has dropped to <180/100 mmHg the patient can be discharged, with a recommendation for salt-free diet and reevaluation by the family doctor

Drugs for the parenteral treatment of hypertensive emergencies

1) Sodium nitroprusside (Nitropress, Niptide)

Shows immediate action (within a few seconds) via vasodilation of the arteries and veins (equal effect on arteries and veins). The effect continues for 2-3 min after administration is stopped.

Dosage: 0.25-10 µg/kg/min, starting with 0.25 µg/kg/min and increasing by 0.2 µg/kg/min every 5 min until the desired result is achieved.

Because of its photosensitivity, the injection solution should be wrapped in aluminum foil and replaced after 4 h with a new solution. Its administration requires great caution in patients with liver or kidney failure. Nitroprusside is metabolized inside red blood cells to cyanides, which are subsequently converted in the liver to thiocyanates that are eliminated by the kidneys (half-life ~7 days). The risk of developing cyanide toxicity (convulsions, confusion) from the accumulation of cyanides increases when it is given in doses >7 µg/kg/min or over a long period (>48 h) and/or there is concomitant kidney or liver failure. Should it become necessary to titrate up to the maximum dosage of 10 µg/kg/min, the infusion duration should be <10 min. Cyanides inhibit oxidative phosphorylation in mitochondria and divert the metabolism to anaerobic with consequent lactic acidosis. Cyanide toxicity is treated with sodium nitrite (10 mL of 3% solution over 3-5 min IV) followed by an infusion of sodium thiosulfate (12.5 g in 50 mL of D/W 5% over 10 min IV).

Preparation of solution and infusion: 50 mg nitroprusside are dissolved in 100 mL D/W 5%, and in an individual weighing 70 kg the infusion begins at a rate of 2 mL/h (~0.25 µg/kg/min) with a gradual increase in dosage by about 2 mL/h every 5 min, depending on the response (more in Chapter 23).

2) Nitroglycerin (Nitro-Bid, Tridil)

This is less effective than nitroprusside as regards BP reduction. It is preferred in cases with myocardial ischemia. It causes vasodilation of the veins and to a lesser degree the arteries (including the coronary arteries). Its effect starts within 2-5 min and the half-life in plasma is ~3 min.

Dosage: 5-200 µg/min IV, starting with 5-10 µg/min and increasing by 5-10 µg/min every 5-10 min until the therapeutic goal is achieved or the maximum dose of 200 µg/min is reached.

Adverse effects: headache and rarely methemoglobinemia*, which

---

*Methemoglobin is an oxidized form of hemoglobin (contains ferric iron [Fe^{3+}]) which has a decreased ability to transport oxygen. It is normally present in a proportion of <1% of total hemoglobin. At levels >10-15% cyanosis, dyspnea, etc. may appear. Symptomatic patients or patients with methemoglobin levels >30% despite being asymptomatic should be treated with methylene blue (1-2 mg/kg IV within 5 min).

may be observed when nitroglycerin is administered for >48 h or in large doses.

Preparation of solution and infusion: 25 mg nitroglycerin are dissolved in 250 mL D/W 5% (solution concentration 100 μg/mL). The infusion begins at a rate of 3-6 mL/h (5-10 μg/min), subsequently increasing by 3-6 mL/h every 5-10 min, depending on the patient's response. The maximum dosage is 120 mL/h (200 μg/min). For more information see Chapter 23.

3) Enalaprilat (Vasotec)

This is an angiotensin-converting enzyme inhibitor. Its action starts within 15 min and lasts 6-12 h. The dosage is 0.625-5 mg IV every 6 h administered over 5 min.

The advantage of this drug is the shifting of the autoregulation curve towards lower BP levels, avoiding cerebral ischemia due to a large drop in BP.

4) Labetalol (Trandate)

This has a combined alpha- and beta-blocker action. During intravenous administration the ratio of β- to α-receptor blockade is 7:1. It may be given:

- By repeated bolus IV injections: initial dose of 20 mg over 2 min and repeated doses of 40-80 mg every 15 min until the therapeutic result is achieved (maximum cumulative or daily dose is 300 mg).
- By continuous IV administration: start with 1-2 mg/min (titrated up to 10 mg/min if required) [maximum cumulative or daily dose is 300 mg].

Its action starts within 5-10 min and lasts 3-6 h. The half-life is ~5.5 h. Because of its long half-life, administration in repeated bolus injections is preferable.

Adverse effects: bronchospasm, orthostatic hypotension, bradycardia, etc.

Contraindications: as for beta-blockers.

Preparation of solution for continuous infusion: 200 mg labetalol (available in vials of 20 and 40 mL containing 100 and 200 mg labetalol, respectively) are added to 160 mL D/W 5% (the resultant solution has a concentration of 1 mg/mL) and given at initial rate of 60-120 mL/h (1-2 mg/min).

5) Phentolamine (Regitine, OraVerse)

This blocks the α-adrenergic receptors. It is given in a dose of 5-15 mg IV. Its effect starts within 1-2 min and lasts 10-30 min.

The main indication is hypertensive pheochromocytoma crisis.

Warning! Beta-blockers are never given as monotherapy for hypertensive pheochromocytoma crisis because they cause further worsening of hypertension by unopposed stimulation of the α-receptors. They may be given, however, provided that alpha-blockers have been administered first, for the treatment of any tachyarrhythmias.

6) Hydralazine (Apresoline)

This has a powerful vasodilatory action on the arteries. Its effect starts within 10-20 min and lasts for 3-8 h. It is given IV in a dose of 10-20 mg over 1-2 min, repeated every 30 min until the desired result is achieved.

Hydralazine causes reflex tachycardia. Because of its prolonged and unpredictable antihypertensive action, it is rarely used today for the treatment of hypertensive crisis. It is a second choice agent for treating severe preeclampsia.

7) Fenoldopam (Corlopam)

This causes peripheral vasodilation by stimulating the dopaminergic D_1 receptors. It has the unique advantage of mediating vasodilation of the renal arteries, by acting on the dopaminergic D_1 receptors of the proximal and distal tubules (10 times more potent than dopamine), and it impedes the reabsorption of sodium, promoting natriuresis and diuresis.

Its effect starts within 5 min and lasts 30-60 min. It is given IV in an initial dose of 0.1 µg/kg/min, increasing every 15 min until control of the hypertension is achieved (maximum dose 0.3 µg/kg/min).

Fenoldopam should be administered with caution in patients with coronary artery disease (causes reflex tachycardia) and in patients with glaucoma (increases intraocular pressure). No rebound of hypertension is observed when administration is stopped.

8) Nicardipine (Cardene)

This is a second-generation dihydropyridine calcium antagonist with high selectivity for vessels. It has a powerful vasodilator effect on the cerebral and coronary vessels, which reduces cerebral and myocardial ischemia.

Its effect starts within 5-15 min and lasts for 4-6 h. It is given IV in an initial dose of 5 mg/h, and the administration rate is increased by 2.5 mg/h every 5 min until the desired BP reduction is achieved (maximum dose 15 mg/h).

9) Esmolol (Brevibloc)

This is an ultra-short-acting cardioselective beta1-blocker with a half-life of 9 min and duration of action 10-20 min after administration is stopped. Its effect starts within 1-2 min.

It is given in a loading dose of 500 µg/kg over 1 min, followed by a maintenance dose of 50-300 µg/kg/min.

For continuous IV administration there are ready–made solutions of esmolol in 250 mL (10 mg/mL) and 100 mL (20 mg/mL) bags of NaCl 0.9%.

The method of administering esmolol is described in detail in Chapter 23.

Table 11.4 shows the dosage schemes of the drugs administered for hypertensive emergencies, and Table 11.5 shows the particularization of antihypertensive treatment based on the underlying disease.

TABLE 11.4	Antihypertensive drugs used for the treatment of hypertensive emergencies.		
Drug	**Dose**	**Onset of action**	**Duration of action**
Enalaprilat	0.625-5 mg over 5 min every 6 h	15 min	6-12 h
Esmolol	500 µg/kg over 1 min, initial infusion 50 µg/kg/min, increasing by 50 µg/kg/min every 4 min up to a maximum dose of 300 µg/kg/min	1-2 min	10-20 min
Fenoldopam	0.1-0.3 µg/kg/min	<5 min	30-60 min
Hydralazine	10-20 mg over 1-2 min, repeat every 30 min until the desired result is achieved	10-20 min	3-8 h
Labetalol	• 20 mg over 2 min, 40-80 mg repeated every 15 min (maximum cumulative or daily dose is 300 mg) • start with 1-2 mg/min and then titrate up to 10 mg/min if required (maximum cumulative or daily dose is 300 mg)	5-10 min	3-6 h
Nicardipine	5-15 mg/h	5-15 min	4-6 h
Nitroglycerin	5-10 µg/min, increasing by 5-10 µg/min every 5-10 min up to a maximum dose of 200 µg/min	2-5 min	5-10 min
Nitroprusside	0.25 µg/kg/min, increasing by 0.2 µg/kg/min every 5 min up to a maximum dose of 10 µg/kg/min	Immediate	2-3 min
Phentolamine	5-15 mg IV	1-2 min	10-30 min

TABLE 11.5	Specific antihypertensive drugs for hypertensive emergencies

Disease	Preferred drug	Comments
Acute pulmonary edema	Nitroglycerin, nitroprusside	Administration of nitroprusside at the lowest effective dose to avoid cyanide toxicity
Acute coronary syndrome	Nitroglycerin, beta-blocker	Avoid nitroprusside because of the risk of causing coronary steal phenomenon
Acute aortic dissection	Esmolol ± nitroprusside, labetalol	Target systolic BP ~100-120 mmHg within 10 min. The beta-blocker precedes the nitroprusside
Hypertensive encephalopathy	Labetalol, nicardipine, fenoldopam, nitroprusside	
Acute ischemic stroke	Labetalol, nicardipine	Administered in the acute phase only if the BP is >220/120 mmHg or >185/100 mmHg when fibrinolysis is to be given
Pheochromocytoma crisis	Phentolamine ± beta-blocker, labetalol, nitroprusside	Avoid beta-blockers unless alpha-blocker is given first
Severe preeclampsia or eclampsia	Labetalol (first choice), hydralazine	Magnesium sulfate is also given for the prevention/treatment of convulsions. If it fails, diazepam is given
Cessation of clonidine	Labetalol	
Cocaine overdose	Benzodiazepine ± nitroglycerin, benzodiazepine ± phentolamine	Avoid beta-blocker (risk of worsening hypertension and causing coronary artery spasm)
Postoperative hypertension	Labetalol, nitroglycerin, esmolol, nicardipine	

BP: blood pressure

Key points

■ The term hypertensive crisis refers to both hypertensive emergencies and hypertensive urgencies.

■ A sudden and marked increase in BP (usually diastolic BP >120-130 mmHg and/or systolic BP >200 mmHg) is classified as:
  a) a hypertensive emergency if it is accompanied by acute or rapidly progressive end-organ damage or
  b) a hypertensive urgency if it is not accompanied by acute or rapidly progressive end-organ damage.

■ In hypertensive emergencies BP reduction (but not to normal levels) needs to be achieved within 30-60 min with IV antihypertensive agents and hospital admission is always required.

■ In hypertensive urgencies BP reduction (to "near normal" levels) needs to be achieved gradually within 12-24 h with oral antihypertensive agents and admission is not required as far as follow up care is ensured.

■ The criterion for the rate of BP reduction in an acute elevation in BP is the degree to which target organs are affected (the most important factor), the BP level, the presence of symptoms, the rate of BP increase, and the previous history of hypertension.

■ The main hypertensive emergencies that require immediate treatment, even if BP levels do not meet the definition, are acute pulmonary edema, acute coronary syndrome, acute aortic dissection, and severe preeclampsia or eclampsia.

■ In a hypertensive emergency apart from the case of acute aortic dissection, immediate BP reduction to normal levels should not be sought: the reduction should rather take place gradually (reduction of BP to levels ~160/100 mmHg within 30-60 min).

■ In acute ischemic stroke BP reduction should be sought only if it is >220/120 mmHg, or >185/100 mmHg if fibrinolysis is to be administered.

■ A pregnant woman with BP ≥170/110 mmHg needs emergency treatment.

Key points - *continued*

- Hypertensive pseudocrisis is the most common type of acute (but not marked) elevation in BP encountered in the Emergency Room. It is a usually asymptomatic increase in BP (systolic BP ~180-220 mmHg and/or diastolic BP ~100-120 mmHg) without associated acute target organ damage. In this case the main goal of treatment is to reassure the patient and, if the hypertension persists (>180/100 mmHg), captopril is given in a dose of 25 mg po.

- The goal in the treatment of hypertensive pseudocrisis is to achieve a systolic BP <180/100 mmHg within few hours.

- In the treatment of hypertensive urgencies or hypertensive pseudocrises administration of nifedipine in a capsule form should be avoided, because of the risk of causing cerebral or myocardial ischemia due to a sudden drop in BP.

- The administration of nitroprusside for the treatment of hypertensive emergencies in doses >7 µg/kg/min significantly increases the risk of developing cyanide toxicity. Administration of the maximum dose of 10 µg/kg/min should not be continued for longer than 10 min.

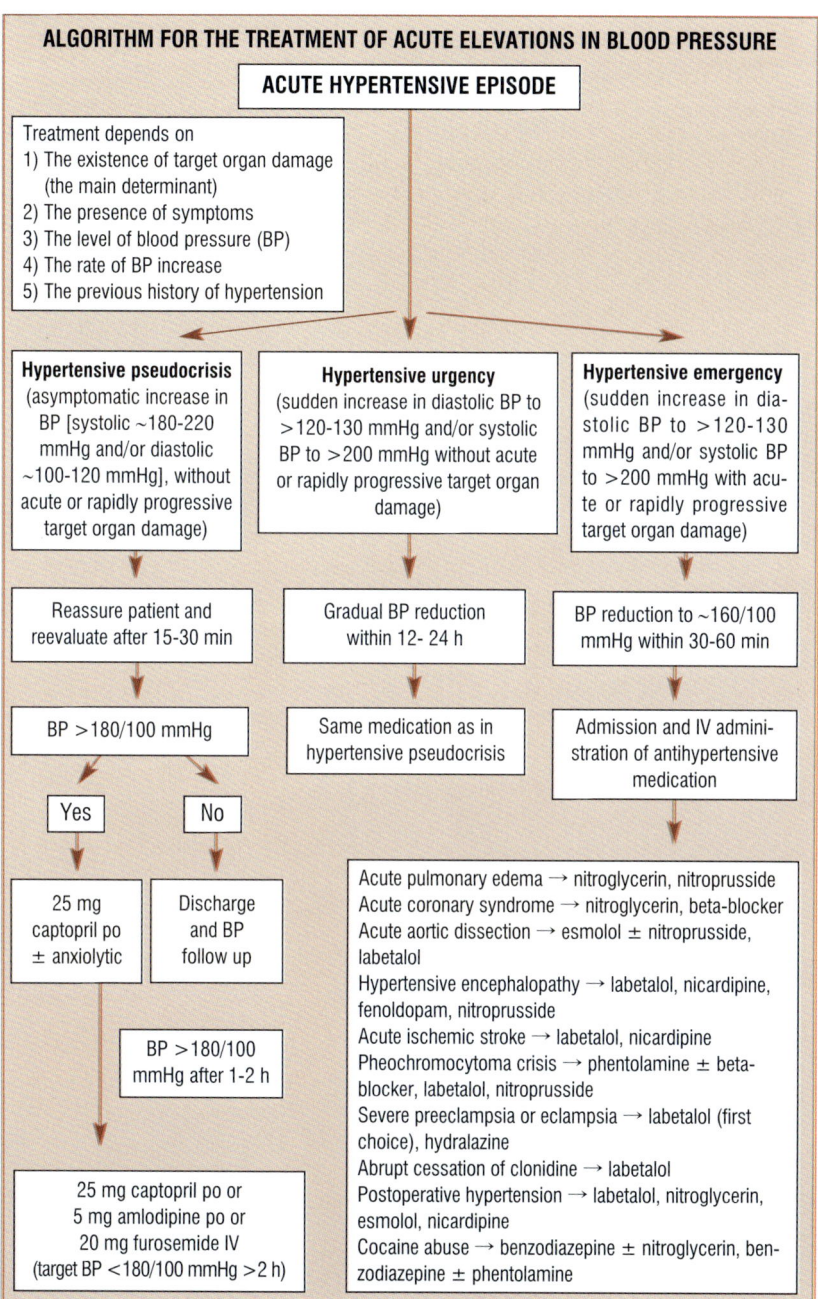

ALGORITHM FOR THE TREATMENT OF ACUTE ELEVATIONS IN BLOOD PRESSURE

ACUTE HYPERTENSIVE EPISODE

Treatment depends on
1) The existence of target organ damage
   (the main determinant)
2) The presence of symptoms
3) The level of blood pressure (BP)
4) The rate of BP increase
5) The previous history of hypertension

Hypertensive pseudocrisis
(asymptomatic increase in BP [systolic ~180-220 mmHg and/or diastolic ~100-120 mmHg], without acute or rapidly progressive target organ damage)

Hypertensive urgency
(sudden increase in diastolic BP to >120-130 mmHg and/or systolic BP to >200 mmHg without acute or rapidly progressive target organ damage)

Hypertensive emergency
(sudden increase in diastolic BP to >120-130 mmHg and/or systolic BP to >200 mmHg with acute or rapidly progressive target organ damage)

Reassure patient and reevaluate after 15-30 min

Gradual BP reduction within 12-24 h

BP reduction to ~160/100 mmHg within 30-60 min

BP >180/100 mmHg

Same medication as in hypertensive pseudocrisis

Admission and IV administration of antihypertensive medication

Yes   No

25 mg captopril po ± anxiolytic

Discharge and BP follow up

BP >180/100 mmHg after 1-2 h

Acute pulmonary edema → nitroglycerin, nitroprusside
Acute coronary syndrome → nitroglycerin, beta-blocker
Acute aortic dissection → esmolol ± nitroprusside, labetalol
Hypertensive encephalopathy → labetalol, nicardipine, fenoldopam, nitroprusside
Acute ischemic stroke → labetalol, nicardipine
Pheochromocytoma crisis → phentolamine ± beta-blocker, labetalol, nitroprusside
Severe preeclampsia or eclampsia → labetalol (first choice), hydralazine
Abrupt cessation of clonidine → labetalol
Postoperative hypertension → labetalol, nitroglycerin, esmolol, nicardipine
Cocaine abuse → benzodiazepine ± nitroglycerin, benzodiazepine ± phentolamine

25 mg captopril po or
5 mg amlodipine po or
20 mg furosemide IV
(target BP <180/100 mmHg >2 h)

BP limits should not be taken as absolute criteria and should be individualized

12

Hypokalemia

The term "**hypokalemia**" refers to a drop in serum potassium levels to <3.5 mEq/L. Hypokalemia is not always the same as kaliopenia, because the fall in potassium may be due to intracellular shifting (as in the case of alkalosis), with no significant change in the overall amount of potassium in the body. Generally, a decrease in serum potassium level by 1 mEq/L corresponds to a potassium deficit of ~300 mEq, if the blood pH is normal. Ninety-eight percent of the body's potassium is located intracellularly. The average daily requirements for potassium are 50-100 mEq. Ninety percent of dietary potassium is eliminated by the kidneys and the remaining 10% by the intestine.

The transmembrane movement of potassium ions depends on the following factors:

- The sodium pump (Na^+/K^+-ATPase), which imports two potassium ions (K^+) and exports three sodium ions (Na^+) from the cell and which is activated through the β_2-receptors. These receptors are activated by catecholamines, insulin and β_2-agonist-type bronchodilators, such as salbutamol.
- The hydrogen ion (H^+) concentration. Alkalosis can cause hypokalemia, as the H^+ moving from the intracellular to the extracellular space in order to "normalize" the pH are replaced by an inflow of K^+ into the cells.

The causes of hypokalemia are listed in Table 12.1. The use of diuretics is the most common cause of hypokalemia. Of the thiazide diuretics, chlorthalidone (Hygroton) is the one that causes the most severe hy-

TABLE 12.1	Causes of hypokalemia

1) Kidney disease: acute tubular necrosis (increased potassium elimination during recovery phase), etc.

2) Use of diuretics (the most common cause): thiazides (e.g. hydrochlorothiazide, chlorthalidone, metolazone), loop diuretics (e.g. furosemide, bumetanide, torsemide).

3) Use of mineralocorticoids: corticosteroids, etc.

4) Increased secretion of aldosterone: Conn's syndrome, secondary hyperaldosteronism (heart failure, dehydration, liver failure), etc.

5) Intracellular influx of potassium ions: metabolic alkalosis, β_2-receptor activation (catecholamines, insulin or salbutamol-type bronchodilators), etc.

6) Gastrointestinal loss of potassium: diarrhea (70-80 mEq/L eliminated), vomiting (5-10 mEq/L eliminated), etc.

7) Reduced dietary intake of potassium

pokalemia because it has the longest duration of action (48-72 h). In order to avoid hypokalemia, doses >12.5 mg daily should be avoided.

Symptoms – Signs

Cases of moderate or severe hypokalemia (potassium levels <3.0 mEq/L) will present with muscle weakness, fatigue, muscle cramps, palpitations due to ventricular extrasystolic arrhythmia (particularly when there is concurrent administration of digoxin, since hypokalemia potentiates the effect of digoxin and arrhythmogenesis in cases of digitalis toxicity) and gastrointestinal disorders (constipation, ileus).

ECG

Flat or inverted T waves, prominent U waves, ST-segment depression, prolonged QT (actually QU) and PR intervals, 2nd degree atrioventricular block, complete atrioventricular block (rarely) and arrhythmogenesis (especially on a substrate of acute myocardial ischemia) that may lead to the development of ventricular tachycardia and ventricular fibrillation.

Laboratory tests

Urea, creatinine, glucose, sodium, potassium, magnesium serum levels and complete blood count (to exclude anemia in case of fatigue). If alkalosis is suspected then the pH should be determined (arterial blood gases measurement).

Treatment

- With mild (potassium levels 3.0-3.4 mEq/L) or moderate (potassium levels 2.5-2.9 mEq/L) hypokalemia, it is usually sufficient to recommend potassium-rich foods (for example, one banana contains 10 mEq, one orange 9 mEq of potassium). Potassium supplements may also be administered as adjunctive oral treatment, e.g. potassium gluconate syrup, potassium chloride effervescent tablets, etc. In addition, loop diuretics (e.g. 40 mg furosemide tablets) are replaced by potassium-sparing diuretics (e.g. 40 mg furosemide + 5 mg amiloride tablets). In cases of hyperaldosteronism, spironolactone (Aldactone) is administered (25-100 mg/day). Lastly, in hospitalized cardiac patients who are susceptible to arrhythmias (e.g. patients with acute myocardial ischemia), faster correction of potassium levels is sought with IV administration of potassium solutions (see below).
- In cases of severe hypokalemia (potassium levels <2.5 mEq/L), or less severe hypokalemia associated with digitalis toxicity or occurrence of arrhythmias or patients unable to take potassium orally, potassium solutions are administered intravenously. Discovery of severe hypokalemia in an Emergency Room patient is grounds for hospitalization. Table 12.2 presents the conditions for safe IV administration of potassium solutions.

Practical instructions for IV administration of potassium

If 10 mL ampoules of 10% KCl are used (each ampoule contains ~13.5 mEq of potassium), then 4 ampoules of KCl are added to 1000 mL of 0.9% NaCl (or to 1000 mL of 5% D/W for cardiac patients, e.g. patients with congestive heart failure, hypertension, etc.). The resulting solution has a concentration of 54 mEq/L and can be administered at a rate of 100 mL/h (equivalent to 5.4 mEq/h). In cases of very severe hypokalemia or hypokalemia complicated by arrhythmia, more concentrated solutions may be

TABLE 12.2	Conditions for safe IV administration of potassium solutions

1) Prepare a 40-60 mEq/L potassium solution (concentrations of 60-100 mEq/L are also used on rare occasions)
2) The rate of infusion of the potassium solution should be <20 mEq/h. If hypokalemia is associated with ECG abnormalities or neuromuscular complications, then the solution may be administered at a rate of up to 40 mEq/h
3) Continuous ECG monitoring (especially for infusion rates >10 mEq/h) and frequent measurement of potassium levels (e.g. at 4 h after starting the infusion) are required

used, e.g. 4 ampoules of KCl in 500 mL of 0.9% NaCl or 5% D/W (concentration 108 mEq/L), and administered at a rate of 100-150 mL/h (~11-16 mEq/h). At the end of the infusion, potassium levels are measured and are used to determine further administration. Generally, administration of potassium in normal saline is preferable to administration in a glucose drip, because glucose can cause a transient decrease in serum potassium by stimulating the secretion of insulin.

Hypomagnesemia

The term hypomagnesemia describes a fall in serum magnesium levels to <1.5 mEq/L. Daily requirements for magnesium are ~20 mEq; this is eliminated renally. For cardiac patients, the most common cause of hypomagnesemia is the use of diuretics and therefore hypokalemia is often present as well.

In cases of severe hypomagnesemia (magnesium levels <1.0 mEq/L), magnesium is replenished by IV administration. This is usually given as a magnesium sulfate solution, at a rate of 1 mEq/kg of magnesium IV over the first 24 h. Therefore, a 70 kg person will receive 70 mEq, which are equivalent to ~9 g of magnesium sulfate (1 g of hydrated magnesium sulfate contains 8 mEq of magnesium). Magnesium sulfate for IV administration is available in various concentrations, i.e. 25% in 10 mL ampoules (provides 2 mEq/mL of Mg), 50% in 10 mL ampoules (provides 4 mEq/mL of Mg), etc. If we use the 25% ampoules, then 4 ampoules are added to 1000 mL of 0.9% NaCl or 5% D/W and the resulting solution is administered at a rate of 40 mL/h.

Table 12.3 lists the "cardiology settings" where magnesium is administered intravenously.

TABLE 12.3	"Cardiology settings" in which IV magnesium is administered

1) Severe hypomagnesemia (magnesium levels <1.0 mEq/L): 1 mEq/kg of IV magnesium over the first 24 h (4 ampoules* of magnesium sulfate in 1000 mL of 0.9% NaCl or 5% D/W at a rate of 40 mL/h)
2) Ventricular arrhythmias due to digitalis toxicity: 2 g of magnesium sulfate (~1 ampoule*) over 2 min (if anti-digoxin antibodies, the treatment of choice, are not immediately available)
3) Torsades de pointes: 2 g of magnesium sulfate (~1 ampoule*) over 2 min and, if arrhythmia persists, repeat after 10 min
4) Severe preeclampsia or eclampsia (prevention or treatment of seizures): 4-6 g (2 ampoules* of magnesium sulfate in 100 mL of 0.9% NaCl or 5% D/W) over 20 min, followed by a maintenance dose of 1-2 g/h

10 mL ampoule of 25% magnesium sulfate

Warning! In cases of hypokalemia, serum magnesium levels should always be examined as well. Furthermore, hypokalemia refractory to replacement therapy should be grounds to suspect magnesium depletion.

 Key points

- The most common cause of hypokalemia in cardiac patients is the use of diuretics (thiazide or loop).

- In cases of moderate or mild hypokalemia, potassium replenishment is achieved through the consumption of potassium-rich foods or oral potassium supplements.

- In cases of severe hypokalemia (potassium <2.5 mEq/L), potassium levels are corrected by IV administration of potassium solutions. The same treatment is used in cases of moderate or mild hypokalemia in hospitalized cardiac patients who are susceptible to arrhythmias, e.g. because of acute myocardial ischemia.

- For IV administration of potassium solutions, the concentration should be <60 mEq/L and the rate of infusion should be <20 mEq/h.

- Hypokalemia is often accompanied by hypomagnesemia.

ALGORITHM FOR THE TREATMENT OF HYPOKALEMIA

HYPOKALEMIA
(serum potassium <3.5 mEq/L)

Initial actions
- Determination of Na, K, Mg, creatinine, urea, glucose and pH (if alkalosis is suspected)
- Record ECG
- Gross neurological assessment

Major causes
- Use of diuretics (most common cause)
- Hypersecretion of aldosterone
- Metabolic alkalosis
- Diarrhea, vomiting

Mild or moderate hypokalemia
(potassium = 2.5-3.5 mEq/L)

Severe hypokalemia
(potassium <2.5 mE/L)
or
Hypokalemia + arrhythmias

- Potassium-rich foods
- PO administration of potassium supplements
- Discontinue diuretics and replace with potassium-sparing diuretics
- Spironolactone in case of hyperaldosteronism
- In hospitalized cardiac patients, usually IV KCl solution

IV administration of KCl solution

- The solution should have a potassium concentration <60 mEq/L (or 60-100 mEq/L in special cases)
- The infusion rate must be <20 mEq/h (or 20-40 mEq/h in special cases)

Continuous ECG monitoring

- 4 ampoules of 10% KCl in 1000 mL of 0.9% NaCl (or 5% D/W in cardiac patients) at a rate of 100 mL/h or
- 4 ampoules of 10% KCl in 500 mL of 0.9% NaCl or 5% D/W at a rate of 100-150 mL/h in cases of arrhythmogenic complications

13 Hyperkalemia

The term "**hyperkalemia**" refers to an increase in serum potassium levels to >5.5 mEq/L, caused by:
- Inability to eliminate potassium by the kidneys (the primary route of elimination), or
- Potassium efflux from the cells due to:
  - transmembrane exchange with H^+ in cases of acidosis (export of K^+ and import of H^+) or
  - cellular destruction.

The possibility of pseudohyperkalemia should be ruled out; this might occur in cases of:
- Excessive thrombocytosis (platelets $>10^6/mm^3$) or leukocytosis (leukocytes >50,000/mm^3), caused by release of potassium in the serum during *in vitro* coagulation (degranulation of platelets or white cell lysis, respectively).
- Hemolysis of the blood sample.

The causes of hyperkalemia are listed in Table 13.1. Hyperkalemia is classified as mild (potassium=5.5–6.0 mEq/L), moderate (potassium=6.1–6.9 mEq/L) or severe (potassium ≥7.0 mEq/L).

Symptoms – Signs
Muscle weakness, weakened or abolished reflexes, paresthesias and cardiac arrhythmias.

ECG
- Potassium levels 6.0-7.0 mEq/L: peaked and tall T waves, more prominent in the precordial leads V_2-V_4 (the earliest change).

TABLE 13.1	Causes of hyperkalemia

1) Renal failure (chronic or acute)

2) Metabolic acidosis (reduction of the pH by 0.1 units will cause an increase in potassium by 0.7 mEq/L)

3) Addison's disease (primary adrenal insufficiency)

4) Cellular destruction and release of potassium (hemolysis, burns, chemotherapy, rhabdomyolysis, muscle contusions)

5) Use of potassium-sparing drugs (amiloride, spironolactone, eplerenone, angiotensin-converting enzyme inhibitors, angiotensin II receptor blockers) and especially in cases of renal failure

6) Digitalis toxicity

7) Pseudohyperkalemia (note that plasma concentration of potassium is normal)

- Potassium levels 7.0-8.0 mEq/L: PR interval prolongation, followed by disappearance of P waves.
- Potassium levels >8.0 mEq/L: QRS complex widening, 2nd or 3rd degree atrioventricular block, ventricular fibrillation and asystole (Figure 13.1).

Warning! The ECG is not very sensitive in detecting hyperkalemia. Almost 50% of patients with potassium levels >6.5 mEq/L do not present ECG changes characteristic of hyperkalemia. This happens most often when hyperkalemia develops slowly.

Laboratory tests

Urea, creatinine, glucose, sodium, potassium, aspartate aminotransferase (to rule out pseudohyperkalemia), creatine kinase (in cases of suspected rhabdomyolysis), digoxin serum levels (in cases of suspected digitalis toxicity) and complete blood count. If acidosis is suspected then the pH should be determined (arterial blood gases measurement).

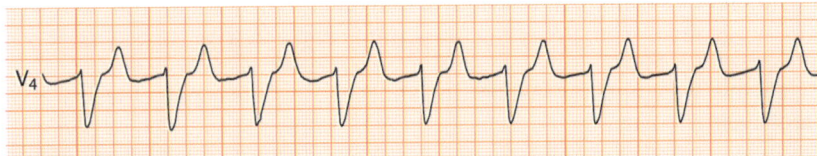

Figure 13.1. ECG (lead V_4) showing widening of QRS complexes (~240 ms) and disappearance of P waves in an 80-year-old woman with severe hyperkalemia secondary to acute severe renal failure (serum potassium levels = 8.3 mEq/L and creatinine levels = 6.9 mg/dL).

Treatment

- Discontinue potassium-sparing drugs.
- Administer the potassium exchange resin, sodium polystyrene sulfonate (Kayexalate, available in vials containing 454 g of powder for suspension), in a dose of 15-30 g in 50-100 mL 20% sorbitol either orally or by enema in nonemergency situations. This may be repeated every 6 h, if necessary. Note that enema should be retained in the intestine for at least 30-60 min. Each gram binds ~1 mEq of potassium and releases 1-2 mEq of sodium in the intestine. Great care is needed in individuals with congestive heart failure (risk of sodium overload). Due to the concern that sorbitol may increase the risk of intestinal necrosis, solutions with sorbitol should be used with great caution.
  Onset of action >1 h and duration of action 4-6 h.
- Administer 250 mL of a 10% D/W solution or 50 mL of a 50% D/W solution to which 10 units of regular insulin have been added, over 15-30 min. Insulin promotes the cellular uptake of potassium by activating the sodium pump (Na^+/K^+-ATPase; imports 2 K^+ and exports 3 Na^+).
  Onset of action >15-30 min and duration of action 4-6 h.
- Inhaled β_2-agonists. Nebulized salbutamol (US: albuterol) in a dose of 10-20 mg over 15 min. It is particularly useful for renal patients who should not ingest liquids, but must be avoided in coronary patients because it causes tachycardia. The decrease in potassium is achieved through β_2-receptor activation, which leads to activation of the sodium pump and stimulation of insulin secretion. It can usually reduce potassium levels by 0.5-1 mEq/L.
  Onset of action >15-30 min and duration of action 2-3 h.
- Administer calcium gluconate (10 mL of a 10% solution) or calcium chloride (~3 mL of a 10% solution) IV over 5 min if potassium levels are ≥6.5 mEq/L and there are concomitant ECG changes, i.e. disappearance of P waves, QRS complex widening, etc. If the ECG changes do not improve the same dose can be repeated every 10 min until the ECG normalizes. The 10 mL ampoule of 10% calcium gluconate contains 4.6 mEq of calcium, whereas the 10 mL ampoule of 10% calcium chloride contains 13.6 mEq of calcium; this means that one calcium chloride ampoule has three times the amount of calcium as an ampoule of calcium gluconate.

Warning! When an IV calcium solution is administered, the physician should give clear instructions as to the type of solution (gluconate or chloride) and the precise amount, rather than just ordering "an ampoule of calcium".

TABLE 13.2	IV administration of agents for immediate or rapid correction of severe hyperkalemia			
Agent	**Dosage**		**Onset of action**	**Duration of action**
Protection of the myocardium (if potassium ≥6.5 mEq/L + ECG changes)				
• Calcium gluconate or	• 10 mL of 10% calcium gluconate over 5 min		• <5 min	• 30-60 min
• Calcium chloride	• ~3 mL of 10% calcium chloride over 5 min		• <5 min	• 30-60 min
Inflow of potassium into the cells				
• Glucose + regular insulin	• 250 mL of 10% D/W or 50 mL of 50% D/W + 10 U of regular insulin over 15-30 min		• 15-30 min	• 4-6 h
• Sodium bicarbonate (if potassium ≥6.5 mEq/L + severe metabolic acidosis)	• ~50 mEq over 5-10 min		• 15-30 min	• 1-2 h
Elimination of potassium by the kidneys (provided there is no renal failure)				
• Furosemide	• 20-80 mg		• >30 min	• 4 h

Administration is performed under continuous ECG monitoring. When the ECG findings of hyperkalemia disappear or bradycardia develops, the administration is discontinued. Great care is needed in individuals receiving digoxin (may enhance its arrhythmogenic effect) and the same IV line should not be used for bicarbonate solutions (water-insoluble calcium salts will form). Note that calcium solutions do not affect potassium levels, but only antagonize its effect on the myocardium.

Onset of action <5 min and duration of action 30-60 min.

• Consider administering ~50 mEq sodium bicarbonate ($NaHCO_3$) IV over 5-10 min only if elevated potassium levels (i.e. ≥6.5 mEq/L) are associa-

ted with severe metabolic acidosis (i.e. pH <7.2). The decrease in potassium is a result of transmembrane exchange of H^+ (outflow) with K^+ (inflow). In patients with renal failure there is a risk of hypernatremia.
Onset of potassium decrease >15-30 min and duration 1-2 h.

- Administer 20-80 mg furosemide IV (in cases of good renal function) to promote potassium elimination from the kidneys.
- Hemodialysis or peritoneal dialysis in cases of acute renal failure or decompensation of chronic renal failure.
- Admission for cardiac monitoring and continuation of treatment if hyperkalemia is:
  - symptomatic
  - associated with ECG changes other than peaked T waves
  - severe (potassium levels ≥7.0 mEq/L)
  - associated with other severe medical conditions, i.e. acute worsening of renal failure.

Table 13.2 lists the agents that are administered IV for the immediate or rapid treatment of severe hyperkalemia.

✓ Key points

- The most common cause of hyperkalemia in cardiac patients is the use of potassium-sparing drugs with (more commonly) or without coexistent renal failure.

- In order to decrease potassium levels in cases of severe hyperkalemia, the goal is:
  - to increase the inflow of potassium into the cells (glucose drip with regular insulin, inhaled β_2-agonists, sodium bicarbonate in cases of severe metabolic acidosis), and
  - to promote potassium elimination by the kidneys (furosemide IV) or the intestine (ion-exchange resin, administered orally or by retention enema).

- If high potassium levels (i.e. ≥6.5 mEq/L) are associated with ECG changes, the first drug to be administered IV should be calcium (gluconate or chloride) because of its rapid onset of action and ability to stabilize myocyte electrical activity.

- Routine use of sodium bicarbonate in hyperkalemia is not recommended. Consider it only if elevated potassium levels are associated with severe metabolic acidosis.

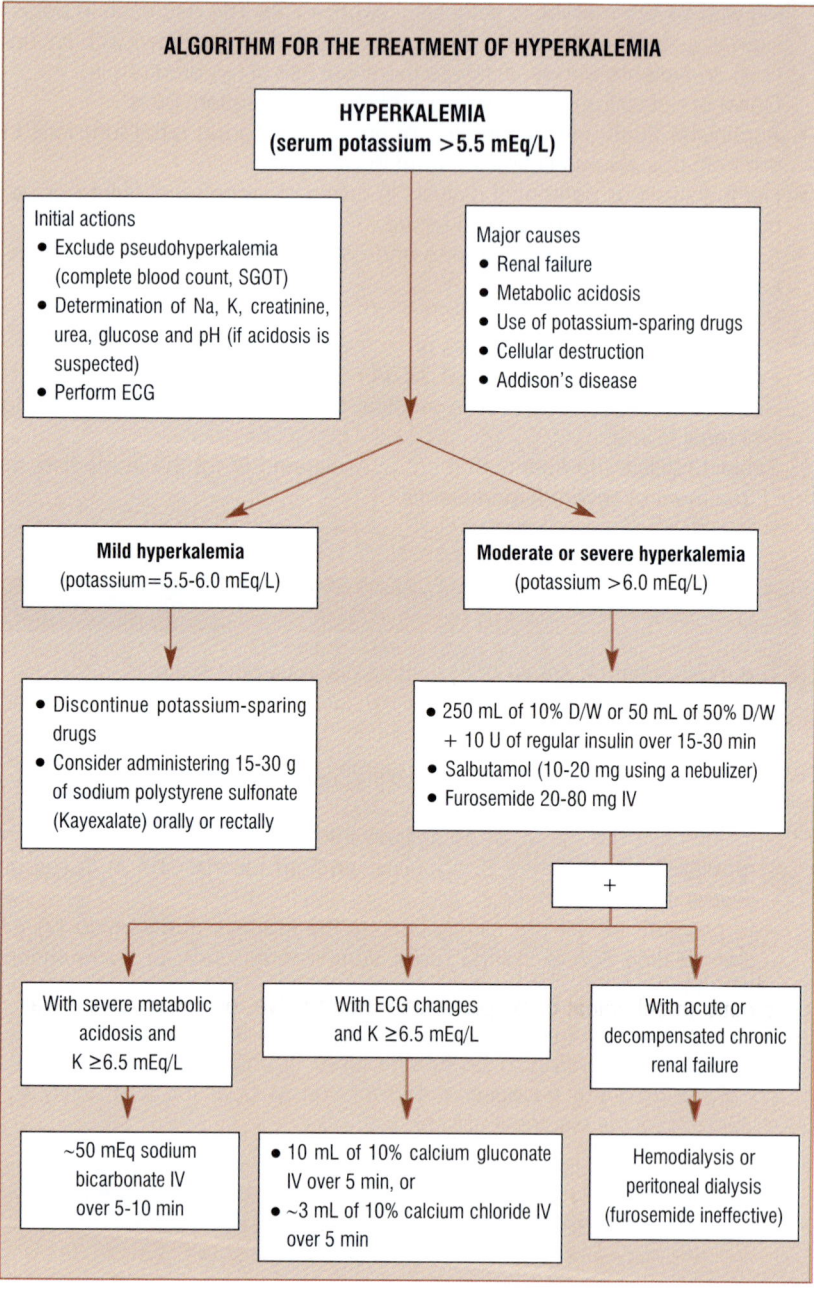

ALGORITHM FOR THE TREATMENT OF HYPERKALEMIA

HYPERKALEMIA
(serum potassium >5.5 mEq/L)

Initial actions
- Exclude pseudohyperkalemia (complete blood count, SGOT)
- Determination of Na, K, creatinine, urea, glucose and pH (if acidosis is suspected)
- Perform ECG

Major causes
- Renal failure
- Metabolic acidosis
- Use of potassium-sparing drugs
- Cellular destruction
- Addison's disease

Mild hyperkalemia
(potassium=5.5-6.0 mEq/L)

Moderate or severe hyperkalemia
(potassium >6.0 mEq/L)

- Discontinue potassium-sparing drugs
- Consider administering 15-30 g of sodium polystyrene sulfonate (Kayexalate) orally or rectally

- 250 mL of 10% D/W or 50 mL of 50% D/W + 10 U of regular insulin over 15-30 min
- Salbutamol (10-20 mg using a nebulizer)
- Furosemide 20-80 mg IV

+

With severe metabolic acidosis and K ≥6.5 mEq/L

With ECG changes and K ≥6.5 mEq/L

With acute or decompensated chronic renal failure

~50 mEq sodium bicarbonate IV over 5-10 min

- 10 mL of 10% calcium gluconate IV over 5 min, or
- ~3 mL of 10% calcium chloride IV over 5 min

Hemodialysis or peritoneal dialysis (furosemide ineffective)

14

Atrial fibrillation

Atrial fibrillation (AF) is the most common sustained cardiac arrhythmia. Its incidence increases with advancing age and varies between 5-10% in people aged >70 years. It is characterized by chaotic electrical activity in the atria that leads to a loss of atrial systole. The ventricular response is completely irregular and usually varies between 100-160 beats/min in people who are not taking bradycardic medication and have normal atrioventricular conduction. The main complication of this arrhythmia is ischemic stroke, the most serious embolic complication, and systemic embolism caused by detachment of thrombi that are usually created within the left atrial appendage as a result of increased stasis and pooling of blood. The risk of ischemic stroke in people with nonvalvular permanent AF is five to seven times greater compared with people who do not have this arrhythmia. Table 14.1 shows the main causes of AF.

Warning! Nonvalvular AF is used to imply AF in the absence of rheumatic mitral valve stenosis (the most thromboembolic native valvulopathy), a prosthetic (mechanical or bioprosthetic) heart valve, or mitral valve repair (January CT, et al. Circulation 2014;130:e199-e267).

Depending on its duration, AF is classified as paroxysmal, persistent, or permanent (Table 14.2).

Clinical presentation
- Palpitations (due to rapid and irregular rhythm), weakness, and dyspnea on effort (due to a reduction in cardiac output because of loss of the atri-

TABLE 14.1	Major causes of atrial fibrillation (AF)

1) Hypertension
2) Coronary artery disease
3) Heart failure
4) Heart valve disease (most commonly of the mitral valve)
5) Cardiomyopathies
6) Pericarditis
7) Acute pulmonary embolism
8) Chronic obstructive pulmonary disease
9) Hyperthyroidism (occurs in ~10% of cases with hyperthyroidism)
10) High alcohol consumption
11) After cardiac surgery (primarily heart valve surgery) [occurs in 30-50% of postsurgical cases]
12) Atrial septal defect
13) Sick sinus syndrome
14) Pulmonary infections
15) Idiopathic or lone AF (accounts for 5-10% of cases)

al kick and shortening of the diastolic ventricular filling period). This is the most common manifestation.

- Angina, acute pulmonary edema, and/or syncope (usually when the ventricular response is >150 beats/min and there is concomitant organic heart disease).
- Ischemic stroke. Approximately 20-25% of all ischemic strokes are due to a detached embolus, usually from the left atrial appendage, on a substrate of AF. Although an ischemic stroke in a patient with AF is most likely to be due to embolism of thrombus from the left atrium, up to 25% of strokes may be due to intrinsic cerebrovascular diseases or other cardiac or aortogenic (atheromatous proximal aorta) sources of embolism.
- Absence of symptoms (discovery of this arrhythmia on chance examination). This occurs when the ventricular response is <100 beats/min and there is usually no severe organic heart disease.

Warning! Patients with permanent AF and a persistent rapid ventricular rate (>100 beats/min) may develop tachycardia-induced cardiomyopathy (tachycardiomyopathy). This type of left ventricular dysfunction is partially or completely reversible once the tachycardia is controlled.

TABLE 14.2	Atrial fibrillation classification by duration

1) Paroxysmal: converts automatically to sinus rhythm (usually ≤48 hours, rarely <7 days)

2) Persistent: lasting >7 days or terminated by electrical or pharmaceutical cardioversion

3) Permanent: its presence is accepted by the patient and the treating physician (rhythm control is not attempted)

Clinical examination
- 1st heart sound of variable intensity.
- Irregular heart sounds.
- Irregular jugular venous pulses and absence of a waves.

Warning! The heart rate should be estimated by auscultating the heart and not by palpating the radial artery, because when there is a rapid ventricular response some cardiac systoles produce low stroke volume insufficient to generate a palpable radial pulse (pulse deficit). Therefore, the heart rate will be underestimated if the peripheral pulses are counted.

ECG (Figure 14.1)
- Absence of P waves. Instead, there are small waveforms, of varying size,

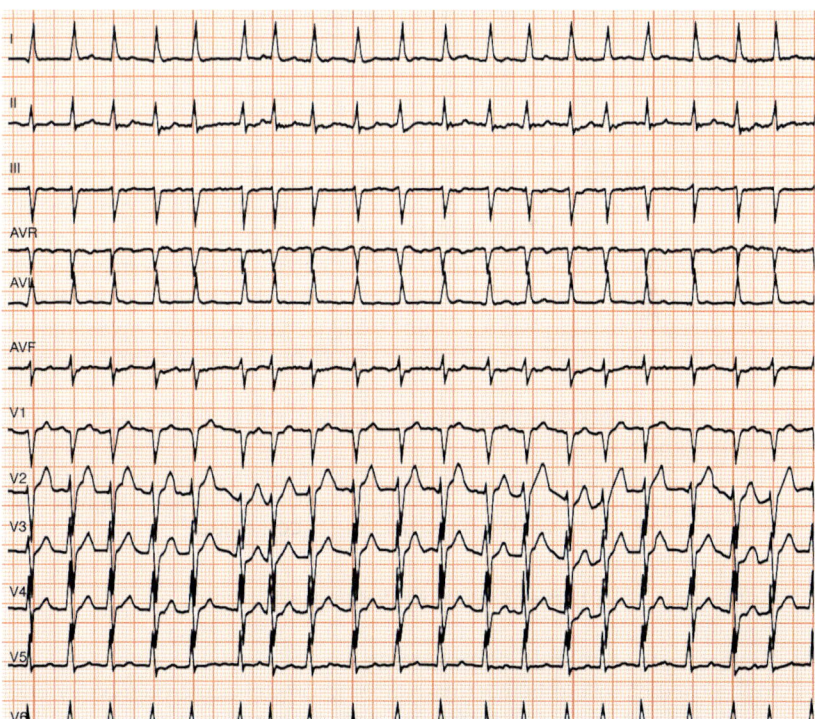

Figure 14.1. ECG of a patient with recent-onset atrial fibrillation. It is characterized by the absence of P waves and by irregular QRS complexes with a rate of ~150 beats/min.

morphology, and frequency (350-600/min) that are called fibrillatory "f" waves. Sometimes these waves are not visible.
- Completely irregular QRS complexes ("irregularly irregular"). When, however, the ventricular rate is very fast or very slow, it appears regular and needs careful measurement and comparison of the R-R intervals.
- If the QRS complexes are widened, consider the possibility of preexisting bundle branch block, aberrant conduction or an accessory pathway. Note that a very fast ventricular response (>200 beats/min) and QRS complexes of varying width usually suggest the existence of an accessory pathway.

Warning! If a patient with AF becomes regular, the probable explanations are: a) conversion to sinus rhythm (most likely); b) development of atrial flutter with constant atrioventricular conduction; c) occurrence of complete atrioventricular block with a junctional or ventricular escape rhythm (usually there is bradycardia); and d) appearance of ventricular tachycardia (rarely). Consequently, if there is a clinical indication of "conversion" of AF, ECG confirmation is always needed.

Basic examinations for the investigation of AF

Complete blood count, basic biochemical tests, inflammation testing (C-reactive protein, if infection/inflammation is suspected), chest X-ray, D-dimers (if acute pulmonary embolism is suspected), thyroid examination (to rule out hyperthyroidism), and echocardiogram. In patients with AF and signs or complaints suggestive of myocardial ischemia, further investigation, e.g. coronary angiography, is necessary to rule out coronary artery disease.

Factors that determine the management of patients with AF in the Emergency Room

Table 14.3 shows the basic questions that must be answered in order to plan the management of patients who present to the Emergency Room with AF.

Management of a patient with AF lasting <48 hours

1) Severe hemodynamic compromise

In the case of severe hemodynamic compromise (acute pulmonary edema, angina, heart rate >200 beats/min, fall in systolic blood pressure [BP] to <90 mmHg), direct current (DC) cardioversion (i.e. delivery of synchronized shock) is performed (first shock at 200 J, followed by 360 J → 360 J for monophasic current or 120 J → 200 J → 200 J for biphasic current if ini-

TABLE 14.3	Questions which need to be answered before deciding on the management of a patient with atrial fibrillation

1) Is there any hemodynamic compromise (angina, dyspnea, systolic arterial blood pressure drop to <90 mmHg)?
2) When did it begin (<48 or ≥48 h)?
3) Is there a triggering factor (e.g. respiratory tract infection, alcohol intake, etc.)?
4) Is there an underlying disease (hypertension, coronary artery disease, chronic pulmonary disease, etc.)?
5) Is the patient receiving anticoagulation?
6) Is it preferable to perform cardioversion (rhythm control) or to control the heart rate (rate control)?

tial shocks fail). A patient who is still conscious should first be sedated. It should be noted that biphasic shocks are preferred because they require less energy for AF cardioversion and the success rate is higher.

2) Moderate or mild hemodynamic compromise

Heart rate control should be performed initially and then cardioversion of the arrhythmia should be attempted:

a) *Heart rate control:*

- **Diltiazem** (Cardizem): administered in a dose of 15-20 mg IV over 2 min, and if there is no response then a further 20-25 mg after 10 min. It has the advantage of rapid action (3-5 min) and simple administration. It may be followed by a continuous IV drip of diltiazem solution in a dose of 5-15 mg/h (see page 126).
- **Verapamil** (Isoptin): initial dose of 5-10 mg IV over 2 min, additional 10 mg if no response after 30 min, and then 5 µg/kg/min continuous infusion.
- **Esmolol** (Brevibloc): initial dose of 500 µg/kg IV over one min followed by continuous infusion at 50-300 µg/kg/min (see Chapter 23).
- **Propranolol** (Inderal): initial dose of 1 mg IV over 2 min, repeated every 5 min up to a maximum dose of 5 mg.
- **Amiodarone** (Cordarone, 1 ampoule contains 150 mg/3 mL): apart from cardioversion, it may be given to control the heart rate in the setting of heart failure or hypotension in patients without Wolf-Parkinson-White syndrome.

Warning! The IV administration of digoxin has no place in the rapid control of heart rate (except in patients with heart failure or hypotension), cause of its relatively delayed onset of action (usually >15-30 min).

b) **Pharmaceutical cardioversion:** Through the administration of appropriate antiarrhythmic medication, cardioversion to sinus rhythm can be achieved in up to 60-90% of cases. Given, however, that the spontaneous conversion rate of recent-onset AF within the first 24 h is 40-60%, the net conversion rate from the administration of antiarrhythmics is 20-30%. Immediately prior to the initiation of pharmacological cardioversion, unfractionated heparin (UFH) is given IV (5000 U), followed by subcutaneous low-molecular-weight heparin (LMWH) [e.g. enoxaparin in a dose of 1 mg/kg x 2/day]. The main antiarrhythmic drugs used for cardioversion are:

- **Amiodarone*** (Cordarone): administered in a dose of 5 mg/kg IV over 60 min (usually 300 mg of amiodarone added to 100 mL D/W 5% and administered over 60 min). If cardioversion is unsuccessful, amiodarone is continued in a dose of 50 mg/h IV until either cardioversion is achieved or 48 h elapse from the onset of arrhythmia (usually 900 mg amiodarone added to 500 mL D/W 5% and administered at a rate of ~25 mL/h). If cardioversion is not accomplished by 48 h after the onset of the arrhythmia, attempts at pharmaceutical cardioversion stop and the practice described below is followed (see page 201).
  Generally, the action of amiodarone is only manifested after a delay (usually >8 h). The conversion rate at 24 h is 70-90%. The advantage of amiodarone is that it slows the atrioventricular conduction and can be given to individuals with left ventricular dysfunction, including acute myocardial infarction. When it is given IV for more than 24 h, it is preferable to administer it via a central line because of the increased risk of thrombophlebitis.

- **Propafenone:** given in a dose of 600 mg po (450 mg in subjects weighing <70 kg or aged >75 years). If the patient is tachycardic (>80 beats/min), 0.5 mg IV digoxin (ampoules Lanoxin, 0.5 mg/2 mL) within 15 min diluted in 50 mL D/W 5% or NaCl 0.9% or another bradycardic medication (e.g. 15-20 mg diltiazem IV within 2 min) is usually given first. This prevents rapid atrioventricular conduction if the patient falls into atrial flutter, which is a rare complication of propafenone administration. A prerequisite for giving propafenone is the absence of coronary artery disease or significant structural heart disease, and there should not be any history of severe obstructive pulmonary disease. The cardioversion rate for recent onset AF is 45% within 3 h and 80% within

---

*Also, many recommend the following IV regimen: 150 mg over 10 min, followed by 1 mg/min x 6 h, and then 0.5 mg/min x 18 h.

8 h (mean conversion time ~3 h). Alternatively, propafenone may be given IV in a dose of 2 mg/kg over 10 min.

- **Flecainide** (Tambocor): given in a dose of 200-300 mg po. It belongs to the same class of antiarrhythmics as propafenone (class IC) and therefore the same conditions apply regarding its administration. Alternatively, it may be given IV in a dose of 2 mg/kg over 10 min.

- **Ibutilide** (Corvert, 1 vial contains 1 mg/10 mL): given in a dose of 1 mg (or 0.01 mg/kg in subjects weighing <60 kg) over 10 min, and if conversion has not been achieved after 10 min the same dose is repeated over 10 min. It belongs to the same category of antiarrhythmics as amiodarone (class III). It is given only when the patient can be hospitalized in the short-term, with continuous ECG monitoring for 4 h, because of the risk of arrhythmias, mainly polymorphic ventricular tachycardia on a substrate of prolonged QT interval (torsades de pointes) with an incidence of ~2-4%. Its administration should be avoided in the case of hypokalemia (potassium levels <4 mEq/L; electrolyte levels should always be checked before administration), a corrected QT (QTc) interval >440 ms, or severe heart failure. The conversion rate to sinus rhythm ranges between 55-75% and conversion usually occurs 10-30 min after administration of the drug. If conversion has not been achieved after 60 min, electrical cardioversion can be applied. It should be noted that the success rate of electrical cardioversion increases after pretreatment with ibutilide.

- **Vernakalant** (Brinavess, 1 vial contains 500 mg/25 mL): given by initial IV infusion of 3 mg/kg over 10 min; if conversion has not been achieved after 15 min, infusion is repeated in a dose of 2 mg/kg over 10 min. Vernakalant has been approved by the European Medicines Agency (EMA) for the rapid conversion of recent onset AF (≤7 days for nonsurgical patients and ≤3 days for postcardiac surgery patients). It has faster action and a higher successful conversion rate compared with amiodarone (50-55% conversion within 90 min). It is contraindicated in patients with systolic BP <100 mmHg, severe aortic stenosis, class III or IV heart failure, acute coronary syndrome within the previous 30 days, or QT interval prolongation.

  A practical guide to vernakalant administration: for individuals weighing ≤100 kg, one vial of Brinavess is dissolved in 100 mL D/W 5% or NaCl 0.9% (final solution volume 125 mL and concentration 4 mg/mL). For an individual weighing 70 kg, 52.5 mL of solution are given IV over 10 min, and in the case of nonconversion after 15 min a repeat dose of 35 mL is given IV over 10 min.

Table 14.4 shows the dosage regimens for drugs available for the cardioversion of recent onset AF.

TABLE 14.4	Dosage of drugs for the cardioversion of recent-onset atrial fibrillation	
Drug	**Starting dose**	**Repeat dose (if the first is ineffective)**
Amiodarone	• 5 mg/kg IV over 1 h	50 mg/h IV until conversion is achieved or 48 h have passed since the arrhythmia was established
Flecainide	• 200-300 mg po • 2 mg/kg IV over 10 min	
Ibutilide	• 1 mg IV over 10 min	1 mg IV over 10 min after waiting for 10 min
Propafenone	• 450-600 mg po • 2 mg/kg IV over 10 min	
Vernakalant	• 3 mg/kg IV over 10 min	2 mg/kg IV over 10 min after waiting for 15 min

The usual practice in the Emergency Room, when pharmaceutical conversion of AF is not achieved within 6-10 h (admission to short-term hospitalization unit), is for the patient to be admitted to the cardiology department for IV administration of amiodarone. This applies whether amiodarone is given as first antiarrhythmic, or as secondary antiarrhythmic after a failed attempt to convert using another drug, e.g. propafenone. At the same time, the anticoagulant treatment is continued (e.g. enoxaparin in a dose of 1 mg/kg x 2/day, subcutaneously).

If the AF is converted within 48 h of its onset, and the patient does not have risk factors for thromboembolism, there is no need for postcardioversion oral anticoagulants other than the pericardioversion administration of heparin.

Finally, if AF occurs on a substrate of hyperthyroidism (seen in ~10% of cases) no cardioversion should be performed unless the patient has previously been rendered euthyroid. AF often converts spontaneously to sinus rhythm with the restoration of thyroid function. Note that for the control of heart rate, the treatment of choice is beta-blockers.

Warning! Digoxin administration does not convert the AF, but simply slows the ventricular response. Furthermore, while sotalol has a good effect in maintaining sinus rhythm after the conversion of AF, it has low effectiveness in converting the arrhythmia itself.

Management of the patient with AF lasting ≥48 hours

If the patient does not show severe hemodynamic compromise, which is the most usual scenario, heart rate control is attempted. More specifically, if the patient is asymptomatic or oligosymptomatic, a beta-blocker, diltiazem or verapamil, is given po. Appropriate dose titration of these drugs can achieve heart rate control both at rest and on exercise. Digoxin used to be given (see Chapter 18) for rate control. It should be stressed, however, that digoxin as monotherapy is unable to control the heart rate on exercise, and will need to be combined with a beta-blocker, diltiazem or verapamil. Digoxin, however, continues to have an indication in symptomatic systolic heart failure in cases of intolerance to beta-blockers, or in combination with them for better heart rate control.

If the patient shows mild or moderate symptomatology, diltiazem IV may be given initially for the rapid control of the ventricular response. The goal is to maintain the heart rate at 60-80 beats/min at rest and <110 beats/min on moderate exercise. Subsequently, two different strategies may be followed: cardioversion (rhythm control), or noncardioversion (rate control).

1) Cardioversion strategy (rhythm control)

a) **Conventional practice (delayed cardioversion):** vitamin K antagonists (VKAs) are administered to achieve a desired international normalized ratio (INR) of 2.0-3.0, and electrical cardioversion is scheduled after three weeks. The INR should be checked every week, and on the day before the cardioversion. If the INR levels are within therapeutic range, electrical cardioversion may be performed without a previous transesophageal echocardiogram (TEE). In actual practice, however, many patients present subtherapeutic INR levels. In this case, they should undergo a TEE before cardioversion in order to rule out the presence of a thrombus within the left atrium (usually in the appendage). If electrical cardioversion is unsuccessful, a second attempt can be made after administering 1 mg of ibutilide IV. The administration of ibutilide significantly increases the chances of a successful second attempt at electrical cardioversion.

b) **Early cardioversion under transesophageal echocardiographic guidance** (see algorithm on page 202): 5000 U of UFH are administered by bolus IV and a TEE is performed. Provided there is no thrombus in the left atrial cavity or left atrial appendage (as occurs in 10-15% of cases), then electrical cardioversion is attempted after a 6-h fast. Electrical cardioversion is preferable to pharmaceutical cardioversion because of its greater success rate (~90%). After the initial administration of IV UFH, LMWH is commenced (e.g. enoxaparin in a dose of 1 mg/kg x 2/day, subcutaneously) concurrently with VKA administration. The LMWH is

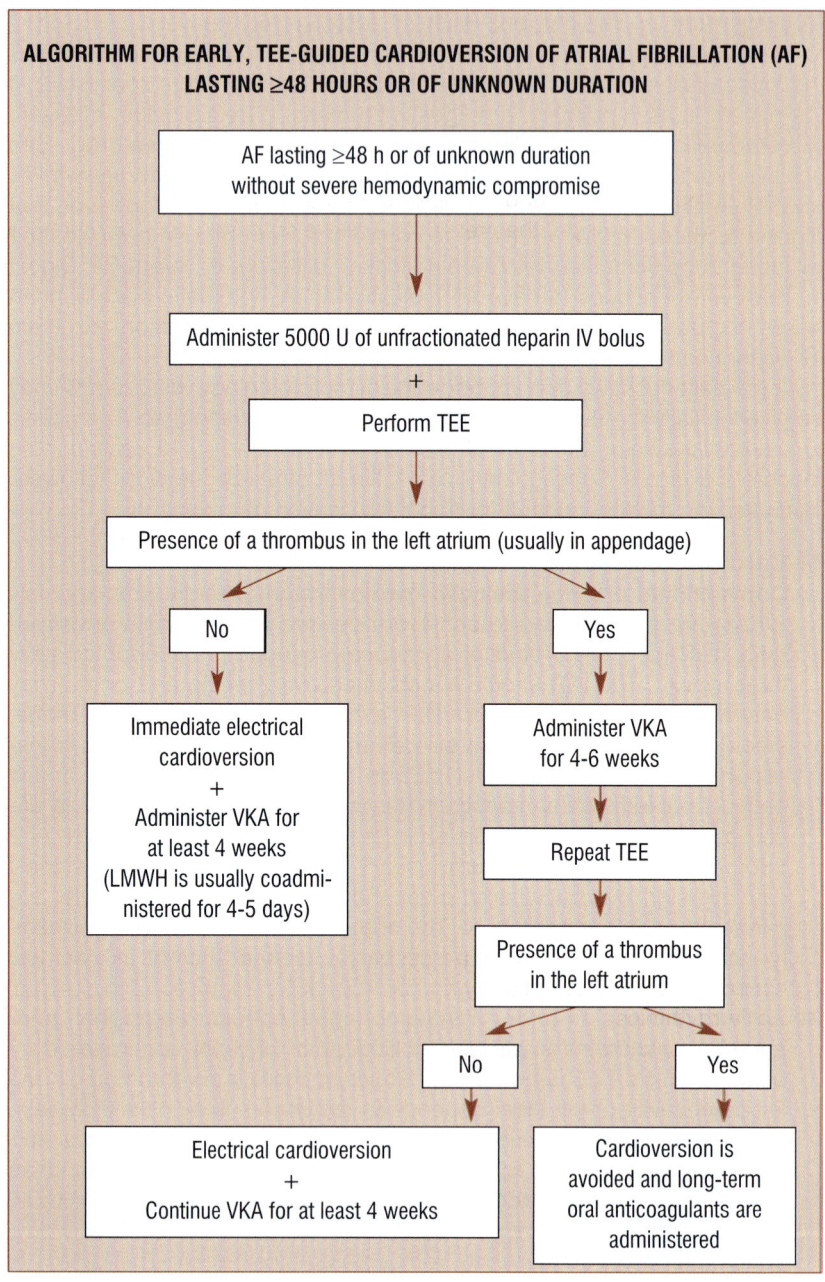

ALGORITHM FOR EARLY, TEE-GUIDED CARDIOVERSION OF ATRIAL FIBRILLATION (AF) LASTING ≥48 HOURS OR OF UNKNOWN DURATION

AF lasting ≥48 h or of unknown duration without severe hemodynamic compromise

↓

Administer 5000 U of unfractionated heparin IV bolus
+
Perform TEE

↓

Presence of a thrombus in the left atrium (usually in appendage)

No → Immediate electrical cardioversion
+
Administer VKA for at least 4 weeks
(LMWH is usually coadministered for 4-5 days)

Yes → Administer VKA for 4-6 weeks

↓

Repeat TEE

↓

Presence of a thrombus in the left atrium

No → Electrical cardioversion
+
Continue VKA for at least 4 weeks

Yes → Cardioversion is avoided and long-term oral anticoagulants are administered

LMWH: low-molecular-weight heparin, TEE: transesophageal echocardiogram, VKA: vitamin K antagonists

continued until therapeutic INR levels are achieved (usually for 4-5 days).

If thrombus is seen, cardioversion is not attempted and a new TEE is conducted after 4-6 weeks of anticoagulation treatment. If the thrombus has disappeared in the follow-up TEE, then electrical cardioversion is attempted. If the thrombus persists, then cardioversion is not attempted and the patient is kept under long-term oral anticoagulation.

Some authors consider the presence of dense spontaneous echo contrast in left atrium or left appendage, a condition associated with high risk for thrombus formation, as a contraindication for the performance of TEE-guided cardioversion.

It should be noted that, for both management approaches, anticoagulation is continued for another 4 weeks after successful cardioversion in order to reduce the risk of new thrombus creation due to temporary mechanical atrial dysfunction (stunning). The duration of atrial dysfunction might last up to 4 weeks and depends mostly on the duration of AF. If a thrombus forms or preexists, it could detach at the moment when the mechanical function of the atria is fully restored.

Both cardioversion practices described above are equally safe with regard to the incidence of thromboembolic episodes ($<1\%$). Remember that $>90\%$ of thromboembolic episodes after successful cardioversion occur within 10 days of cardioversion. TEE-guided early cardioversion is superior to the conventional cardioversion strategy because of its lower rate of hemorrhagic manifestations (3% versus 5.5%), which is due to the fact that the duration of anticoagulation is ~3 weeks shorter.

After successful cardioversion, and provided this is the first episode of AF, the current trend is to refrain from prescribing chronic antiarrhythmic medication. Also, antiarrhythmics are usually not used when AF episodes are very infrequent, e.g. <2 per year, and are well tolerated. In other cases, they are given in order to increase the chances of maintaining sinus rhythm (Table 14.5). Therefore, while the percentage of patients who maintain sinus rhythm per year without antiarrhythmics is 30-50%, it increases to 50-70% with antiarrhythmics.

Amiodarone is the most effective antiarrhythmic agent in maintaining sinus rhythm, but because of its toxicity it should only be used when other agents have failed or are contraindicated. If amiodarone is administered, thyroid testing should always be performed beforehand (free T_4, free T_3 and TSH levels, and anti-TPO antibodies) and repeated every six months (TSH levels), because long-term administration causes hypo- or hyperthyroidism in 5-10% of cases (hypothyroidism >hyperthyroidism). Note that serum T_4 levels can be slightly elevated in the absence of hyperthyroidism because

TABLE 14.5	Selection of antiarrhythmic drug* to prevent atrial fibrillation

1) In case of absent or minimal organic heart disease (ejection fraction >50%, absence of active ischemia and history of myocardial infarction)
   - Propafenone, sotalol, flecainide, dronedarone, dofetilide** (1st choice)
   - Amiodarone (2nd choice)

2) In case of heart failure
   - Amiodarone, dofetilide

3) In case of coronary artery disease
   - Sotalol, dronedarone, dofetilide**(1st choice)
   - Amiodarone (2nd choice)

4) In case of hypertension and severe left ventricular hypertrophy ($\geq$14 mm)
   - Dronedarone (1st choice)
   - Amiodarone (2nd choice)

5) In case of hypertension without severe left ventricular hypertrophy (<14 mm)
   - Propafenone, sotalol, flecainide, dronedarone (1st choice)
   - Amiodarone (2nd choice)

The daily dosage of the antiarrhythmics is: amiodarone 200 mg x 2 or x 3 for 2-4 weeks followed by 100-200 mg x 1, dofetilide 125-500 μg x 2, dronedarone 400 mg x 2, flecainide 50-200 mg x 2, propafenone 150-300 mg x 3, sotalol 40-160 mg x 2.

**Recommended by the American Guidelines for Atrial Fibrillation (January CT, et al. Circulation 2014;130:e199-e267).*

amiodarone inhibits the peripheral conversion of T_4 to T_3. Therefore, the diagnosis of hyperthyroidism is based on the measurement of TSH (low) and free T_3 (high). Tests for hepatic enzymes (increase in 10-20% of cases) should also be performed every six months, and a chest X-ray yearly because of the risk of pneumonitis/pulmonary fibrosis (dose-dependent side effect, potentially life-threatening, occurring very rarely when daily amiodarone doses $\leq$200 mg are administered). Other side effects include: corneal microdeposits (>90%, without clinical significance), anorexia/nausea (10-30%), photosensitivity (10-30%), bradycardia (~3%), torsades de pointes (<1%), peripheral neuropathy (<1%), etc.

Warning! If new arrhythmia appears in a patient on chronic treatment with amiodarone, exclude hyperthyroidism (measure free T_3 and TSH levels), while if the patient develops nonproductive cough and progressive dyspnea, exclude pneumonitis/pulmonary fibrosis (request chest-X-ray to look for patchy interstitial infiltrates ± pulmonary function tests)

The indications for antithrombotic treatment after successful cardioversion depend on the patient's risk of thromboembolism (more details are given below).

Lastly, in cases with frequent, highly symptomatic recurrence of AF despite optimal medication, the physician should consider using intervention techniques such as:

- Left atrial ablation (usually pulmonary vein isolation). This technique is the most promising and involves the delivery of radiofrequency energy around the pulmonary veins, the area where the centers that trigger the AF are frequently located, thus achieving electrical isolation of the arrhythmogenic sites. This procedure is successful in maintaining sinus rhythm over the next year in 70-80% of patients. Its complications include cardiac tamponade (<1.5%), stroke or transient ischemic attack (<1%), atrioesophageal fistula (<0.1%, late complication), death (~0.15%), etc.
- Atrioventricular node ablation and creation of complete atrioventricular block with simultaneous implantation of a permanent pacemaker.
- Surgical ablation (maze procedure) of AF should be considered in patients who are undergoing cardiac surgery.

2) No-cardioversion strategy (heart rate control)

It is said that all patients with AF deserve at least one attempt at cardioversion, but this is usually avoided:

- When the AF is well tolerated and its duration is >1 year or the size of the left atrium is >60 mm.
- In elderly patients who have a good ventricular response without taking bradycardic medication, because of a concurrent disorder in atrioventricular conduction.
- In individuals with frequent AF episodes despite antiarrhythmic medication.

It should be noted that there is no difference in survival between patients who remain in AF and receive anticoagulants and heart rate control medication, and patients who are cardioverted and receive long-term antiarrhythmic treatment. Therefore, the decision should always be individualized by the treating physician. In order to control the ventricular response, a beta-blocker, diltiazem or verapamil is administered po. In patients with systolic heart failure, as mentioned earlier, digoxin may be administered in case of intolerance to beta-blockers or in combination with a beta-blocker in order to achieve better heart rate control (see page 268).

Warning! If a patient with permanent AF presents to an Emergency Room complaining of a rapid and irregular heart rate (e.g. >120 beats/min), then acute causes of compensatory increase in heart rate should be ruled out. These are: acute pulmonary embolism, blood loss, respiratory tract infection, decompensated heart failure, etc.

AF and Wolff–Parkinson–White syndrome

In the case of AF with wide and variable QRS complexes and usually a rate of >200 beats/min, we should suspect Wolff-Parkinson-White (WPW) syndrome [Figure 14.2]. If a patient with WPW syndrome and an accessory pathway with a short refractory period (~25% have a refractory period <250 ms) develops AF, then the stimuli descend primarily through the accessory pathway and excite the ventricles together with the stimuli descending through the atrioventricular node. This leads to wide QRS complexes of variable morphology, depending on the timing of ventricular stimulation through the two routes.

If pharmaceutical cardioversion is attempted (when there is no severe hemodynamic compromise), then procainamide or ibutilide is administered IV. The IV administration of amiodarone (January CT, et al. Circulation 2014;130:e199-267), digoxin, verapamil, diltiazem, beta-blockers, adenosine or lidocaine is contraindicated because these drugs reduce the accessory pathway's refractory period, facilitating the rapid descent of stimuli through the pathway, and there is a risk of the arrhythmia degenerating into ventricular fibrillation.

Indications for long-term antithrombotic treatment in AF

The indications for administration of antithrombotic treatment are determined primarily by the presence of risk factors for thromboembolic

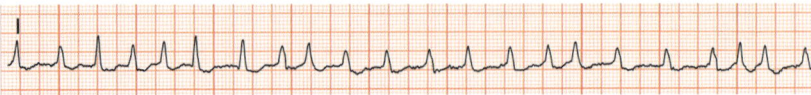

Figure 14.2. ECG (lead I) of a patient with known Wolff-Parkinson-White syndrome who developed atrial fibrillation. The QRS complexes are irregular, wide, with variable morphology and a heart rate of ~190/min.

TABLE 14.6	Assessment of thromboembolism risk in patients with nonvalvular AF	
Letter	**Risk factor**	**Score**
C	**C**ongestive heart failure / Ejection fraction ≤40%	1
H	**H**ypertension	1
A	**A**ge ≥75 years	2
D	**D**iabetes mellitus	1
S	**S**troke/Transient ischemic attack/Thromboembolism	2
V	**V**ascular disease (prior myocardial infarction, peripheral artery disease, aortic plaque)	1
A	**A**ge 65-74 years	1
Sc	**S**ex category (i.e. female sex)	1
		9 (maximum)

episodes and by weighing its benefit against the risk of hemorrhagic complications. In addition, the ability to perform regular INR testing after VKA administration is taken into account. According to the European Guidelines for the Management of AF (Camm AJ, et al. Eur Heart J 2010;31:2369-429) the assessment of thromboembolic risk in a patient with nonvalvular AF is based on the study of risk factors, expressed by the acronym CHA_2DS_2-VASc, as presented in Table 14.6. The greater the score, the greater the risk of thromboembolic event, particularly a stroke. Table 14.7 lists the indications for antithrombotic therapy depending on the patient's score. Thus, pa-

TABLE 14.7	Suggested antithrombotic treatment for the prevention of thromboembolism in nonvalvular AF, based on the CHA_2DS_2-VASc score
CHA_2DS_2VASc score	**Suggested antithrombotic treatment**
≥2	Vitamin K antagonists (target INR = 2.0-3.0)
1* (male)	Vitamin K antagonists (target INR = 2.0-3.0)
0 (male) or 1 (female)	No antithrombotic treatment

*The latest American Guidelines for AF (January CT, et al. Circulation 2014;130:e199-e267) do not encourage the administration of antithrombotic treatment in patients with nonvalvular AF and CHA_2DS_2-VASc score =1. In particular, for patients with nonvalvular AF and a CHA_2DS_2-VASc score = 1, no antithrombotic therapy or treatment with oral anticoagulant or aspirin may be considered

tients with AF and a score of 1 for men or ≥2 (regardless of gender) should take VKAs (target INR=2.0-3.0). On the contrary, for men with a score of 0 or for women with a score of 1 no antithrombotic therapy is necessary. This category includes men aged <65 years with no risk factors for thromboembolism (i.e. idiopathic or lone AF) [score 0] or women aged <65 years with no risk factors for thromboembolism, despite the fact that they have a score of 1 because of their gender. Note that antithrombotic treatment is recommended in patients with hypertrophic cardiomyopathy and AF even with CHA_2DS_2-VASc score 0.

Lastly, for patients who refuse to take VKAs or any of the non-VKA oral anticoagulants (NOACs), the coadministration of aspirin (75-100 mg/day) with clopidogrel (75 mg/day), or alternatively monotherapy with aspirin (75-325 mg/day; less effective) is recommended.

Warning! Patients with paroxysmal AF have indications for antithrombotic therapy similar to patients with persistent or permanent AF (Table 14.7).

When antithrombotic therapy is administered, the risk of hemorrhagic events should be taken into account. The risk of hemorrhage can be assessed by calculating the HAS-BLED score, which is based on the patient's clinical features (Table 14.8). Patients with a HAS-BLED score ≥3 are considered to have increased risk of hemorrhage.

In such cases:
- The VKA anticoagulation effect (INR) should be checked frequently.
- An INR value in the lower therapeutic range (~2.0) should be sought.
- Any factors which increase the hemorrhagic risk should be strictly controlled, e.g. by effective control of any arterial hypertension, avoidance of nonsteroidal antiinflammatory drugs, etc.

Patients with stable coronary artery disease who develop AF should be given a VKA. In such cases, the concurrent use of aspirin provides no additional protection while increasing the risk of hemorrhage; it is therefore preferable to administer VKAs only.

Non-VKA oral anticoagulants (NOACs)

1) **Dabigatran** (Pradaxa). This is a direct thrombin inhibitor which acts both on free and on clot-bound thrombin. It is a prodrug, activated in the liver without the involvement of cytochrome P450, which explains the lack of significant interaction with other drugs. Its half-life is 12-17 h and its peak plasma level is achieved in ~2 h. Eighty percent of the dose is eliminated by the kidneys and therefore it is contraindicated in patients with creati-

Letter	Risk factor	Score
	Clinical characteristics that determine the hemorrhagic risk based on the HAS-BLED score (TABLE 14.8)	
H	**H**ypertension (systolic BP >160 mmHg)	1
A	**A**bnormal kidney (creatinine >2.3 mg/dL) or liver function (transaminases >3 x ULN)*	1 or 2
S	**S**troke	1
B	**B**leeding (previous bleeding and/or predisposition to bleeding)	1
L	**L**abile INRs (unstable / high or low INRs)	1
E	**E**lderly (age >65 years)	1
D	**D**rugs (antiplatelets or NSAIDs) or alcohol*	1 or 2
		9 (maximum)

*one point each
BP = blood pressure, NSAIDs = nonsteroidal antiinflammatory drugs, ULN=upper limit of normal
INR = international normalized ratio

nine clearance <30 mL/min. The RE-LY study (Connolly SJ, et al. N Engl J Med 2009;361:1139-51), which compared it to warfarin in patients with nonvalvular AF and increased risk of stroke, showed that the 150 mg x 2 daily dose was associated with fewer ischemic strokes and systemic emboli and with the same risk of major hemorrhages compared to warfarin. Dabigatran given at a dose of 110 mg x 2 daily was associated with similar rates of ischemic stroke and systemic embolism but lower rates of major hemorrhage compared to warfarin.

Based on the results of RE-LY, dabigatran has been approved by both the U.S. Food and Drug Administration (FDA) and the European Medicines Agency (EMA) for the prevention of stroke and systemic embolism in patients with nonvalvular AF (Table 14.9). It is given at a dosage of 150 mg x 2 daily. There are also data suggesting that elective cardioversion of AF can be safely performed with the administration of NOACs (dabigatran, rivaroxaban or apixaban) for 3 weeks prior to cardioversion and for a minimum of 4 weeks postcardioversion. If compliance with NOACs can be reliably confirmed, conversion can be performed without TEE guidance.

No monitoring of its anticoagulation effect with laboratory assays or dose titration is necessary. The INR is minimally affected by dabigatran, and it appears that the most reliable techniques for evaluating its anticoagulation effect are the thrombin time (TT) and the ecarin clotting time

(ECT). Its administration also prolongs the activated partial thromboplastin time (aPTT). Recently (October 2015), FDA approved idarucizumab for use in patients on dabigatran in case of life-threatening bleeding or emergency surgery. Idarucizumab (Praxbind, 1 vial contains 2.5 g/50 mL) is given in a dose of 5 g IV bolus and within minutes selectively neutralizes the anticoagulant effect of dabigatran.

Warning! At trough, i.e. 12-24 h after the previous administration of dabigatran, an aPTT >2 x upper limit of normal (ULN) or an ECT $\geq$3 x ULN suggests excess bleeding risk

2) Direct factor Xa inhibitors

- **Rivaroxaban** (Xarelto). The ROCKET-AF study (Patel MR, et al. N Engl J Med 2011;365:883-91), which randomized patients with nonvalvular AF and an elevated risk of stroke to treatment with rivaroxaban (20 mg daily) or warfarin, showed that rivaroxaban was not inferior to warfarin in preventing stroke or systemic embolism, and that there was no difference with regard to major hemorrhagic episodes. Based on the results of ROCKET-AF, rivaroxaban has been approved by both the FDA and the EMA for the prevention of stroke and systemic embolism in patients with nonvalvular AF (Table 14.9). It is given at a dosage of 20 mg daily. Rivaroxaban should be taken with food since it results in better absorption and high bioavailability of the drug.
- **Apixaban** (Eliquis). The ARISTOTLE study (Granger CB, et al. N Engl J Med 2011;365:981-92), in which patients with nonvalvular AF and at

TABLE 14.9	Indications for non-VKA oral anticoagulants as alternative to vitamin K antagonists for prevention of thromboembolism in nonvalvular AF, based on the CHA$_2$DS$_2$-VASc score
CHA$_2$DS$_2$-VASc score	**Suggested antithrombotic treatment**
$\geq$2	Dabigatran, rivaroxaban, apixaban or edoxaban
1* (male)	Dabigatran, rivaroxaban, apixaban or edoxaban
0 (male) or 1 (female)	No antithrombotic treatment

*The latest American Guidelines for AF (January CT, et al. Circulation 2014;130:e199-e267) do not encourage the administration of antithrombotic treatment in patients with nonvalvular AF and CHA$_2$DS$_2$-VASc score =1. In particular, for patients with nonvalvular AF and a CHA$_2$DS$_2$-VASc score=1, no antithrombotic therapy or treatment with oral anticoagulant or aspirin may be considered

least one additional risk factor for stroke were randomized to apixaban (5 mg x 2 daily) or warfarin, showed fewer strokes (ischemic or hemorrhagic) or systemic embolisms, fewer major hemorrhages and lower overall mortality in the apixaban group. Apixaban has been approved by both the FDA and the EMA for the prevention of stroke and systemic embolism in patients with nonvalvular AF (Table 14.9). It is administered in a dose of 5 mg x 2 daily.

- **Edoxaban** (Savaysa, Lixiana). Recently, both FDA and EMA approved edoxaban for the prevention of stroke and systemic embolism in patients with nonvalvular AF (Table 14.9) based on the results of the ENGAGE AF-TIMI 48 trial (Giugliano RP, et al. N Engl J Med 2013;369: 2093-104). This trial, in which patients with nonvalvular AF and an elevated risk of stroke were randomized to edoxaban or warfarin, showed that edoxaban (60 mg daily) was not inferior to warfarin in preventing ischemic stroke or systemic embolism, and was associated with significantly lower rates of hemorrhagic stroke and death from cardiovascular causes. Edoxaban is administered in a dose of 60 mg daily.

Warning! All NOACs should be given with great caution in patients with renal failure and the creatinine clearance should always be calculated (Cockcroft–Gault formula) before their administration begins. In particular, if creatinine clearance is <30 mL/min dabigatran is contraindicated, while rivaroxaban, apixaban and edoxaban are contraindicated if creatinine clearance is <15 mL/min.

Table 14.10 shows the characteristics of the NOACs, and Table 14.11 presents the preoperative management of patients taking NOACs. Postoperatively, the NOACs are usually resumed 24 h after a minor surgery or 48 h after a major surgery or spinal anesthesia.

When are NOACs preferred over VKAs for the prevention of thromboembolism in nonvalvular AF?

NOACs are at least as effective as warfarin for thromboembolism prevention in nonvalvular AF and have a lower risk of intracranial bleeding. Their advantages are that they are administered in fixed doses, there is no need for anticoagulation monitoring, they have a rapid onset of action and they have few drug–drug or drug–food interactions. Their main disadvantages are the lack of specific antidotes for quick and effective reversal of their action (with the exception of dabigatran), the lack of widely available tests for measuring the anticoagulant effect (check of adherence or in case of major bleeding), their higher cost, their renal dependence, and the lack of long-term data.

TABLE 14.10 Characteristics of non-VKA oral anticoagulants *(Heidbuchel H, et al. Europace 2013;15:625-51)*

	Dabigatran	Rivaroxaban	Apixaban	Edoxaban
Mechanism	Direct thrombin inhibitor	Direct factor Xa inhibitor	Direct factor Xa inhibitor	Direct factor Xa inhibitor
Bioavailability	3-7%	66% without food >80% with food	50%	62%
Prodrug	Yes	No	No	No
Plasma peak levels (hours after ingestion)	2	2-4	1-4	1-2
Plasma trough levels (hours after ingestion)	12-24	16-24	12-24	12-24
Half-life (hours)	12-17	5-9 (young) 11-13 (elderly)	12	9-11
Excretion	80% renal 20% liver	65% liver 35% renal	73% liver 27% renal	50% liver 50% renal
Metabolism via CYP3A4	No	Yes	Yes	Minimal
Permeability glycoprotein (P-gl)* substrate	Yes	Yes	Yes	Yes
Daily dose	150 mg x 2	20 mg x 1	5 mg x 2	60 mg x 1

	Dabigatran	Rivaroxaban	Apixaban	Edoxaban
Special considerations on dose	110 mg x 2 in cases of • age ≥80 years • HAS-BLED score ≥3 • CrCl 30–49 mL/min • concomitant use of verapamil, amiodarone	15 mg x 1 in cases of CrCl 15–49 mL/min	2.5 mg x 2 if at least 2 of the following exist • age ≥80 years • weight ≤60 kg • serum creatinine ≥1.5 mg/dL	30 mg x 1 in cases of • CrCl 15–49 mL/min • weight ≤60 kg • concomitant use of verapamil, dronedarone
Contraindicated in combination with	Dronedarone, azole antifungals (ketoconazole, itraconazole, etc.), rifampicin, anticonvulsants (phenytoin, carbamazepine, etc.)	Azole antifungals (ketoconazole, itraconazole, etc.), HIV protease inhibitors	Azole antifungals (ketoconazole, itraconazole, etc.), rifampicin, anticonvulsants (phenytoin, carbamazepine, etc.)	Azole antifungals (ketoconazole, itraconazole, etc.), HIV protease inhibitors
Not recommended if	CrCl <30 mL/min	CrCl <15 mL/min	CrCl <15 mL/min	CrCl >95 mL/min or CrCl <15 mL/min

CrCl: creatinine clearance

P-gl is a protein of cell membrane that mediates the export of drugs from cells located in the small intestine, hepatocytes, kidney proximal tubules, and blood brain barrier

P-gl inhibitors (amiodarone, dronedarone, quinidine, verapamil, etc.) may increase levels of P-gl substrates while P-gl inducers (rifampicin, carbamazepine, phenytoin, etc.) may decrease levels of P-gl substrates when coadministered

Based on all the available data, NOACs appear to have several advantages over VKAs and provide an attractive alternative for many patients with nonvalvular AF. Appropriate patient selection is critical for the optimal use of NOACs. In particular, NOACs should be preferred in patients with nonvalvular AF, if at least one of the following applies:

1) Inadequate access to laboratory monitoring or patient's preference not to be monitored
2) Poor INR control despite evidence that the patients are complying with VKA medication
3) Resistance to VKA treatment
4) Need for frequent use of medications that interact with VKAs.

A prerequisite for the administration of NOACs is the absence of severe renal impairment, i.e. creatinine clearance <30 mL/min for dabigatran or <15 mL/min for rivaroxaban, apixaban and edoxaban. In addition, it is prudent for patients who are receiving NOACs to have regular assessment of kidney function, i.e. every 6 to 12 months, as a worsening of renal function might warrant a change in the dose of NOACs, or switching from a NOAC to a VKA.

Table 14.12 presents the main differences between warfarin and NOACs.

Warning! Noncompliance with VKAs is not an indication for initiating therapy with NOACs since many of the causes of noncompliance with VKAs may also result in noncompliance with NOACs, e.g. chaotic lifestyle. It should be noted that missing one or two doses of NOACs may have much more devastating consequences than omitting one or two doses of VKA, because the rapid offset of their anticoagulant effect means that the patient will be exposed to the risk of thromboembolism >12-24 h.

Guidelines for pharmaceutical cardioversion of AF at home ("pill-in-the-pocket" approach)

In carefully selected cases, conversion of recent-onset (<48 h, preferably <12 h) AF may be attempted at home by the patient, provided that the efficacy and safety of the treatment has been tested previously in the hospital and the episodes are not frequent (>1/month). In this way, the stressful and time-consuming visit to hospital and stay in the Emergency Room can be avoided. This is particularly important considering the recurrent nature of this arrhythmia. The rate of successful cardioversion in such selected cases is >80%.

Pharmaceutical cardioversion at home is attempted with a single oral dose of 600 mg of propafenone (450 mg in patients weighing <70 kg) given 15 min after the onset of palpitations. Alternatively, flecainide may be given

TABLE 14.11	Suggested preoperative management of patients taking non-VKA oral anticoagulants *(modified from Douketis J, et al. Can Fam Physician 2014;60:997-1001)*		
Drug	**Renal function**	**Minor surgery (low bleeding risk)**	**Major surgery or spinal anesthesia (high bleeding risk)**
Dabigatran (twice daily)	• Normal renal function or mild impairment (eGFR >50 mL/min) • Moderate renal impairment (eGFR 30-50 mL/min)	• Last dose: 2 days before surgery (skip 2 doses) • Last dose: 3 days before surgery (skip 4 doses)	• Last dose: 3 days before surgery (skip 4 doses) • Last dose: 4-5 days before surgery (skip 6-8 doses)
Rivaroxaban (once daily)	• Normal renal function or mild to moderate renal impairment (eGFR >30 mL/min)	• Last dose: 2 days before surgery (skip 1 dose)	• Last dose: 3 days before surgery (skip 2 doses)
Apixaban (twice daily)	• Normal renal function or mild to moderate renal impairment (eGFR >30 mL/min)	• Last dose: 2 days before surgery (skip 2 doses)	• Last dose: 3 days before surgery (skip 4 doses)
Edoxaban (once daily)	• Normal renal function or mild to moderate renal impairment (eGFR >30 mL/min)	• Last dose: 2 days before surgery (skip 1 dose)	• Last dose: 3 days before surgery (skip 2 doses)

eGFR: estimated glomerular filtration rate

TABLE 14.12	Main differences between warfarin and non-VKA oral anticoagulants	
	Warfarin	**Non-VKA oral anticoagulants**
Mechanism	Disrupts production of vitamin K-dependent clotting factors II, VII, IX, X and proteins C and S	Dabigatran: direct thrombin inhibitor Rivaroxaban, apixaban, edoxaban: direct factor Xa inhibitor
Half-life	Warfarin: 36-42 h Acenocoumarol: 10-24 h	5-17 h
Onset of action	Slow (full effect >few days)	Rapid (full effect >few hours)
Routine coagulation monitoring	Required	Not required under normal circumstances
Tests for measuring anticoagulant effect	Available	Not widely available
Dietary interaction	Foods rich in vitamin K should be avoided	Minimal
Drug interaction	Many	Few
Specific antidote in case of bleeding	Vitamin K_1	Recently, FDA approved idarucizumab for dabigatran. Under development is andexanet for direct factor Xa inhibitors
Dose adjustment in renal disease	None required (hepatic metabolism)	Required Avoid if CrCl <30 mL/min (dabigatran) or <15 mL/min (rivaroxaban, apixaban, edoxaban)
Management of major bleeding complications	• Vitamin K_1 • Fresh frozen plasma • 4-factor PCC	• Activated charcoal (in overdose) • Idarucizumab for dabigatran • Potential role (insufficient data) for 4-factor PCC, recombinant factor VIIa (rFVIIa)
Perioperative bridging anticoagulation	Usually required	Not required
Cost	Low	High

CrCl: creatinine clearance, PCC: prothrombin complex concentrate

TABLE 14.13	Prerequisites for safe cardioversion of recent-onset atrial fibrillation at home

1) Previous successful cardioversion with propafenone or flecainide in a hospital setting

2) Absence of hemodynamic impairment during the episode i.e. dyspnea, chest pain, systolic blood pressure <100 mmHg

3) Resting heart rate >50 beats/min

4) Age ≤75 years (insufficient data for patients aged >75 years)

5) Absence of coronary artery disease, cardiomyopathy, severe valve disease, WPW syndrome, known bundle branch block, Brugada or long-QT syndrome, a history of sinus node or atrioventricular conduction disorders

6) Absence of severe extracardiac disease, e.g. chronic renal or hepatic failure

7) No history of previous thromboembolic episodes

8) The patient should not be taking prophylactic antiarrhythmic treatment on a long-term basis

in a dose of 300 mg (200 mg in patients weighing <70 kg). In anxious individuals, concurrent use of an anxiolytic is recommended, such as 1.5 mg of bromazepam. Many physicians recommend also the administration of low-dose beta-blocker (e.g. 40 mg propranolol po) before administering propafenone or flecainide in order to avoid atrial flutter with 1:1 conduction (a rare complication). The mean time until cardioversion is ~3 h. If cardioversion of AF has not been achieved >6 h, the patient should report to an E-mergency Room. While waiting for cardioversion, the patient is instructed to stay in bed or remain seated and, if a fainting tendency, dyspnea, chest pain or a sense of a rapidly accelerated heartbeat or bradycardia (<50 beats/min) develops, they should report to an on-duty hospital.

For safe cardioversion of recent-onset AF at home, the prerequisites listed in Table 14.13 should be met.

Key points

■ AF is a recurrent arrhythmia with thromboembolic episodes as its major complication.

■ Basic hematology and biochemistry tests, thyroid panel tests and echocardiography should be performed even for single episodes of AF.

■ For AF lasting >48 h, cardioversion is "prohibited" before anticoagulation therapy has been administered po for 3 weeks or unless the early, TEE-guided cardioversion approach is followed.

■ For scheduled cardioversion of AF lasting >48 h, the total duration of po anticoagulation therapy should be at least 7 weeks, i.e. 3 weeks before scheduled cardioversion and at least 4 weeks after successful cardioversion.

■ Administration of antithrombotic therapy to a patient with nonvalvular AF (paroxysmal, persistent or permanent) is determined by the patient's risk of thromboembolism, which is assessed by the CHA_2DS_2-VASc score. For patients with a score of:
   ● ≥2, VKAs should be administered
   ● 1 for men, VKAs should be administered
   ● 0 for men or 1 for women, no antithrombotic therapy is required.

■ NOACs are at least as effective as warfarin for thromboembolism prevention in nonvalvular AF and have a lower risk of intracranial bleeding. In selected patients with nonvalvular AF, NOACs can be given as an alternative to VKAs according to patients CHA_2DS_2-VASc score as follows:
   ● ≥2, dabigatran, rivaroxaban, apixaban or edoxaban should be administered
   ● 1 for men, dabigatran, rivaroxaban, apixaban or edoxaban should be administered
   ● 0 for men or 1 for women, no antithrombotic therapy is required.

■ NOACs should be preferred over VKAs in case of:
   ● inadequate access to laboratory monitoring or patient's preference not to be monitored
   ● poor INR control despite evidence that the patients are complying with VKA medication
   ● resistance to VKA treatment or
   ● need for frequent use of medications that interact with VKAs.

Key points - *continued*

- In patients (both males and females) aged <65 years with lone AF, chronic antithrombotic treatment is not recommended because of the low thromboembolic risk.

- For cardioversion of recent-onset AF (<48 h) in the absence of moderate or severe organic heart disease, propafenone, ibutilide, flecainide or vernakalant may be given; amiodarone is given in cases with organic heart disease.

- Digoxin does not convert recent-onset AF, it merely slows atrioventricular conduction.

- For rapid slowing of the ventricular response in recent-onset AF, the drug of choice is diltiazem IV because of its rapid onset of action. Alternatively, esmolol IV is given.

- AF with wide variable QRS complexes and a rate of >200 beats/min raises suspicion of WPW syndrome. In this case, IV administration of amiodarone, digoxin, verapamil, diltiazem, adenosine, lidocaine and beta-blockers is contraindicated and IV procainamide or ibutilide may be given.

- In selected patients, pharmaceutical cardioversion of recent-onset AF (<48 h, preferably <12 h) with propafenone or flecainide may be attempted at home.

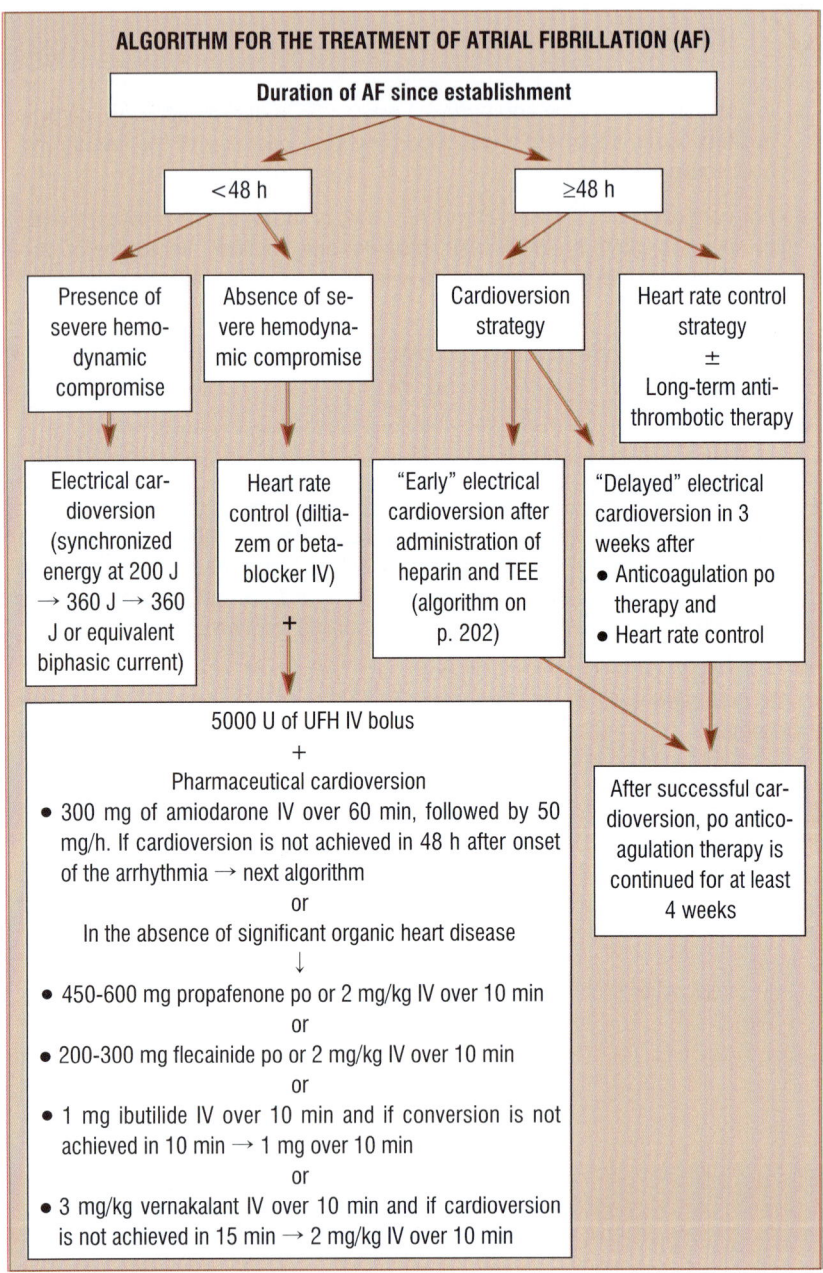

ALGORITHM FOR THE TREATMENT OF ATRIAL FIBRILLATION (AF)

Duration of AF since establishment

<48 h   ≥48 h

| Presence of severe hemo-dynamic compromise | Absence of severe hemodyna-mic compromise | Cardioversion strategy | Heart rate control strategy ± Long-term anti-thrombotic therapy |

Electrical cardioversion (synchronized energy at 200 J → 360 J → 360 J or equivalent biphasic current)

Heart rate control (diltia-zem or beta-blocker IV)
+

"Early" electrical cardioversion after administration of heparin and TEE (algorithm on p. 202)

"Delayed" electrical cardioversion in 3 weeks after
• Anticoagulation po therapy and
• Heart rate control

5000 U of UFH IV bolus
+
Pharmaceutical cardioversion
• 300 mg of amiodarone IV over 60 min, followed by 50 mg/h. If cardioversion is not achieved in 48 h after onset of the arrhythmia → next algorithm
or
In the absence of significant organic heart disease
↓
• 450-600 mg propafenone po or 2 mg/kg IV over 10 min
or
• 200-300 mg flecainide po or 2 mg/kg IV over 10 min
or
• 1 mg ibutilide IV over 10 min and if conversion is not achieved in 10 min → 1 mg over 10 min
or
• 3 mg/kg vernakalant IV over 10 min and if cardioversion is not achieved in 15 min → 2 mg/kg IV over 10 min

After successful cardioversion, po anticoagulation therapy is continued for at least 4 weeks

TEE: transesophageal echocardiogram, UFH: unfractionated heparin

15

Regular supraventricular tachycardia

The most common types of regular supraventricular tachycardia (usually with narrow QRS complexes) encountered in the emergency cardiology clinic are atrioventricular nodal reentrant tachycardia (AVNRT), atrioventricular reentrant tachycardia (AVRT), and atrial flutter. Note that the most common type of regular tachycardia, with rates of 100-150 beats/min (or up to 200 beats/min in younger individuals during strenuous exercise) is **sinus tachycardia,** which does not require special medication beyond the correction of the underlying cause (Table 15.1). Sinus tachycardia has a gradual onset and offset.

A rare form of sinus tachycardia is **inappropriate sinus tachycardia,**

TABLE 15.1	Major causes of sinus tachycardia

1) Anxiety, pain

2) Fever

3) Hypotension or shock

4) Myocardial ischemia or heart failure

5) Exercise

6) Anemia

7) Overconsumption of coffee, tea, cola-type beverages

8) Hyperthyroidism

9) Hypoxemia

10) Medication (e.g. salbutamol, sympathomimetic drugs, inotropic drugs, atropine)

11) Acute pulmonary embolism

which is characterized by an elevated heart rate (>100 beats/min at rest) with no secondary cause for this increase. In patients with symptomatic inappropriate sinus tachycardia ivabradine (Procoralan, 2.5-7.5 mg x 2 daily) or beta-blockers (less effective) can be given.

1) Atrioventricular nodal reentrant tachycardia (AVNRT)

This is the most common type of supraventricular regular tachycardia (~60% of all cases of regular supraventricular tachycardia, excluding sinus tachycardia). It is caused by a reentry mechanism at the level of the atrioventricular (AV) node, where two pathways with different conduction speeds are found: the **slow pathway,** with a short refractory period, and the **fast pathway,** with a prolonged refractory period. Tachycardia is triggered by a premature atrial impulse (extrastimulus) that is usually conducted anterogradely to the ventricles through the slow pathway (typical form), since the fast pathway is still in its refractory period and will not conduct. The circuit closes with the retrograde conduction of the extrastimulus through the fast pathway (slow-fast conduction), causing atrial stimulation.

It is characterized by sudden onset and termination; the heart rate usually ranges between 150 and 250 beats/min. It usually occurs in individuals with no underlying organic heart disease. Symptoms range from palpitations and nervousness to angina, dyspnea and (more rarely) syncope. Polyuria may coexist, due to oversecretion of the atrial natriuretic peptide because of increased intraatrial pressures.

ECG
Characterized by regular tachycardia with narrow QRS complexes (except in the case of preexisting bundle branch block or if functional aberrant conduction develops). P waves are usually not visible because they coincide with the QRS complexes (simultaneous excitation of the atria and the ventricles) [Figure 15.1].

Treatment
1) If the patient does not present significant hemodynamic compromise, which is the most likely scenario, then vagal maneuvers are attempted as a first step (achieve cardioversion in ~50% of cases); if these fail, medication is administered.
   a) Vagal maneuvers:
      • **Valsalva maneuver:** the patient exhales forcefully with mouth and nose sealed, for about 15 s (patient is asked to exert pressure as when defecating).
      • **Carotid sinus massage:** before massage, both carotids should be

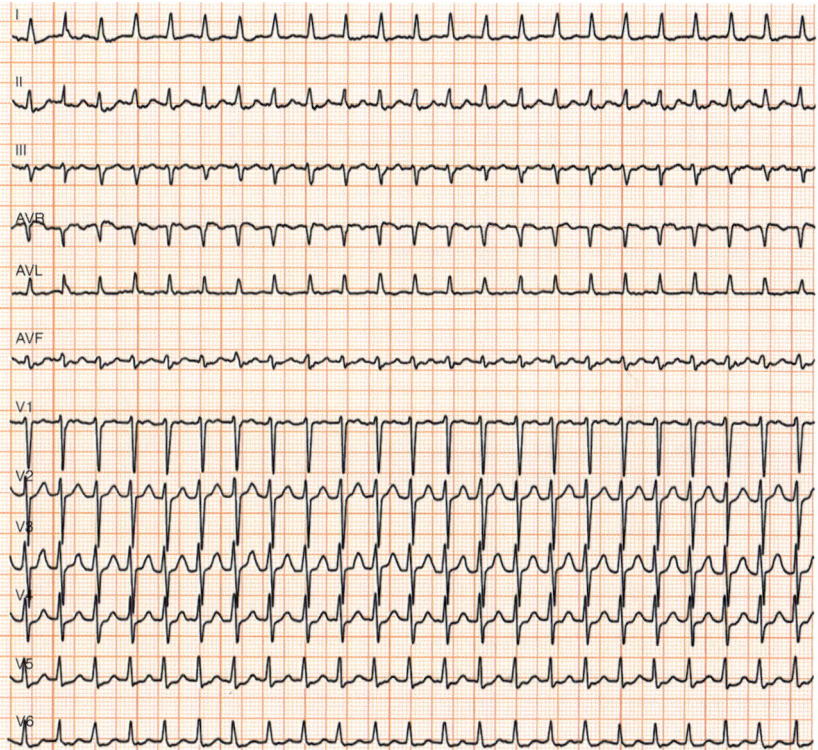

Figure 15.1. ECG of a patient with atrioventricular nodal reentrant tachycardia. This is a case of regular tachycardia at a rate of 180 beats/min, with narrow QRS complexes and no visible P waves.

auscultated and massage should be avoided if a bruit is heard or if there is a history of cerebrovascular accident within the last three months. Duration should be ~5 s. If massaging one sinus is not effective, then massaging the contralateral sinus should be attempted after a wait of 2 min so that the AV node will have time to produce acetylcholine. Table 15.2 presents the preconditions for a safe massage of the carotid sinus.

Warning! Massage should always be performed under ECG monitoring. If asystole occurs, the patient is asked to cough and/or a precordial thump is delivered. If these are not effective, IV atropine is administered.

TABLE 15.2	Preconditions for safe massage of the carotid sinus

1) Place a peripheral line
2) The patient is placed in a supine position
3) Avoid massage if a carotid bruit is detected or there is a history of cerebrovascular accident within the last three months. It is also prudent to avoid massage in persons older than 70 years
4) Never massage both carotid sinuses simultaneously
5) Using two fingers (index and middle), firmly but gently massage (do not apply so much pressure to occlude carotid artery) the area just below the angle of the jaw and in front of the sternocleidomastoid muscle, at the position where the carotid pulse is felt most strongly (Figure 15.2)
6) Massage for ~5 s
7) Monitor the ECG throughout the massage
8) Atropine in syringes should be available for IV administration in case of prolonged asystole not responding to cough and/or to precordial thump

- **Pressure on the eyes:** should not be performed because of the risk of retinal detachment. It is also very painful.

b) If the vagal maneuvers fail, then the patient is treated with medication using:
  - **Adenosine** (Adenocard, Adenocor): this is the drug of choice for cardioversion, since it interrupts the reentry circuit. With regard to its effects on the cardiovascular system, it acts mostly on the AV node by reducing its conductivity, and relaxes the vascular smooth muscle fibers (vasodilation). It has a short half-life (<10 s). It is administered by rapid IV injection (bolus), followed by immediate flushing with 10 mL of normal saline so that the drug will move quickly to the target organ (heart) before it is removed from the circulation (through uptake, mostly by vascular endothelial cells and erythrocytes). For 2 min after the infusion the patient is monitored continuously by ECG. The starting dose is 6 mg. If cardioversion is not achieved in 2 min (usually occurs within 1 min), another 12 mg are administered and may be repeated if the arrhythmia persists: the administration sequence is 6 → 12 → 12 mg. The rate of successful cardioversion is >90%. Adenosine's rapid and very short duration of action permits its administration even in cases where severe hemodynamic compromise dictates electrical cardioversion,

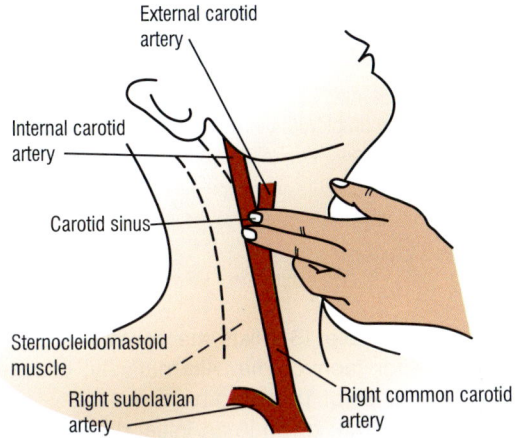

Figure 15.2. Site for carotid sinus massage.

which will of course be performed if the tachycardia is not cardioverted pharmaceutically.

Adenosine is contraindicated in individuals with a history of bronchial asthma. If the patient has taken dipyridamole (which inhibits adenosine uptake by endothelial cells, and therefore its metabolism and inactivation), the dose of adenosine should be halved, because its effect is increased (risk of hypotension). Lower doses are also given to elderly individuals because of the possibility of concurrent sinus node disease, in heart transplant recipients and if administration is via a central line. On the other hand, if the patient has received theophylline or caffeine, which antagonize adenosine uptake by cellular receptors, then a larger dose of adenosine will be required.

At the moment of cardioversion, the patient will feel temporary lightheadedness because adenosine causes transient asystole (usually <5 s). Other side effects (which last <1 min) are flushing, chest pain, headache and dyspnea. In individuals with a history of asthma or chronic respiratory failure, a bronchial asthma attack can be triggered, which may last up to 30 min. In rare cases (<3%), it causes atrial fibrillation due to shortening of the atrial myocardium's refractory period.

- **Verapamil** (Isoptin): administered if adenosine fails or is contraindicated (history of bronchial asthma), in a dose of 5 mg over 1-2 min, and can be repeated after 5 min at the same dose if cardioversion

TABLE 15.3	Contraindications to the administration of verapamil for the treatment of regular tachycardia

1) Hypotension (systolic blood pressure <100 mmHg)
2) Widened (>120 ms) QRS complexes, because it can cause shock in the setting of ventricular tachycardia or in persons with WPW syndrome
3) Known left ventricular dysfunction (ejection fraction <40%), because it can cause acute left heart failure due to its negative inotropic effect
4) Concurrent use of beta-blockers

is not achieved. Table 15.3 lists the contraindications to verapamil administration for tachycardia. Alternatively, diltiazem can be administered at a dose of 15-20 mg IV.
- **Propranolol** (Inderal): given in an initial dose of 1 mg IV, and then repeated every 5 min up to a maximum dosage of 5 mg (usually 2-4 mg are sufficient). Alternatively, esmolol IV can be administered (for the dosage regimen, see Chapter 23).

Warning! Digoxin IV is not administered for cardioversion of AVNRT because of its delayed effect (usually >60 min).

2) In case of severe hemodynamic compromise, synchronized electrical (direct current or DC) cardioversion is attempted (20-50 J are usually sufficient). This is rarely done today because, as mentioned previously, adenosine can be administered even in cases of severe hemodynamic compromise and electrical cardioversion will be performed only if this fails.
3) In case of severe hemodynamic compromise and contraindication for electrical cardioversion, i.e. previous administration of large doses of digoxin, programmed atrial pacing can be performed through a temporary transvenous atrial electrode.

Advice on discharge from the Emergency Room for individuals with cardioverted atrioventricular nodal reentrant tachycardia
- Avoid smoking and overconsumption of alcohol, coffee, tea and cola-type drinks.
- Check thyroid function (to rule out hyperthyroidism) and obtain an echocardiogram (to rule out organic heart disease).
- If the episodes are infrequent (<3 per year), brief and well tolerated, then no prophylactic medication is prescribed.
- If the episodes are frequent or prolonged, then prophylaxis is pre-

scribed: verapamil (40-120 mg x 3/day), diltiazem (60 mg x 3/day), beta-blockers or, if there is no left ventricular dysfunction, propafenone (150 mg x 3/day).

- If the episodes are not controlled with medication or the patient does not wish to take long-term pharmacological treatment, then the patient is referred to specialist centers for radiofrequency ablation (usually of the slow pathway) [success rate >95%].

- If the patient presents infrequent and prolonged episodes that are well tolerated, and also has no history of organic heart disease (e.g. previous myocardial infarction or cardiomyopathy) or Wolff-Parkinson-White (WPW) syndrome, then they may attempt to cardiovert the tachycardia at home with 120 mg diltiazem + 80 mg propranolol po (pill-in-the-pocket).

2) Atrioventricular reentrant tachycardia (AVRT)

This accounts for 15-30% of all cases of regular supraventricular tachycardia. In this type of tachycardia, an accessory pathway (or bypass tract) is always involved. Accessory pathways are myocardial tracts with different electrophysiological properties (i.e. stimulus conduction speed and refractory period) compared to the myocardium. They are located around the AV valve annuli (most commonly in the free left lateral wall of the left ventricle) and can permit the conduction of stimuli from the atria to the ventricles (AV conduction) and/or from the ventricles to the atria (ventriculoatrial conduction). Therefore, an accessory pathway can be:

a) **Apparent** through the observation of preexcitation in the resting ECG. This means that it conducts stimuli from the atria to the ventricles, which are stimulated before the arrival of the stimulus that follows the normal pathway, so that the widened QRS complex results from the fusion of the ventricular depolarizations through the two different pathways (the accessory pathway and the normal pathway). The term "WPW syndrome" refers to individuals with characteristic preexcitatory ECG changes (Table 15.4) as well as a history of paroxysmal tachycardia.

b) **Concealed,** capable of retrograde (ventriculoatrial) conduction; therefore preexcitation is not apparent in the ECG, which is normal. The concealed accessory pathway is diagnosed only through an electrophysiological study.

The most common type of tachycardia (~95%) in individuals with an accessory pathway is orthodromic AVRT. In this case, the stimulus descends anterogradely to the ventricles through the AV node and returns to the atria through the accessory pathway. The QRS complex is normal (except in cases of aberrant conduction or preexisting bundle branch block), since the sti-

TABLE 15.4	ECG characteristics in WPW syndrome with visible preexcitation

1) Narrow PR interval (<120 ms)
2) Presence of a delta wave (this is the first part of the QRS complex, of slow ascent or descent type, and is caused by preexcitation)
3) Widened QRS complex (>120 ms) [due to the presence of the delta wave]
4) ST-segment/T wave changes (directed opposite to the major delta wave and QRS complex)

mulus is conducted through the AV node. In ~5% of cases, the tachycardia is antidromic, because the stimulus descends through the accessory pathway and returns through the AV node. In this case, the QRS complex is widened and ventricular tachycardia should be included in the differential diagnosis. Orthodromic and antidromic AVRT are characterized by sudden onset and termination.

When should we suspect that a narrow QRS complex tachycardia is concealing an accessory pathway?

- The ECG during tachycardia may show visible inverted P waves after the QRS complexes (RP interval is usually >70 ms) in the inferior wall leads (whereas these are almost never visible in AVNRT).
- The heart rate is usually >200 beats/min (whereas in AVNRT it is usually between 150 and 200 beats/min).

Treatment

- In cases of regular narrow QRS complex tachycardia, the treatment is similar to AVNRT, i.e. vagal maneuvers, **adenosine** (drug of choice), or **verapamil.** In cases of severe hemodynamic compromise, DC cardioversion (i.e. delivery of shock synchronized to the QRS complex) is attempted.

Warning! Adenosine is the drug of choice for the cardioversion of AVNRT and AVRT that occurs in a pregnant woman.

- In cases of regular tachycardia with wide QRS complexes in a person with known WPW syndrome, which needs to be differentiated from ventricular tachycardia, the drug of choice is procainamide. **Procainamide** (Pronestyl, injection solution of 1000 mg/10 mL) is given in a dose of 100 mg over 2 min and is repeated in the same 100 mg dose every 5 min until cardioversion is achieved (maximum dosage 1000 mg in the first hour) or until hypotension develops or the QRS complex widens by more than 50%. In cases of severe hemodynamic compromise (systolic blood pressure [BP] <90 mmHg, angina or acute pulmonary edema), DC cardioversion is performed under sedation (if there is time).

What is the appropriate management for a patient who presents ECG findings consistent with WPW syndrome after tachycardia cardioversion?

- The patient is referred to a specialized center for an electrophysiological study and possible therapeutic intervention (catheter ablation of the accessory pathway), if findings indicating a high risk of sudden death, such as an accessory pathway with a refractory period <250 ms, are identified. Some centers recommend an electrophysiological study even in asymptomatic patients who have ECG findings consistent with preexcitation syndrome.

- If ablation of the accessory pathway is not performed (success rate ~95%) and medication is preferred for tachycardia prevention, amiodarone, sotalol, propafenone or flecainide may be given. The administration of verapamil, diltiazem or digoxin is contraindicated, because if atrial fibrillation develops there is a risk of ventricular fibrillation.

3) Atrial flutter

This is less common than atrial fibrillation. It is due to a macroreentry mechanism through a circuit most commonly located within the right atrium. The reentrant wavefront typically travels in a circular loop behind the tricuspid valve, involving the cavotricuspid isthmus (area between the inferior vena cava and the tricuspid valve). Atrial flutter is an unstable arrhythmia and often degenerates into atrial fibrillation. It develops more commonly on a substrate of organic heart disease. The causes of atrial flutter are listed in Table 15.5.

We distinguish two types of atrial flutter:

1) The **typical or the cavotricuspid isthmus-dependent atrial flutter:** originates in the right atrium, involves the cavotricuspid isthmus, and the circuit rotates around the tricuspid valve in either counterclockwise (more common) or clockwise direction

2) The **atypical or the noncavotricuspid isthmus-dependent atrial flutter:** does not involve the cavotricuspid isthmus, can originate in both the right and left atria, and is usually due to reentry around atrial scars (e.g. after cardiac surgery or ablation for atrial fibrillation).

The ventricular rate in atrial flutter can be:
- Regular (usually) if the AV conduction is constant. If the AV conduction is 2:1 or 4:1, then the ventricular rate is ~150 or 75 beats/min, re-

TABLE 15.5	Causes of atrial flutter

1) Coronary artery disease
2) Mitral or tricuspid valve diseases
3) Cardiomyopathies
4) Pericarditis
5) Acute myocarditis
6) Acute pulmonary embolism
7) Hyperthyroidism
8) Overconsumption of alcohol
9) Postcardiac surgery
10) Respiratory tract infections and chronic obstructive pulmonary disease

spectively. In rare pediatric cases with preexcitation syndrome or hyperthyroidism, AV conduction may be 1:1 and the ventricular rate may be ~300 beats/min.

- Irregular, if there is a Wenckebach-type AV block or an alternating 2:1, 3:1, or 4:1 AV conduction.

ECG

The typical form is characterized by regular atrial waves (flutter waves) with an atrial rate of ~300 beats/min (in the absence of drug therapy) which have a "sawtooth" appearance between the QRS complexes (no isoelectric line is interposed between them). The counterclockwise atrial flutter shows negative flutter waves in leads II, III, aVF and a positive wave in V_1 (Figure 15.3), while the clockwise atrial flutter has the opposite pattern (positive flutter waves in the inferior leads and a negative wave in V_1).

Differential diagnosis for atrial flutter

Atrial flutter must be distinguished from other forms of supraventricular tachycardia, especially if flutter waves are not clearly visible. This is more difficult in patients who present with regular tachycardia, narrow QRS complexes, heart rate ~150 beats/min and no discernible flutter waves, as these are masked by the QRS complexes. This tachycardia can easily be mistaken for AVNRT or AVRT. In such cases, vagal maneuvers should be performed or adenosine should be administered, which transiently increases the AV block (e.g. from 2:1 to 4:1 AV conduction), the flutter waves can be discerned and the correct diagnosis is established.

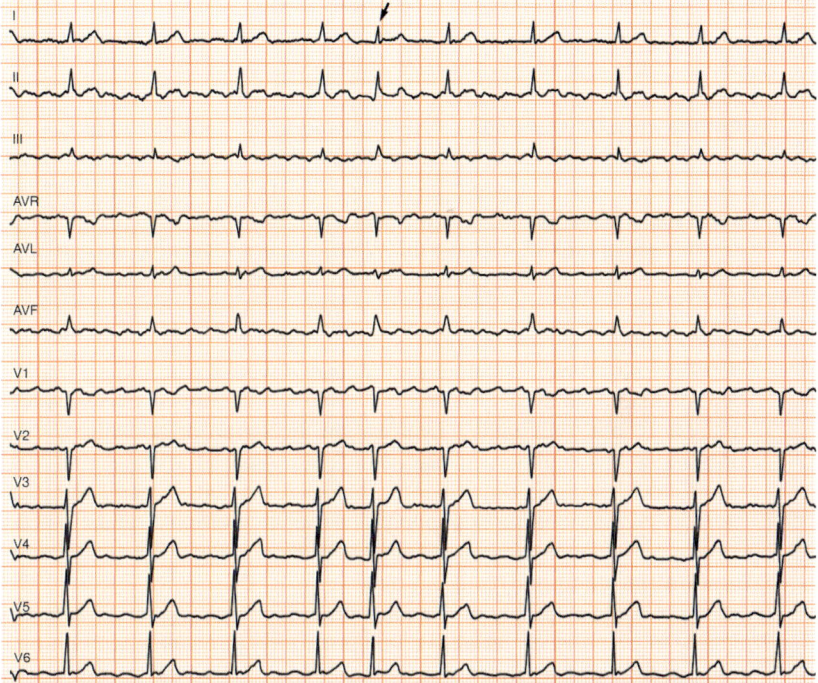

Figure 15.3. This ECG shows a typical counterclockwise atrial flutter with stable atrioventricular (AV) block (4:1 AV conduction). There are visible flutter waves (negative in leads II, III, aVF and positive in V_1) and the QRS complexes are narrow and regular (~75 /min). The exception is the 5th QRS complex (arrow), which occurs sooner because of a 3:1 AV conduction.

Warning! A cardiac patient with a regular narrow QRS complex tachycardia and a heart rate of ~150 beats/min is likely to have atrial flutter with 2:1 AV conduction.

Treatment

1) Severe hemodynamic compromise

In case of severe hemodynamic compromise (acute pulmonary edema, a fall in systolic BP to <90 mmHg, etc.), synchronized DC shock is delivered (with a first shock at 50 or 100 J and then 200 J → 360 J if that fails, if monophasic current is used, or equivalent energy for biphasic current). If, after electrical discharge, atrial flutter converts to atrial fibrillation, then cardioversion with higher energy is attempted.

2) *Mild or moderate hemodynamic compromise*

a) **DC cardioversion** under sedation: This is the treatment of choice because of the low effectiveness of antiarrhythmic drugs (except for ibutilide).

b) **Antithrombotic treatment:** The indications for its administration are similar to those in atrial fibrillation. If the time of onset is <48 h, cardioversion should be attempted after 5000 U of IV unfractionated heparin have been given, followed by subcutaneous administration of low-molecular-weight heparin (LMWH) [e.g. enoxaparin in a dose of 1 mg/kg x 2/day]. After successful cardioversion, provided that there are no risk factors for thromboembolism, anticoagulation medication may be stopped. If the time of onset is ≥48 h, anticoagulation should be administered for 3 weeks before and at least 4 weeks after the scheduled cardioversion. As an alternative to vitamin K antagonists, non-VKA oral anticoagulants (dabigatran, rivaroxaban, apixaban or edoxaban) may be given in cases of nonvalvular atrial flutter. Also, if the onset time of atrial flutter cannot be determined precisely or is ≥48 h, early electrical cardioversion under transesophageal echocardiographic guidance can be attempted (as in the case of atrial fibrillation: page 202).

c) **Rapid atrial pacing:** This is an alternative to DC cardioversion in the setting of digitalis toxicity or in situations in which pacing atrial wires are already in place, such as after cardiac surgery, in patients with permanent pacemaker, etc. By pacing the right atrium with a catheter in it or in the esophagus (e.g. with a burst of atrial pacing at a rate of 400 beats/min), the flutter rate is overdriven, which achieves cardioversion in ~70% of cases.

d) **Pharmaceutical treatment:**
  - **Cardioversion:** may be attempted in stable patients with **ibutilide**, as an alternative to electrical cardioversion. Ibutilide converts atrial flutter to sinus rhythm in ~60% of cases. It is contraindicated in cases of hypokalemia (which should be corrected first – serum potassium must be >4 mEq/L), preexisting QT prolongation and severe left ventricular dysfunction. Also, continuous ECG monitoring of the patient for 4 h (at least) after cardioversion is required, because of the risk of torsades de pointes due to prolongation of the QT interval. Ibutilide (Corvert, ampoule of 1 mg/10 mL) is administered IV at a dose of 1 mg (in individuals weighing <60 kg, the dose is 0.01 mg/kg) over 10 min, and the same dose is repeated after 10 min if cardioversion fails. For the cardioversion of atrial flutter other antiarrhythmics, such as **amiodarone** or **procainamide** IV may be used, but they are less effective (success rate <40%) and therefore ibutilide is the preferred agent for pharmaceutical cardioversion nowadays. In particular, because of procainamide's vagolytic effect and the resultant

increase in AV conductivity, in conjunction with the reduction in a-trial rate it causes (e.g. from 300 to 200 beats/min), it can lead to 1:1 conduction resulting in a rapid ventricular response (e.g. 200 beats/min). Therefore, it should always be preceded by IV adminis-tration of a bradycardic calcium channel blocker (diltiazem or vera-pamil), a beta-blocker, or digoxin, so that the AV block will be in-creased. However, these drugs are never administered when pro-cainamide is given to patients with WPW syndrome, because they can lead to 1:1 conduction and therefore to a rapid ventricular re-sponse. This is caused by the atrial stimuli all descending through the accessory pathway, as these drugs shorten its refractory period and also slow the conduction through the AV node.

Table 15.6 lists the drugs indicated and contraindicated in stable patients with WPW syndrome and wide QRS complex tachycardia (regular or irregular).

Warning! In patients with atrial flutter and suspected WPW syndrome, the treatment of choice is DC cardioversion. If, however, the patient is stable, pharmaceutical cardioversion may be attempted with IV procainamide.

TABLE 15.6	Drugs (IV) that are indicated or contraindicated in stable patients with WPW syndrome and wide QRS complex tachycardia (regular or irregular)

1) WPW syndrome + irregular tachycardia (i.e. AF): drugs **indicated** for the cardioversion:
   - Procainamide
   - Ibutilide

2) WPW syndrome + irregular tachycardia (i.e. AF): drugs **contraindicated** because they reduce the refractory period of the accessory pathway and facilitate the rapid descent of stimuli:
   - Amiodarone
   - Digoxin
   - Verapamil, diltiazem
   - Beta-blockers
   - Adenosine
   - Lidocaine

3) WPW syndrome + regular tachycardia (i.e. antidromic AVRT, atrial flutter or ventricular tachycardia): drug **indicated** for the cardioversion:
   - Procainamide

AF: atrial fibrillation, AVRT: atrioventricular reentrant tachycardia

- **Reduction of the ventricular rate:** For acute control of the ventricular rate in stable patients, the following may be administered (according to the recent American Guidelines for the Management of Supraventricular Tachycardia, Page RL, et al. Circulation 2016;133:e471-505):
  - Verapamil IV at an initial dose of 5-10 mg or diltiazem IV at an initial dose of 15-20 mg
  - Propranolol IV at an initial dose of 1-5 mg or esmolol (initial dose 500 µg/kg over 1 min, followed by infusion at 50-300 µg/kg/min) or
  - Amiodarone IV at an initial dose of ~300 mg within 60 min (see page 198), in the setting of systolic heart failure when beta-blockers are contraindicated or are ineffective.

Warning! In general, heart rate control with drugs in atrial flutter is much more difficult than in atrial fibrillation.

If heart rate control is selected over immediate cardioversion (e.g. if the patient presents >48 h after the onset of the arrhythmia and DC cardioversion is scheduled for 3 weeks later), then a bradycardic calcium channel blocker (diltiazem or verapamil), a beta-blocker or digoxin may be administered po.

e) **Catheter ablation:** should be considered in patients with symptomatic or recurrent atrial flutter without a reversible cause. Catheter ablation (usually radiofrequency) of typical flutter (counterclockwise and clockwise) has an acute success rate of ~90%. Because ablation of atrial flutter is so effective and poses little risk, it can be offered as first line therapy. However, it should be noted that after successful ablation, ~30% of patients will develop atrial fibrillation.

4) Atrial tachycardia

This accounts for 10-15% of supraventricular tachycardias and can be caused by a microreentry mechanism, increased automaticity (automatic atrial tachycardia), or triggered activity (the least common). In most cases, no clear identification of the mechanism can be made, since the clinical features and ECG patterns are overlapping. It is usually seen in individuals with coronary artery disease, heart failure, pulmonary disease, electrolyte disorders, or digitalis toxicity. Atrial tachycardias frequently occur in short recurrent bursts. If atrial tachycardia is incessant, tachycardia-induced cardiomyopathy can result. This type of ventricular dysfunction may be partially or totally reversible by eliminating the tachycardia.

ECG

The atrial rate ranges from 150 to 250 beats/min and the P waves are regular — except for automatic atrial tachycardia which accelerates after its initiation (warm-up phenomenon) — and have a morphology different to that of sinus P waves. In contrast to the atrial flutter ECG, there is an isoelectric line between the P waves. Second-degree AV block (2:1 or 3:1 AV conduction) is a common finding. The response of atrial tachycardia to manipulations causing AV block (vagal maneuvers or administration of adenosine) is variable and depends on the underlying mechanism: automatic atrial tachycardia does not response to vagal maneuvers, while adenosine may slow it transiently but it is unlikely to terminate it.

Treatment

If the atrial tachycardia is caused by digitalis toxicity, digoxin should be discontinued and any hypokalemia should be corrected. In severe cases, infusion of anti-digoxin antibodies may be required. DC cardioversion is contraindicated because it may be complicated by the development of refractory arrhythmia.

For other causes of atrial tachycardia, slowing of AV conduction is attempted through the IV administration of beta-blockers or bradycardic calcium channel blockers. The ability of adenosine, beta-blockers or verapamil to terminate atrial tachycardias is variable. In addition, DC cardioversion is ineffective in automatic atrial tachycardia. It should be noted that, in all these cases, it is very important to treat any underlying triggering cause (e.g. respiratory insufficiency) at the same time. If the tachycardia persists, the preferred therapy is catheter ablation.

An uncommon type of atrial tachycardia is **multifocal (chaotic) atrial tachycardia (MAT).** The mechanism appears to be increased automaticity or triggered activity. It is characterized by atrial rates between 100 and 130 beats/min, P waves of at least three distinct morphologies, and totally irregular P-P, PR and R-R intervals. Because the ventricular rate is irregular, this arrhythmia is most likely to be mistaken for atrial fibrillation. MAT is usually observed in older patients with chronic obstructive pulmonary disease and associated hypoxia. It can degenerate into atrial fibrillation. Treatment is directed primarily at the underlying disease, with antiarrhythmics playing only a minor role. Verapamil or amiodarone IV may be useful. Maintenance of the potassium and magnesium balance may suppress the tachycardia. DC cardioversion is contraindicated (ineffective and may precipitate dangerous arrhythmias).

Table 15.7 lists the most common causes of narrow QRS complex regular tachycardia and their most important differences.

| TABLE 15.7 | The most common causes of regular narrow QRS complex tachycardia |

Type of arrhythmia	Ventricular rate (beats /min)	P waves on the ECG	Carotid sinus massage	Treatment of choice
Sinus tachycardia	100-150	Visible, precede each QRS complex	Slight transient slowing	Treatment of the underlying disease
Atrioventricular nodal reentrant tachycardia	150-250	Usually not visible	Sudden cardio-version or no effect ("all or nothing" response)	Adenosine IV
Atrioventricular reentrant tachycardia (orthodromic)	150-250 (usually >200)	May appear inverted after the QRS complexes	Sudden cardio-version or no effect ("all or nothing" response)	Adenosine IV
Atrial flutter	65-175	Usually visible sawtooth atrial waves	Sudden tran-sient slowing because of an increase in atrioventricular block (unmasking of flutter waves)	Electrical cardioversion or ibutilide IV
Atrial tachycardia	150-250	Visible with an isoelectric line between them	Variable response depending on the underlying mechanism	Treatment of the triggering cause Little role of drugs

Key points

- A patient presenting to the Emergency Room with regular tachycardia with a rate ≥150 beats/min and narrow QRS complexes will probably have:
  - AVNRT (the most common)
  - AVRT (orthodromic)
  - atrial flutter with stable 2:1 AV conduction (~150 beats/min), or
  - atrial tachycardia.

- IV adenosine can be a diagnostic and therapeutic tool in patients with a regular, narrow QRS complex tachycardia: If, after adenosine administration:
  - the tachycardia is cardioverted, then the cause is AVNRT or AVRT
  - the heart rate decreases and atrial flutter waves emerge, then the cause is atrial flutter.

- Adenosine should be administered by rapid IV bolus and then flushed with normal saline so that it is transported as quickly as possible to its target organ, the heart (half-life <10 s).

- A patient with WPW syndrome who develops regular tachycardia with:
  - narrow QRS complexes: should be treated in the same way as for AVNRT (the drug of choice is adenosine)
  - wide QRS complexes: since it is usually impossible to determine the mechanism of the tachycardia in the Emergency Room (orthodromic AVRT with aberrant conduction or preexisting bundle branch block, antidromic AVRT, atrial flutter with anterograde conduction via the accessory pathway, or most importantly ventricular tachycardia) the preferred treatment is DC cardioversion. In stable patients cardioversion can be attempted with IV procainamide.

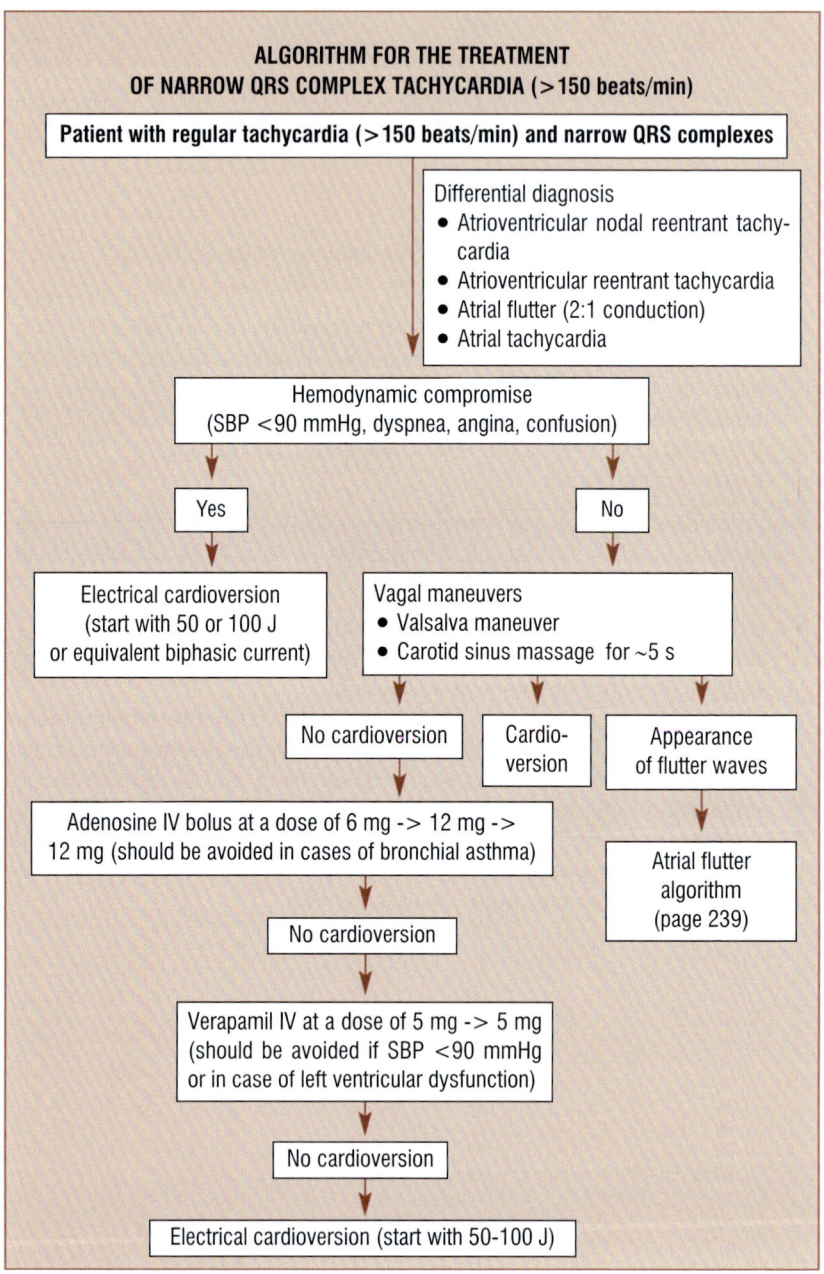

**ALGORITHM FOR THE TREATMENT
OF NARROW QRS COMPLEX TACHYCARDIA (>150 beats/min)**

Patient with regular tachycardia (>150 beats/min) and narrow QRS complexes

Differential diagnosis
- Atrioventricular nodal reentrant tachy-cardia
- Atrioventricular reentrant tachycardia
- Atrial flutter (2:1 conduction)
- Atrial tachycardia

Hemodynamic compromise
(SBP <90 mmHg, dyspnea, angina, confusion)

Yes

No

Electrical cardioversion
(start with 50 or 100 J
or equivalent biphasic current)

Vagal maneuvers
- Valsalva maneuver
- Carotid sinus massage for ~5 s

No cardioversion

Cardio-version

Appearance
of flutter waves

Adenosine IV bolus at a dose of 6 mg -> 12 mg ->
12 mg (should be avoided in cases of bronchial asthma)

Atrial flutter
algorithm
(page 239)

No cardioversion

Verapamil IV at a dose of 5 mg -> 5 mg
(should be avoided if SBP <90 mmHg
or in case of left ventricular dysfunction)

No cardioversion

Electrical cardioversion (start with 50-100 J)

SBP: systolic blood pressure

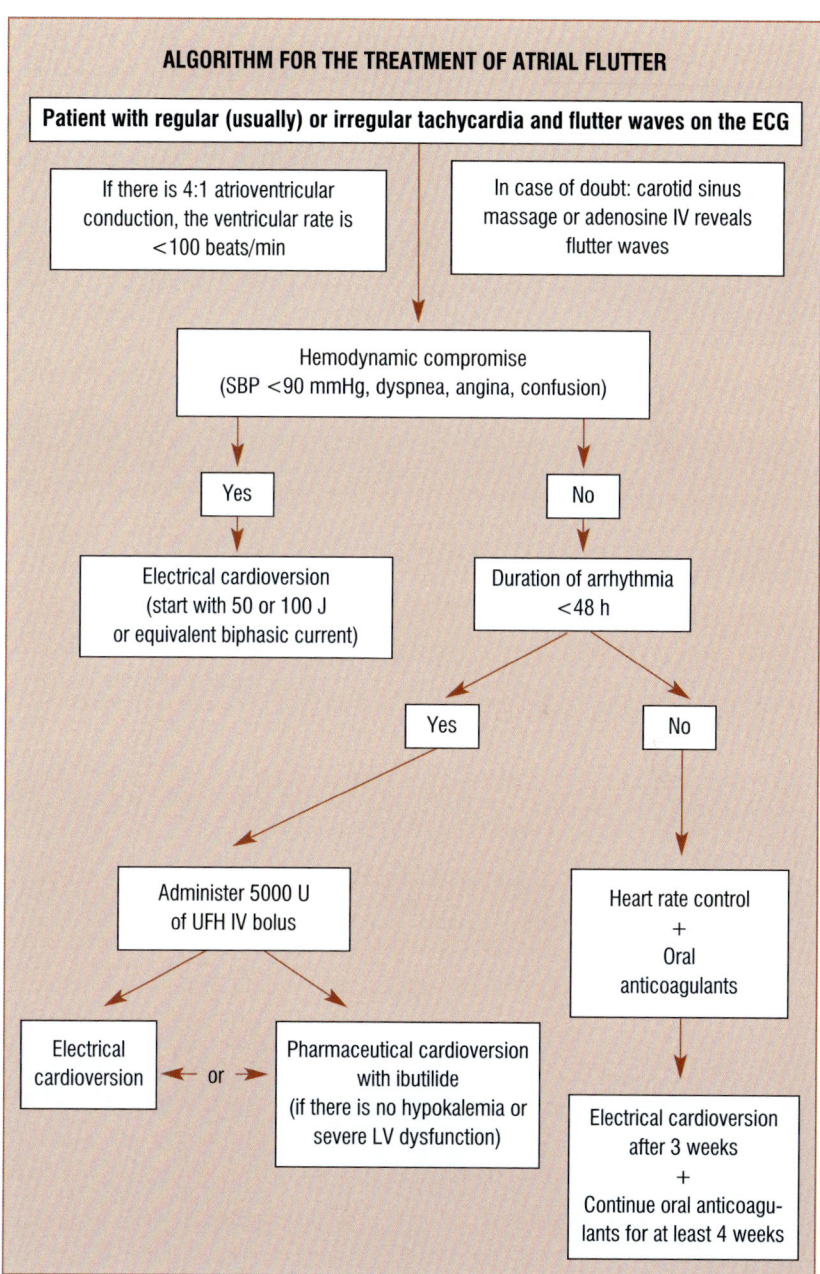

ALGORITHM FOR THE TREATMENT OF ATRIAL FLUTTER

Patient with regular (usually) or irregular tachycardia and flutter waves on the ECG

If there is 4:1 atrioventricular conduction, the ventricular rate is <100 beats/min

In case of doubt: carotid sinus massage or adenosine IV reveals flutter waves

Hemodynamic compromise (SBP <90 mmHg, dyspnea, angina, confusion)

Yes

No

Electrical cardioversion (start with 50 or 100 J or equivalent biphasic current)

Duration of arrhythmia <48 h

Yes

No

Administer 5000 U of UFH IV bolus

Heart rate control + Oral anticoagulants

Electrical cardioversion ← or → Pharmaceutical cardioversion with ibutilide (if there is no hypokalemia or severe LV dysfunction)

Electrical cardioversion after 3 weeks + Continue oral anticoagulants for at least 4 weeks

SBP: systolic blood pressure, UFH: unfractionated heparin, LV: left ventricular

16

Ventricular tachycardia

Ventricular tachycardia (VT) is defined as ≥3 successive ventricular complexes with a rate of >100 beats/min. VT is a potentially lethal arrhythmia and is classified as either:

- sustained, when it lasts for ≥30 s, or regardless of duration if it is accompanied by hemodynamic compromise, or
- nonsustained, when it terminates spontaneously in <30 s.

Causes of ventricular tachycardia

Table 16.1 shows the main causes of VT. The most common of all (>70% of tachycardias) is coronary artery disease (CAD). The tachycardia appears either in the phase of acute ischemia (usually abnormal automaticity within the ischemic border zone) or in chronic CAD (mainly in patients

TABLE 16.1	Main causes of ventricular tachycardia (VT)
1) Coronary artery disease	6) Arrhythmogenic right ventricular cardiomyopathy
2) Cardiomyopathy (dilated or hypertrophic)	7) Electrolyte disorders (mainly hypokalemia)
3) Long-QT syndrome (mainly responsible for polymorphic VT)	8) Surgically corrected tetralogy of Fallot
4) Acute myocarditis	9) Brugada syndrome (mainly responsible for polymorphic VT)
5) Idiopathic (absence of organic heart disease)	

with an old myocardial infarction and impaired left ventricular function, where it is usually due to a reentry mechanism in the region of the scar).

Clinical presentation

This depends on the duration, the rate, and the underlying cardiac disease. It may manifest itself in the form of palpitations, but it more often causes hemodynamic compromise (dyspnea, angina, hypotension, confusion from cerebral hypoperfusion, syncope or arrest).

The hemodynamic compromise is not a sure criterion for the differential diagnosis from wide QRS complex supraventricular tachycardia. Relatively slow VT in individuals who do not have severe left ventricular dysfunction may be well tolerated, while a rapid supraventricular tachycardia may be symptomatic, especially in patients with organic heart disease.

In general, VTs with a rate <150 beats/min may be well tolerated if they are of short duration, even in patients with organic heart disease, while VTs of >200 beats/min are almost always symptomatic. VT does not respond to vagotonic maneuvers, with the exception of a rare form of idiopathic VT that appears in normal hearts.

Clinical signs

- Signs of atrioventricular dissociation: variable intensity of the 1st heart sound and jugular a waves of varying sizes independent of ventricular systoles. When the right atrial systole coincides with the right ventricular systole, i.e. right atrial contraction against a closed tricuspid valve, large a waves (**cannon a waves**) occur, which are irregular.
- When there is retrograde conduction and the atria are activated by ventricular stimuli (~25%) there are regular large jugular a waves (cannon a waves) that are due to the simultaneous systole of right atrium and right ventricle.

ECG (Figure 16.1)

This is characterized by wide regular QRS complexes at a rate of >100 beats/min (an exception is polymorphic VT, which is irregular and is covered at the end of this chapter). The following features are suggestive of VT:

1) QRS duration >140 ms with a right bundle branch block (RBBB) morphology and >160 ms with a left bundle branch block (LBBB) morphology.
2) QRS complexes with a left (-30° to -90°) or indeterminate axis deviation (-90° to ±180°).
3) Positive or negative concordance of QRS complexes from leads V_1 to V_6 (specificity >90%, sensitivity ~20%). While the presence of negative QRS complexes strongly suggests VT, positive complexes in all pre-

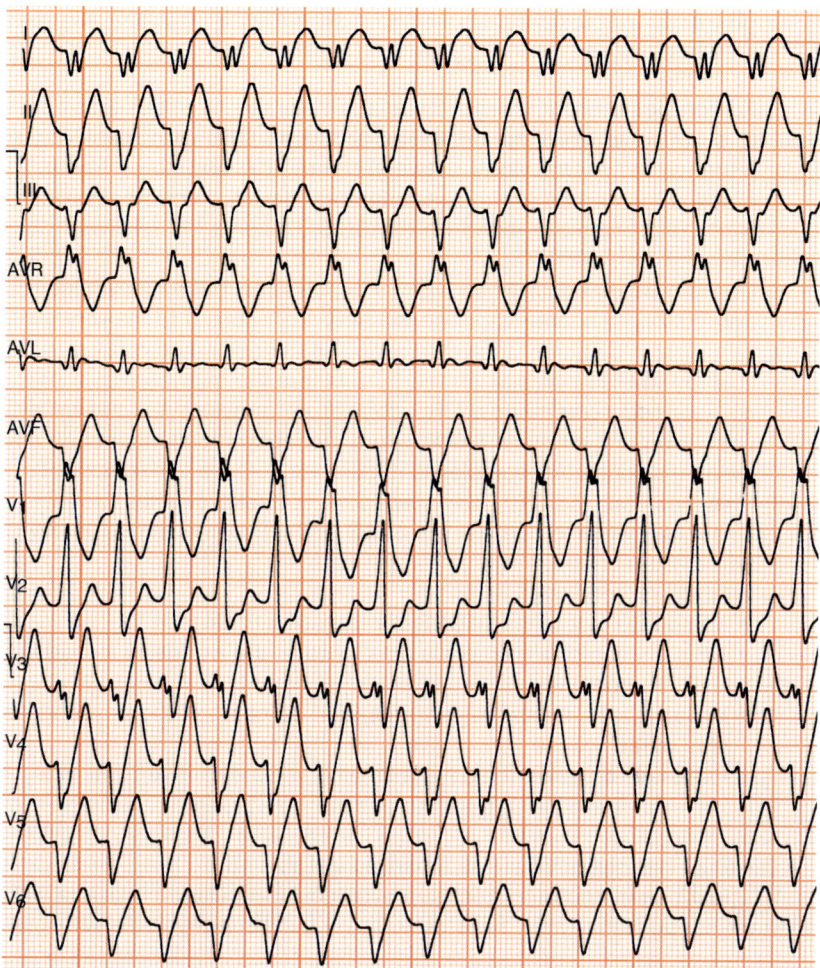

Figure 16.1. The ECG shows regular tachycardia (~150 beats/min) with wide QRS complexes (~140 ms) and an indeterminate QRS axis. This is ventricular tachycardia on a substrate of ischemic cardiomyopathy. QRS complexes have a right bundle branch block morphology and in lead V_1 R> R'. In addition, there is an initial R wave in lead aVR (Vereckei criterion).

cordial leads are also observed in the rare form of antidromic (descent of stimulus via a left posterior accessory pathway) atrioventricular reentrant tachycardia in Wolff–Parkinson–White (WPW) syndrome.

4) Atrioventricular dissociation, namely P waves independent of and fewer than the QRS complexes. Specificity is almost 100%, but sensitivity is <50%.

5) **Fusion beats** occur when a sinus and a ventricular impulse coincide to produce a hybrid complex. The produced QRS complexes are of intermediate morphology between ventricular and sinus beats. In practice, some beats with a morphology different from that of most ventricular beats are found on the ECG. Observed in relatively slow VTs.

6) **Capture beats** occur when a sinus impulse reach the atrioventricular node during a nonrefractory period and is conducted to the ventricles (transiently "captures" the ventricles). The conducted complex is identical to the QRS complex on the ECG before the tachycardia. In practice, we find some narrow QRS complexes (provided the patient did not show bundle branch block before the tachycardia) interposed between the ventricular complexes (Figure 16.2). Observed in slow VTs.

7) Presence of an initial R wave in lead aVR (Vereckei criterion).

8) Onset of R wave to deepest point of S wave (R-S interval) >100 ms in any precordial lead.

9) In RBBB morphology:
   • Monophasic or biphasic QRS complex (R >R') in lead V_1.
   • QS or rS complex (namely, a small r wave and a large S) in lead V_6.

10) In LBBB morphology:
   • Wide R wave in lead V_1 (>40 ms) and notching of the descending limb of the S wave.
   • QS or qR complex (namely, a small q wave and a large R) in lead V_6.

The ECG features of VT are summarized in Table 16.2.

VT must be differentiated from supraventricular regular tachycardia with aberrant conduction (Table 16.3) or supraventricular tachycardia with pre-

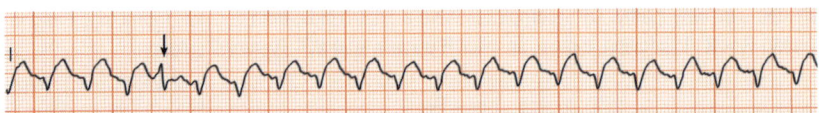

Figure 16.2. ECG lead I showing ventricular tachycardia (~150 beats/min) with a capture beat (5th QRS complex, arrow). This complex has a different morphology from the rest, one similar to that of the ECG after cardioversion of the arrhythmia.

TABLE 16.2	**ECG features of ventricular tachycardia (monomorphic)**

1) QRS duration >140 ms in RBBB and >160 ms in LBBB

2) Left or indeterminate axis deviation (-30° to ±180°)

3) Positive or negative QRS complexes in all precordial leads

4) Atrioventricular dissociation (P waves independent of QRS complexes)

5) Fusion beats (QRS complexes of intermediate morphology between ventricular and sinus beats)

6) Capture beats (QRS complexes of the same morphology as sinus beats)

7) Presence of an initial R wave in lead aVR (Vereckei criterion)

8) R-S interval >100 ms in any precordial lead

9) In case of RBBB morphology:
- Monophasic or biphasic QRS complex (R > R') in lead V_1
- QS or rS complex in lead V_6

10) In case of LBBB morphology:
- Wide R wave in lead V_1 (>40 ms) and notching of the descending limb of the S wave
- QS or qR complex in lead V_6

RBBB: right bundle branch block, LBBB: left bundle branch block

existing bundle branch block. Table 16.4 shows the main causes of wide QRS complex tachycardias.

The role of the ECG in determining the cause of ventricular tachycardia

1) Suspicion of arrhythmogenic right ventricular cardiomyopathy arises when the postcardioversion ECG shows:
- Negative T waves in leads V_1-V_3 (in individuals aged >14 years and in the absence of complete RBBB).
- An epsilon wave (notching in the final section of the QRS complex) in leads V_1-V_3.
- Prolongation of the QRS complex (>110 ms) in leads V_1-V_3.

TABLE 16.3	Differential diagnosis between ventricular tachycardia (monomorphic) and supraventricular regular tachycardia with wide QRS complexes due to aberrant conduction*	
	Ventricular tachycardia	**Supraventricular tachycardia with aberrant conduction**
History	Usually old myocardial infarction or cardiomyopathy	Usually absence of organic heart disease
Vagotonic maneuvers (Valsalva maneuver or carotid massage)	Are not effective (except in idiopathic ventricular tachycardia)	May achieve cardioversion ("all or nothing" response)
Clinical symptoms	Usually symptomatic	Usually well tolerated unless very fast
Clinical signs	• Changing intensity of the 1st heart sound • Irregular cannon a waves (unless there is retrograde ventriculoatrial conduction)	• Steady intensity of the 1st heart sound • Usually regular cannon a waves
ECG	• QRS duration >140 ms • Monophasic or biphasic QRS complexes in lead V_1 • Fusion beats • Capture beats • P waves independent of QRS complexes • Left or indeterminate axis deviation (-30° to ±180°) • Positive or negative QRS complexes in leads V_1-V_6 • QS in lead V_6	• QRS duration <140 ms • Triphasic QRS complexes in lead V_1
Adenosine	No effect (exception is idiopathic ventricular tachycardia)	Conversion rate >90%
Verapamil	Risk of shock	Usually converts

The right branch of the His bundle has a longer refractory period than the left branch. Consequently, an early supraventricular impulse may find the right bundle to be refractory and will be conducted only via the left bundle, leading to aberrant conduction. In this case, the conducted impulse has a right bundle branch block morphology.

TABLE 16.4	Main causes of tachycardias (regular or irregular) with wide QRS complexes (>120 ms)

A) Regular tachycardia

    1) Monomorphic ventricular tachycardia (most common cause of wide QRS complex tachycardias)

    2) Supraventricular tachycardia with aberrant conduction

    3) Supraventricular tachycardia with preexisting bundle branch block

    4) Antidromic atrioventricular reentrant tachycardia with WPW syndrome (rare)

B) Irregular tachycardia

    1) Atrial fibrillation with preexisting bundle branch block

    2) Atrial fibrillation with WPW syndrome

    3) Atrial flutter and variable atrioventricular conduction with preexisting bundle branch block

    4) Polymorphic ventricular tachycardia

During the tachycardia there is an LBBB morphology.

Arrhythmogenic right ventricular cardiomyopathy is a form of cardiomyopathy that leads to dilation and severe impairment of the right (usually) or both ventricles.

2) If the postcardioversion ECG shows a prolonged QT interval (>500 ms), this is likely to have been the triggering cause of the tachycardia. However, a long QT interval is usually involved in causing polymorphic VT (torsades de pointes).

3) If the postcardioversion ECG shows coved-type ST-segment elevation ≥2 mm in more than one right precordial lead (V_1-V_3) followed by negative T waves is diagnostic of Brugada syndrome (type-1 ECG pattern) [more in page 138]. This heritable arrhythmia syndrome is typically complicated by episodes of polymorphic VT that may result in syncope (self-terminating polymorphic VT) or sudden cardiac death (polymorphic VT that degenerates into ventricular fibrillation). Symptoms are more frequent at rest or during sleep.

4) If the postcardioversion ECG shows Q waves indicative of an old myocardial infarction, then the VT was probably caused by a reentry mechanism in the region of the scar. In these patients any existing myocardial ischemia should be corrected.

5) VT with LBBB morphology and a right axis (arrhythmogenic focus in the right ventricular outflow tract) in young people who have no organic heart disease or family history of sudden cardiac death probably denotes idiopathic VT. This is the most common type of idiopathic VT and it may be cardioverted with vagotonic maneuvers, or administration of

adenosine or verapamil IV. It has a good prognosis and may be treated radically with catheter ablation.

Treatment

1) In cases of hemodynamic compromise (angina, dyspnea, systolic blood pressure (BP) <90 mmHg, confusion due to hypoperfusion of the brain), direct current cardioversion is performed. The initial energy supplied is 100 J; if conversion is not achieved, this is increased to 200 J and then to 360 J of monophasic current, or biphasic current with the equivalent energy.

2) If the patient is pulseless, then defibrillation is performed, followed by the algorithm for pulseless VT (Chapter 10).

3) In the absence of hemodynamic compromise, pharmaceutical cardioversion can be attempted. Procainamide appears to be superior to other antiarrhythmic medications and is the drug of first choice. When it is ineffective or the VT recurs in spite of its administration, or when the administration is problematic (severe heart failure or kidney failure) amiodarone is preferred. Lidocaine appears to be effective when the VT develops on a substrate of acute myocardial ischemia.

   - **Procainamide** (Pronestyl): administered in a dose of 100 mg over 2 min and repeated in a dose of 100 mg every 5 min until conversion of the VT (maximum loading dose 1000 mg) or the appearance of hypotension or >50% widening of the QRS complex. After conversion, maintenance therapy is continued with continuous infusion of 2-6 mg/min for at least 24-48 h. Procainamide has a negative inotropic action and BP should be monitored frequently during its administration (risk of hypotension). In addition, its dosage is reduced in cases of renal failure, since ~60% is eliminated by the kidneys.

   Practical instructions for IV administration: procainamide is supplied in vials of Pronestyl, 1000 mg/10 mL. The preparation of the solution for the maintenance therapy involves the addition of two vials of Pronestyl to 230 mL D/W 5% (resulting in a solution of concentration 8 mg/mL), administered at a rate of 15-45 mL/h.

   - **Amiodarone** (Cordarone): administered in an initial dose of 150 mg IV over 10 min, followed by 360 mg over 6 h (i.e. 1 mg/min x 6 h) and then 540 mg over 18 h (i.e. 0.5 mg/min x 18 h). Therefore, the total dose is ~1 g within 24 h. If the initial dose of 150 mg is ineffective, an additional infusion of 150 mg over a 10-min period can be given after 10 min. We should mention that in our daily clinical practice, after the initial infusion of 150 mg (+ 150 mg after 10 min if the initial dose is ineffective), we usually administer amiodarone solution at a constant rate, as described in the following paragraph. Hypotension is the most common side effect during infusion.

Practical instructions for IV administration: amiodarone is supplied in ampoules of Cordarone, 150 mg/3 mL. For the initial administration, 1 ampoule of Cordarone is added to 100 mL D/W 5% and the solution is administered over 10 min. For the remainder of the administration, 6 ampoules of Cordarone (i.e. 360+540=900 mg) are added to 500 mL D/W 5% and the solution is administered at an infusion rate of ~20 mL/h (~37 mg/h) for at least 24-48 h.

- **Lidocaine** (Lidocaine, Xylocaine): administered in an initial dose of 75-100 mg IV (1-1.5 mg/kg) over 2 min, followed by a repeat dose of half the initial quantity 30 min later. The repeated dose is considered essential in order to rapidly achieve therapeutic levels of lidocaine, even if conversion to sinus rhythm has been achieved. If the initial dose is not effective, the same dose (75-100 mg) may be repeated up to twice every 5 min (avoid administration of >300 mg during the first hour). At the same time, any concomitant hypokalemia (serum potassium levels <4 mEq/L) should be corrected, as normal potassium levels enhance lidocaine's action. When conversion is achieved, it is followed by continuous infusion of 1-4 mg/min for at least 24-48 h.

  Lidocaine is metabolized in the liver and the dosage should be reduced to about 50% in case of liver failure, low cardiac output, or in the elderly (>70 years). The main adverse effect (dose-dependent) is neurotoxicity, which is manifested as dizziness, hallucinations, confusion, or convulsions.

  Practical instructions for IV administration: lidocaine is supplied as an injectable solution of 50 mL Xylocaine in a concentration of 2%; namely, each mL contains 20 mg of lidocaine. Two vials of Xylocaine, i.e. 2 x 50 x 20 = 2000 mg, are added to 400 mL D/W 5%, forming a solution with a concentration of 4 mg/mL. For administration of 1-4 mg/min the solution is infused at a rate of 15-60 mL/h.

Throughout the pharmaceutical intervention there should be the capability for direct electrical cardioversion in case severe hemodynamic compromise should arise. In general, when pharmaceutical conversion of hemodynamically stable VT is performed, if one, or at most two of the above antiarrhythmic drugs fail within 30-60 min, electrical cardioversion should be applied.

Considerations when treating wide QRS complex tachycardias

- VT is the most common cause of wide QRS complex tachycardia (~80% of all cases). More specifically, regular tachycardia with a wide QRS complex in individuals with a history of old myocardial infarction or cardiomyopathy is in all probability VT.

- Every wide QRS complex tachycardia, even if the diagnosis is uncertain, should be treated as VT until proven otherwise.
- In wide QRS complex tachycardias verapamil administration should be avoided, because if the tachycardia is ventricular it may cause a precipitous drop in blood pressure.
- If there is doubt in the differential diagnosis between ventricular and supraventricular tachycardia with wide QRS complexes, adenosine may be given as long as the patient is hemodynamically stable. If the tachycardia converts to sinus rhythm, it is most likely supraventricular (atrioventricular nodal reentrant tachycardia, atrioventricular reentrant tachycardia), or more rarely idiopathic VT; if it is not converted it is most probably ventricular, while if temporary atrial activity is revealed (flutter waves) it is atrial flutter.
- In irregular tachycardia with QRS complexes that are wide or have varying morphology and a rate of >200 beats/min, we should consider atrial fibrillation in a patient with WPW syndrome (avoid administering amiodarone, digoxin, verapamil, diltiazem, adenosine, lidocaine, beta-blockers IV). If there is no hemodynamic compromise, the drug of choice is procainamide or ibutilide IV.

Management of patients with ventricular tachycardia that is cardioverted in the Emergency Room

1) The patient is always admitted to the coronary care unit for monitoring during the first 24-48 h.
2) The IV administration of the antiarrhythmic drug used for cardioversion in the Emergency Room is continued for at least 24-48 h and is then discontinued provided that the arrhythmia does not recur. If the patient has undergone electrical cardioversion, IV amiodarone is usually given.
3) Reversible causes are sought and corrected (e.g. myocardial ischemia, electrolyte disturbances, etc.).
4) The attempt to determine the causes of the VT is likely to include one or more of the following examinations:
   - Echocardiography (always performed), mainly for evaluation of left ventricular function, to rule out various forms of cardiomyopathy, such as hypertrophic cardiomyopathy, arrhythmogenic right ventricular cardiomyopathy (needs careful evaluation of right ventricular morphology and function), etc.
   - Myocardial perfusion scintigraphy if necessary to rule out active ischemia.
   - Coronary angiography to show the extent of CAD, if the myocardial perfusion scintigraphy detects ischemia.
   - Cardiac magnetic resonance imaging (MRI), if there is suspicion of arrhythmogenic right ventricular cardiomyopathy or acute myocarditis.

- Electrophysiological study, if the arrhythmogenic focus needs to be located and to guide the antiarrhythmic therapy (pharmaceutical or non-pharmaceutical).

Possible interventions for the treatment of future recurrences of VT are:
- Myocardial reperfusion if the patient has active ischemia.
- Long-term administration of antiarrhythmic drugs.
- Implantable cardioverter defibrillator (e.g. in patients with CAD who have sustained VT after active myocardial ischemia has been ruled out, in patients with Brugada syndrome and sustained VT, etc.).
- Radiofrequency catheter ablation (e.g. for idiopathic VT, etc.).

One special type of VT is polymorphic VT, which requires completely different pharmaceutical management from the monomorphic type described above. It will be discussed below.

Polymorphic ventricular tachycardia

This is a usually spontaneously terminating VT that is characterized on the ECG by a periodic increase and decrease in the QRS complexes that appear to twist around the isoelectric line with a rate of 200 to 250/min. It is a usually irregular, nonsustained (duration 5-30 s), repeated tachycardia that may degenerate into ventricular fibrillation.

Polymorphic VT may appear in patients with a normal (the most common cause is acute myocardial ischemia) or a long QT interval. When it occurs in patients with a long QT interval (corrected QT >440 ms in men or >460 ms in women) it is called torsades de pointes (twisting of the points). Table 16.5 shows the basic points for the measurement of the QT interval and Table 16.6 shows the causes of its prolongation. The drugs that carry the greatest risk for QTc prolongation and torsades de pointes are the class IA antiarrhythmics (1-5% of patients). Drugs associated with an increased QT interval are listed on the following website: www.torsades.org.

Treatment of polymorphic ventricular tachycardia

The treatment of this arrhythmia, apart from immediate defibrillation in the case of hemodynamic compromise, also involves maneuvers to reduce the possibility of recurrence, which is its main feature. In particular, the treatment of polymorphic VT as a consequence of acquired long QT interval includes (Table 16.7):
- Defibrillation in case of hemodynamic compromise.
- Administration of **magnesium sulfate** IV in a dose of 2 g bolus (conversion rate ~75% within 5 min) and, if conversion is not achieved, repetition of the same dose after 5-15 min. Magnesium sulfate for IV adminis-

TABLE 16.5	Basic points for the measurement of the QT interval

1) The QT interval is measured from the start of the Q wave (or from the start of the R wave if there is no Q wave) to the end of the T wave

2) To calculate the corrected QT interval, the longest QT on the ECG is measured (QT_{max}, in ms) and is divided by the square root of the R-R interval (in seconds) that precedes QT_{max} (Bazett formula), thus:

$$\text{corrected QT interval} = QTc = \frac{QT_{max}\ (ms)}{\sqrt{R\text{-}R}\ (s)}$$

3) Practical rule of thumb: if $QT_{max} > 1/2$ the previous R-R interval, then in all likelihood there is prolongation of the QT interval provided the heart rate is <100 beats/min

tration is available in various concentrations, e.g. 25% in 10 mL ampoules (provides 2 mEq/mL of Mg), 50% in 10 mL ampoules (provides 4 mEq/mL of Mg), etc. Magnesium sulfate is also effective in the absence of hypomagnesemia. On its own, it does not shorten the QT interval. If necessary, it may be given in a continuous infusion (3-20 mg/min) until the QT interval is corrected by the treatment of the causes that prolonged it. If ampoules of 25% magnesium sulfate are used then 4 ampoules (4 x 2.5 g, equivalent to ~80 mEq Mg) are added to 1000 mL D/W 5% and are given over 12-24 h. Note that 1 g of hydrated magnesium sulfate contains 8 mEq of magnesium.

TABLE 16.6	Causes of QT interval prolongation (corrected QT >440 ms in men and >460 ms in women)

1) Class IA antiarrhythmic drugs (quinidine, procainamide, disopyramide)

2) Class III antiarrhythmic drugs (sotalol, ibutilide, dofetilide, amiodarone*)

3) Hypokalemia, hypomagnesemia, hypocalcemia

4) Tricyclic antidepressants and phenothiazines

5) Macrolides (erythromycin, clarithromycin), quinolones and azole antifungals

6) Methadone

7) Subarachnoid hemorrhage

8) Severe bradyarrhythmias such as complete atrioventricular block

9) Congenital long-QT syndrome

Amiodarone administration is rarely complicated by torsades de pointes (<1%)

TABLE 16.7	**Treatment of polymorphic ventricular tachycardia as a consequence of acquired long QT interval**

1) If there is hemodynamic compromise: defibrillation

2) Administration of magnesium sulfate IV (initial treatment of choice)

3) Treatment of underlying reversible cause, e.g. correction of hypokalemia, discontinuation of culprit drug, etc.

4) In the presence of bradycardia or pauses: temporary ventricular or atrial pacing at 90-110 beats/min

5) Isoproterenol or atropine IV are given as a bridge to pacing

6) Avoid administration of class IA and III antiarrhythmic drugs

- Treatment of the underlying reversible cause, e.g. correction of hypokalemia, discontinuation of the offending drug, etc. Serum levels of potassium, magnesium, and calcium should always be checked.

- In the presence of bradycardia or pauses, which are common triggering factors of polymorphic VT, **temporary transvenous atrial pacing** is applied (or ventricular in the case of atrioventricular block) at a rate of 90-110 beats/min in order to shorten the QT interval. Until pacing is started, as a bridge therapy, **isoproterenol** (a beta-agonist with $\beta_1 > \beta_2$ action) or **atropine** may be given IV with a view to increasing the heart rate to >90 beats/min. The isoproterenol dose ranges between 1-10 μg/min and is titrated based on the patient's heart rate response. Isoproterenol is supplied in 1 mL ampoule of Isuprel which contains 200 μg. For an initial administration of 1 μg/min, 5 ampoules of Isuprel are added to 250 mL D/W 5% and the solution is administered at a rate of 15 mL/h. Isoproterenol should be given with great caution to patients with stable CAD, because of the risk of ischemia, and is contraindicated in acute myocardial infarction and in congenital long-QT syndrome.

- Avoid administering antiarrhythmic drugs of class IA (e.g. procainamide) and III (e.g. amiodarone) because they may prolong the already long QT interval, worsening the arrhythmia.

Warning! Polymorphic VT in individuals with a normal QT interval, usually on a substrate of acute myocardial ischemia, is treated in the same manner as monomorphic VT.

Table 16.8 briefly presents the drugs given for tachycardias that do not exhibit hemodynamic compromise severe enough to require electrical cardioversion.

TABLE 16.8	Main drugs administered for the treatment of tachycardias without severe hemodynamic compromise
1) Atrial fibrillation:	• Diltiazem, verapamil, beta-blocker (e.g. propranolol, esmolol) to slow the ventricular response • Propafenone, flecainide, amiodarone, ibutilide, vernakalant for cardioversion
2) Atrial flutter:	• Verapamil, diltiazem, beta-blocker to slow the ventricular response • Ibutilide for cardioversion (unless electrical preferred)
3) Supraventricular regular paroxysmal tachycardias (atrioventricular nodal reentrant tachycardia, orthodromic atrioventricular reentrant tachycardia): adenosine (drug of choice), verapamil, beta-blocker	
4) Ventricular tachycardia (monomorphic): procainamide, amiodarone, lidocaine	
5) Torsades de pointes:	• Magnesium sulfate • Correction of direct causes (e.g. hypokalemia) • Temporary pacing (for bradycardia or pauses) • Isoproterenol or atropine as a bridge to pacing
6) Tachycardia in WPW syndrome:	• Regular tachycardia with narrow QRS complex: adenosine • Regular (antidromic atrioventricular reentrant tachycardia, atrial flutter or ventricular tachycardia) or irregular (atrial fibrillation) with wide QRS complexes: procainamide

Key points

- VT is a potentially lethal arrhythmia and requires immediate treatment and full investigation.

- VT is the most common cause of regular tachycardia with a wide QRS complex.

- Any regular wide QRS complex tachycardia, whether accompanied by hemodynamic compromise or not, should be treated as VT until proven otherwise.

- In regular wide QRS complex tachycardia, IV administration of verapamil is "prohibited", because if the tachycardia is ventricular it could cause a precipitous drop in blood pressure.

- In wide QRS complex tachycardia, always consider the possibility that it might be a manifestation of WPW syndrome, in which case if it is irregular it is atrial fibrillation, while if it is regular it may be atrial flutter, antidromic atrioventricular reentrant tachycardia or VT. If there is no severe hemodynamic compromise, procainamide may be given IV.

- Polymorphic VT in stable patients typically terminates on its own but it tends to recur. When the patients are in sinus rhythm, the ECG should be analyzed to determine whether the QT interval is normal or prolonged.

- In polymorphic VT on a substrate of acquired long QT interval, the best antiarrhythmic drug is magnesium sulfate administered IV. At the same time any underlying electrolyte disorders are corrected and if there is concomitant bradycardia or pauses temporary pacing is applied at a rate of 90-110 beats/min.

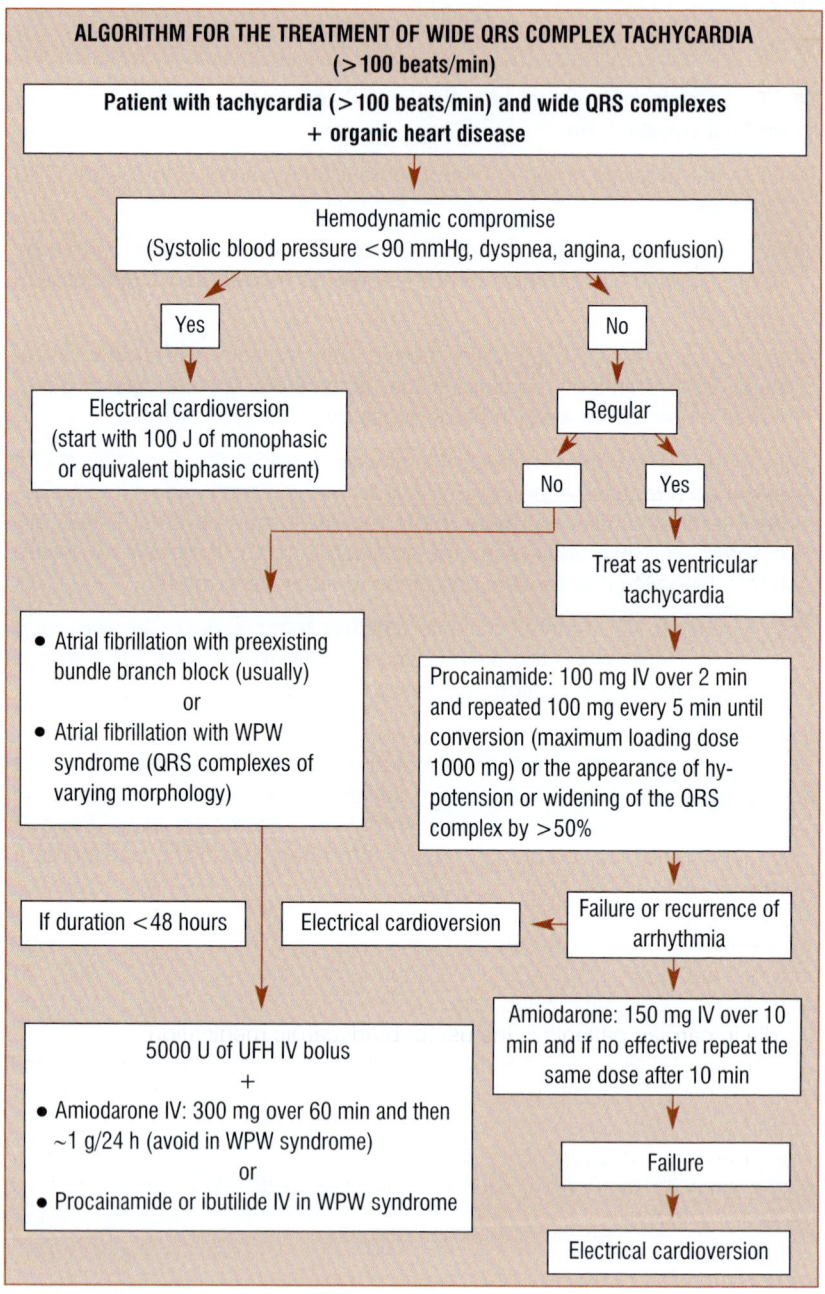

ALGORITHM FOR THE TREATMENT OF WIDE QRS COMPLEX TACHYCARDIA
(>100 beats/min)

Patient with tachycardia (>100 beats/min) and wide QRS complexes
+ organic heart disease

Hemodynamic compromise
(Systolic blood pressure <90 mmHg, dyspnea, angina, confusion)

Yes

No

Electrical cardioversion
(start with 100 J of monophasic
or equivalent biphasic current)

Regular

No   Yes

Treat as ventricular
tachycardia

- Atrial fibrillation with preexisting
  bundle branch block (usually)
  or
- Atrial fibrillation with WPW
  syndrome (QRS complexes of
  varying morphology)

Procainamide: 100 mg IV over 2 min
and repeated 100 mg every 5 min until
conversion (maximum loading dose
1000 mg) or the appearance of hypotension or widening of the QRS
complex by >50%

If duration <48 hours

Electrical cardioversion

Failure or recurrence of
arrhythmia

5000 U of UFH IV bolus
+
- Amiodarone IV: 300 mg over 60 min and then
  ~1 g/24 h (avoid in WPW syndrome)
  or
- Procainamide or ibutilide IV in WPW syndrome

Amiodarone: 150 mg IV over 10
min and if no effective repeat the
same dose after 10 min

Failure

Electrical cardioversion

WPW: Wolff-Parkinson-White, UFH: unfractionated heparin

17

Bradycardia

Bradycardia is defined as a drop in heart rate to below 60 beats/min. This definition does not have any clinical utility since many healthy individuals (e.g. athletes) are naturally bradycardic (markedly so in some cases), while heart disease patients may have a heart rate <60 beats/min because of the therapeutic effect of their medication. When practicing emergency cardiology, our primary concern is to treat pathological bradycardia, i.e. bradycardia that is associated with symptoms or exposes the patient to an increased risk of syncope or cardiac arrest. As a rule, asymptomatic bradycardia — except when caused by atrioventricular (AV) block — rarely requires emergency treatment. The primary causes of bradycardia are summarized below.

1. Sinus bradycardia

Sinus bradycardia is defined as a decrease in heart rate to <60 beats/min while the P waves have normal morphology, each P wave precedes a QRS complex, and the PR interval is stable. Table 17.1 lists the primary causes of sinus bradycardia. The most common cause of sinus bradycardia in cardiac patients is the use of bradycardic medication.

The clinical picture depends on the degree of bradycardia and the individual's activity. Some people may be asymptomatic even with severe bradycardia, while others will develop symptoms ranging from mild to significant weakness or dyspnea on exertion, and syncope in rare cases. Generally, a sinus bradycardia of <40-45 beats/min is associated with symptoms, except in athletes.

TABLE 17.1	Primary causes of sinus bradycardia

1) Normal bradycardia (increased parasympathetic tone, i.e. vagotonia): athletes, sleep

2) Bradycardic medication: beta-blockers, diltiazem, verapamil, digoxin, most antiarrhythmics (e.g. amiodarone, propafenone), etc.

3) Sick sinus syndrome

4) Acute parasympathetic activation: vomiting, common faint, carotid sinus hypersensitivity, etc.

5) Acute inferior myocardial infarction (especially during the first 2 h)

6) Hypothyroidism

7) Increased intracranial pressure: subarachnoid hemorrhage, intracranial tumors, etc.

8) Severe hypoxia

9) Hypothermia

10) Sepsis by Gram-negative bacteria

11) Cholestatic jaundice

Warning! Eye drops for the treatment of glaucoma that contain beta-blockers can cause severe bradycardia in the elderly.

Treatment

1) Absence of symptoms: usually, no intervention is needed. If the heart rate is <50 beats/min and the patient is receiving bradycardic medication, then a reduction in dosage or discontinuation is recommended.

2) Presence of symptoms: **atropine** is administered IV in an initial dose of 0.5 mg, which may be repeated every 3-5 min up to a maximum dose of 3 mg. The action of atropine begins at 1 min and can last for 30-60 min. Atropine is contraindicated in cases of prostate hypertrophy and closed-angle glaucoma. If there is no response, **temporary transvenous pacing** is applied (see Chapter 22). If the cause of symptomatic bradycardia is reversible, e.g. medication, then a normal heart rate is usually restored after 24-48 h and the temporary pacemaker is removed. If this does not occur, then permanent pacing may be considered.

2) Atrioventricular conduction disturbances

A) First-degree atrioventricular block

All stimuli are conducted from the atria to the ventricles, but there is a delay that is reflected in the ECG as a prolonged PR interval (>200 ms). The delay usually occurs at the AV node (usually narrow QRS complexes) or more rarely within the His-Purkinje system (widened QRS complex). Heart auscultation shows a decrease of the 1st heart sound. It may be caused by drugs that slow AV conduction (beta-blockers, diltiazem, verapamil, digoxin, amiodarone, etc.), increased parasympathetic tone (e.g. athletes), inferior acute myocardial infarction (AMI), etc. No specific treatment is necessary. If, however, the PR interval prolongation is caused by medication, then the dosage is reduced or the drug is discontinued.

B) Second-degree atrioventricular block

In this case, not all stimuli are conducted from the atria to the ventricles. This condition is classified into:

- **Mobitz type I atrioventricular block or Wenckebach-type block:** characterized by progressive prolongation of the PR interval (with a reduction in the R-R interval), until a P wave is not conducted to the ventricles (Figure 17.1). This disorder is usually benign and the site of block is almost always within the AV node (intranodal) when a narrow QRS complex is present. It can be caused by vagotonia (e.g. athletes), bradycardic drugs, inferior AMI, etc. If there are no associated symptoms (which is the most common scenario), no treatment is necessary.
- **Mobitz type II atrioventricular block:** characterized by a sudden loss of conductivity (stable or intermittent) of one or more P waves to the ventricles without preceding lengthening of the PR interval. The site of block is almost always below the AV node (infranodal), i.e. within the His bundle in ~30% of cases and within the bundle branches in the remainder. It has a high likelihood of conversion to complete AV block

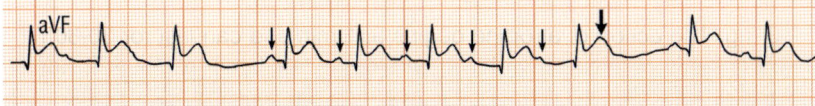

Figure 17.1. ECG showing Mobitz type I atrioventricular block on a substrate of inferior acute myocardial infarction (lead aVF). There is a gradual increase in the PR interval (the small arrows indicate P waves) until the 6th P wave is not conducted. Note that the nonconducted P wave is not recognized because it coincides with the ST-segment (large arrow).

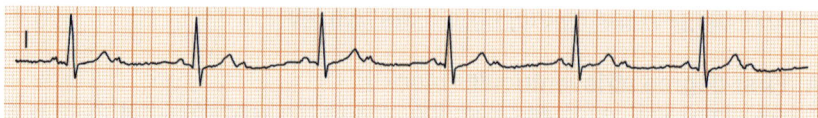

Figure 17.2. ECG showing 2:1 atrioventricular block that may be of Mobitz I or Mobitz II type (lead I). The presence of narrow QRS complexes suggests Mobitz type I atrioventricular block. The heart rate is 42 beats/min.

with a low ventricular rate. The causes of Mobitz type II AV block are anteroseptal AMI, Lev's or Lenègre's disease, and other causes generally similar to those of complete AV block (see below).

A distinct form of heart block is 2:1 AV block, where loss of conduction occurs on every second P wave (Figure 17.2). This type of AV block cannot be classified reliably as Mobitz type I or Mobitz type II, because the absence of 2 successive conducted P waves makes it impossible to study the behavior of the PR interval. In such cases, the presence of narrow QRS complexes is indicative of Mobitz type I AV block, whereas wide QRS complexes suggest Mobitz type II AV block.

Less common AV block types are 3:1 (Figure 17.3), 4:1, etc., which are collectively called high-grade AV blocks and are characterized by a high risk of conversion to complete AV block.

In cases of Mobitz type II AV block, atropine must be avoided because it can cause a paradoxical decrease in heart rate (AV conduction decreases as the atrial rate increases). Isoproterenol infusion may be tried with caution. This type of AV block requires permanent pacing in the absence of reversible causes.

Warning! Atropine does not improve AV conduction in Mobitz type II AV block, and can further aggravate the bradycardia.

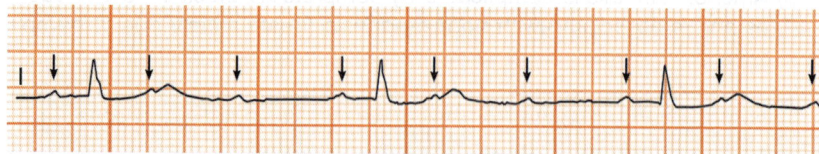

Figure 17.3. ECG showing 3:1 atrioventricular conduction in an 86-year-old woman who was transferred to the Emergency Room because of extreme debility (lead I) [arrows indicate P waves]. The heart rate is 36 beats/min.

C) Third-degree (complete) atrioventricular block

In third-degree AV block, none of the atrial stimuli are conducted to the ventricles, which are therefore excited by independent pacing foci. The level of the block may be located at the AV node, the His bundle or its branches. The atria may be in sinus rhythm, atrial ectopic rhythm, or atrial fibrillation. The rate and pattern of the escape rhythm exciting the ventricles depends on the level of the block. If the escape focus is proximal to the His bundle, the rate will be 40-60 beats/min and the QRS complexes are usually narrow, whereas if the escape focus is more distal to the His bundle the rate will be <40 beats/min and the QRS complexes are wide.

Complete AV block is usually symptomatic. It is characterized by symptoms of low cardiac output, such as weakness, presyncope or syncope. While the AV block is established, an intervening period of ventricular asystole leading to Stokes–Adams attacks may occur (see below for more details).

Clinical examination shows a 1st heart sound of fluctuating intensity, because of changes in the PR interval, and a waves in the jugular veins (caused by right atrial contractions) that have no fixed temporal association with the ventricular contractions. Intermittent large a waves (cannon a waves), caused by contraction of the right atrium against a closed tricuspid valve, and a functional systolic ejection murmur may be noted.

The most important causes of complete AV block are:

- Lev's disease: degenerative disease characterized by fibrosis and calcification of the heart's fibrous scaffold, extending to the cardiac conduction system.
- Lenègre's disease: degenerative disease affecting the cardiac conduction system.
- Acute myocardial ischemia:
    a) Inferior AMI: this is complicated by complete AV block in ~8-10% of cases. It is usually caused by transient ischemia or edema of the AV node, due to obstruction of the AV nodal artery, a branch of the right coronary artery (in ~80% of cases, the AV node is supplied by the right coronary artery). This block is usually transient and is characterized by a stable escape rhythm with a rate of 40-60 beats/min (Figure 17.4).
    b) Anterior AMI: this is complicated by complete AV block in ~3% of cases and is associated with poor prognosis (death mainly due to pump failure). The disturbance is located in the His-Purkinje system (supplied mainly by the anterior descending coronary artery) and is the result of extensive septal necrosis involving the bundle branches. The escape focus is unstable (high risk of asystole) and has a rate of <40 beats/min.
- Bradycardic drugs: beta-blockers, diltiazem, verapamil, digoxin, most antiarrhythmic drugs (e.g. amiodarone), etc. It may be the result of taking

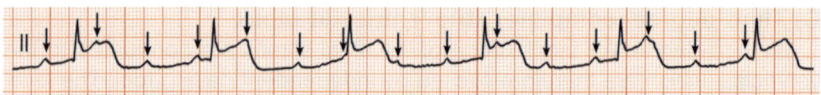

Figure 17.4. ECG showing complete atrioventricular block on a substrate of acute inferior myocardial infarction (lead II). The P waves (arrows) are regular, they have a rate of 120/min and show no temporal association with the QRS complexes, which are regular, narrow and have a rate of 43/min. The site of block is intranodal and a junctional escape rhythm has taken over.

high doses or combinations of such drugs. This pharmaceutical block occurs most commonly in individuals with a preexisting latent disturbance of AV conduction.

- Marked parasympathetic excitation can cause transient complete AV block.
- Electrolyte disturbances: marked hyperkalemia.
- Congenital complete AV block: this is the most common type of AV block in pediatric patients and it is usually located in the AV node.
- Other causes: severe calcification of the aortic valve or the mitral annulus, myocarditis, infiltrative processes (amyloidosis, sarcoidosis, etc.), traumatic causes (e.g. cardiac valve surgery), etc.

The therapeutic management of complete AV block depends on the symptoms and the level of the block:

a) In symptomatic complete AV block located in the AV node, **atropine** is administered at an initial dose of 0.5 mg IV, which may be repeated every 3-5 min up to a maximum dose of 3 mg. If the block persists or does not improve with atropine, **temporary transvenous pacing** is applied and a permanent pacemaker may be implanted, depending on whether the cause is reversible or not.

b) In symptomatic complete AV block located distally to the AV node, atropine is usually ineffective. In such cases **isoproterenol** (Isuprel, 1 mL ampoule contains 200 µg) is administered at a dose of 1-10 µg/min IV (the lowest effective dose is selected), which can accelerate the escape focus. Specifically, 5 Isuprel ampoules (=1000 µg isoproterenol) are added to 250 mL of 5% D/W and the solution (concentration 4 µg/mL) is administered at an initial rate of 15 mL/h (equivalent to 1 µg/min). Caution is needed for patients with stable coronary artery disease; also, the drug should be avoided in cases of acute myocardial ischemia. Therefore, isoproterenol is administered only as bridging therapy until a temporary or permanent pacemaker is placed, depending on the indication. If the complete AV block is a complication of an inferior AMI, then permanent pacing is rarely required.

Warning! Regular bradycardia in an elderly patient with known permanent atrial fibrillation is usually due to the development of complete AV block (Figure 17.5).

Stokes–Adams attacks

In their typical form, Stokes–Adams attacks are episodes of syncope caused by transient ventricular asystole (~90%) or, less commonly, by torsades de pointes. In a more general sense, however, these attacks have a wide range of clinical manifestations, depending on the duration of asystole; these can range from momentary dizziness to loss of consciousness, seizures and sudden death.

The attacks are sudden, unpredictable, often recurring, without warning signs, of varying severity, and regardless of the body's position (even supine). When they manifest as episodes of syncope and the patient is standing, then the patient will fall abruptly to the ground (injuries are frequent); he/she will be pulseless and pallid and, when cardiac function returns (usually within 15-30 s), will recover quickly with no neurological deficits. Typically, the facial hue will return to normal very quickly (postischemic flush) because of relatively well-oxygenated blood entering a systemic circulation vasculature that is dilated because of hypoxia. Note that respiratory motions during a Stokes–Adams attack continue or are labored; the blood is therefore "adequately" oxygenated. If the syncopal episode lasts >15-20 s, then clonic seizures (usually small and arrhythmic) may develop, and the condition will need to be differentiated from an epileptic seizure.

After patient's spontaneous recovery, the ECG may show complete (most often) or Mobitz type II AV block, or less commonly sinus rhythm with a picture of bundle branch block. The period of asystole that causes the

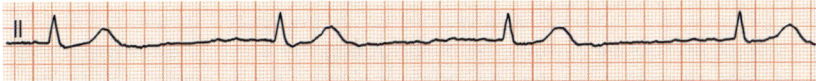

Figure 17.5. ECG showing no organized P waves (atrial fibrillation), with QRS complexes that are wide, regular and have a rate of 32/min (lead II). This is a case of complete atrioventricular block with an escape focus below the atrioventricular node located in the bundle branches of His in a patient with atrial fibrillation.

Stokes–Adams attacks usually corresponds to the time elapsing until a ventricular escape rhythm takes over as complete AV block is established. The most common causes of Stokes–Adams attacks are Lev's disease and Lenègre's disease, which affect the conduction system. Such patients require implantation of a permanent pacemaker.

 Key points

- Although bradycardia is defined as a drop in heart rate to <60 beats/min, in clinical practice only heart rates <50 beats/min (except for athletes) are cause for concern.

- Bradycardia <50 beats/min can be regular (i.e. sinus bradycardia, Mobitz type II AV block, complete AV block, etc.) or irregular (i.e. atrial fibrillation with slow ventricular response, etc.).

- The site of AV block may be:
  – intranodal in first-degree AV block and in Mobitz type I AV block
  – infranodal in Mobitz type II AV block
  – intranodal or infranodal in complete AV block.

- The treatment of bradycardia in the Emergency Room depends on the presence or absence of symptoms. Generally, symptomatic bradycardia is an emergency medical problem and can be complicated by syncope or cardiac arrest.

- In complete AV block, the width and frequency of QRS complexes reflects the level of the block. This means that, when QRS complexes are:
  a. narrow, with a rate of 40-60/min, then the block is located in the AV node (intranodal block) and usually responds to atropine.
  b. wide, with a rate of <40/min, then the block is located below the AV node (infranodal block) and does not respond to atropine (may respond to isoproterenol).

  In both cases, the patient is a candidate for a temporary or permanent pacemaker, depending on whether the disturbance is reversible or not.

- Episodes of syncope in elderly patients, characterized by sudden onset, lack of prodromal symptoms, pallor during the episode and hyperemia immediately after, as well as rapid recovery, usually constitute Stokes–Adams attacks. Such patients require permanent pacing.

- Atrial fibrillation that becomes regular and has a low rate is usually complicated by complete AV block.

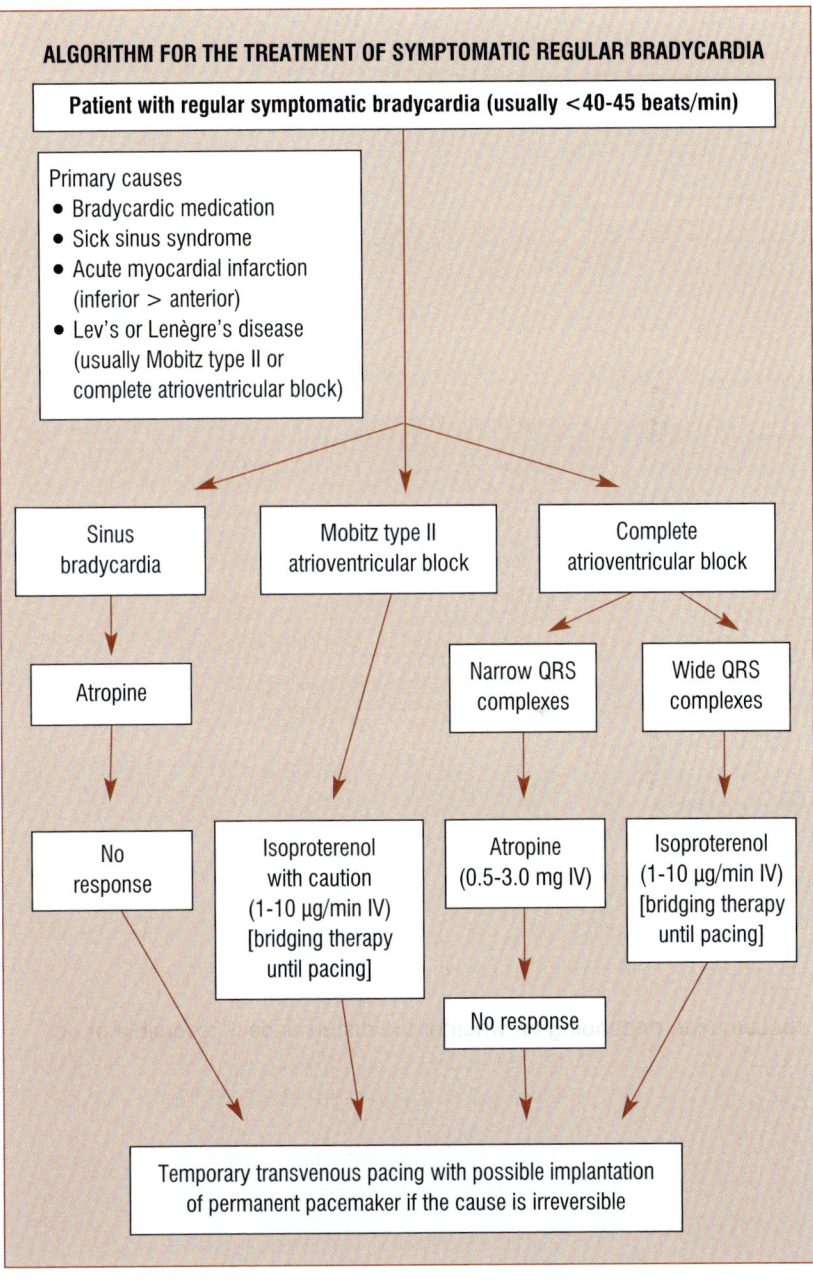

ALGORITHM FOR THE TREATMENT OF SYMPTOMATIC REGULAR BRADYCARDIA

Patient with regular symptomatic bradycardia (usually <40-45 beats/min)

Primary causes
- Bradycardic medication
- Sick sinus syndrome
- Acute myocardial infarction
  (inferior > anterior)
- Lev's or Lenègre's disease
  (usually Mobitz type II or
  complete atrioventricular block)

Sinus bradycardia

Mobitz type II atrioventricular block

Complete atrioventricular block

Atropine

Narrow QRS complexes

Wide QRS complexes

No response

Isoproterenol with caution (1-10 μg/min IV) [bridging therapy until pacing]

Atropine (0.5-3.0 mg IV)

Isoproterenol (1-10 μg/min IV) [bridging therapy until pacing]

No response

Temporary transvenous pacing with possible implantation of permanent pacemaker if the cause is irreversible

18

Digitalis

Digitalis is the only inotropic drug with bradycardic effects (a weaker inotrope than sympathomimetics). Its mechanism of action includes:

- Inhibition of the sodium pump (Na^+, K^+-ATPase) which imports 2 potassium ions and exports 3 sodium ions from the cell. This action leads to an increase in intracellular sodium ions that, by activating the sodium/calcium ion exchange system, increases the intracellular calcium ions. Such an increase of calcium ions in the myocardial cells leads to increased myocardial contractility.
- Stimulation of the parasympathetic nervous system, which causes suppression of sinus node and atrioventricular node function, and
- Inhibition of the sympathetic nervous system.

Digoxin is the most frequently used digitalis product today. When administered orally, 60-80% of the dose of digoxin is absorbed. Its half-life in plasma is 1.5 days and it is eliminated primarily through the renal route (~70%). Another digitalis compound, rarely used nowadays, is digitoxin, which is eliminated via the liver.

Dosage

When the goal is to achieve therapeutic levels relatively quickly, then digoxin is administered:

- Intravenously (Lanoxin, Digoxin). For rapid digitalization it is administered initially in a dose of 0.5 mg and then 0.25 mg IV are given at 12 and 24 h after the initial dose, for a total of 1 mg over the first 24 h. IV administration of digoxin should be performed slowly (0.5 mg of digoxin are added to 50 mL NaCl 0.9% or D/W 5% and are given over

~15 min). Rapid IV infusion may rarely cause vasospasm. Intramuscular administration should be avoided, because it is painful and leads to unpredictable absorption. Note that the action of digoxin after IV administration reaches its maximum after 1-4 h.

- Orally (Lanoxin, Digoxin), in a dose of 0.25 mg x 2 daily for two days, and at a maintenance dose thereafter.

The maintenance dose is usually 0.25 mg po daily. Lower doses (0.125 mg daily or every other day) should be used if the patient is >70 years of age, has impaired renal function, or has a low lean body mass.

Levels of digoxin

The currently recommended therapeutic trough levels of digoxin in serum range between 0.5 and 0.9 ng/mL (associated with fewer heart failure deaths and hospitalizations), lower than previously recommended (Yancy CW, et al. Circulation 2013;128:e240-e327). Blood samples should be taken at least 6-8 h after the last dose. For an accurate assessment of digoxin levels in the morning blood draw, digoxin must be taken in the late afternoon or early evening.

The most important causes of increased digoxin levels are renal failure and use of certain drugs (Table 18.1).

Effects of digoxin on the ECG

Digoxin can cause ST-segment depression, shortening of the QT interval, extrasystolic arrhythmia (usually ventricular extrasystoles, occasionally as bigeminy), atrioventricular conduction disorders, etc.

Indications for digoxin

- Symptomatic heart failure caused by impairment of left ventricular systolic function and persistent/permanent atrial fibrillation (primary indication) for controlling the ventricular rate:
  - in cases of intolerance to beta-blockers (metoprolol, carvedilol, bisoprolol or nebivolol) or

TABLE 18.1	Drugs that increase the levels of digoxin in the blood
Quinidine	Spironolactone
Verapamil, diltiazem	Carvedilol
Amiodarone	Macrolides
Propafenone	Cyclosporine

- in combination with beta-blockers as the preferred second drug in order to improve heart rate control (target heart rate <80 beats/min at rest and <110 beats/min on moderate exercise).
- Symptomatic heart failure caused by impairment of left ventricular systolic function in sinus rhythm may be considered (class IIb recommendation according to the European Guidelines, McMurray JJ, et al. Eur Heart J 2012;33:1787-847):
  - in case of intolerance to beta-blockers. Patients should also receive an angiotensin-converting enzyme inhibitor and spironolactone or eplerenone
  - in case of lack of improvement in symptoms despite treatment with a beta-blocker, angiotensin-converting enzyme inhibitor and spironolactone or eplerenone.
- Persistent/permanent atrial fibrillation without heart failure. This used to be one of the primary indications for digoxin, but today the use of beta-blockers, diltiazem or verapamil is preferred. These drugs can control the heart rate satisfactorily, both at rest and during exercise. Note that digoxin will not control the heart rate satisfactorily during exercise. If such patients are given digoxin, it should be combined with a beta-blocker, diltiazem or verapamil.

Major contraindications for digoxin
- Second or third degree atrioventricular block.
- Hypertrophic obstructive cardiomyopathy: because of its inotropic effect, it can increase the obstruction of the left ventricular outflow tract. Exceptions are the establishment of atrial fibrillation or the development of heart failure because of conversion to dilated-type cardiomyopathy.
- Wolff–Parkinson–White syndrome with atrial fibrillation: risk of accelerated conduction through the accessory pathway and precipitation of ventricular tachycardia or ventricular fibrillation.
- Acute myocardial infarction or acute myocarditis: increased risk of arrhythmogenesis.
- Sick sinus syndrome.
- Exacerbation of chronic obstructive pulmonary disease: risk of hypoxia-induced arrhythmogenesis.
- Diastolic heart failure: no clinical benefit.

Digoxin is no longer administered
- For conversion of recent-onset atrial fibrillation (ineffective).
- For conversion of supraventricular paroxysmal tachycardias, i.e. atrioventricular nodal or atrioventricular reentrant tachycardia (delayed onset of action, less effective than adenosine).
- For prevention of episodes of atrial fibrillation (ineffective).

Key points

■ Digoxin is the only inotrope drug with a bradycardic effect.

■ Its mechanism of action includes inhibition of the sodium pump (Na^+, K^+-ATPase), parasympathetic stimulation, and sympathetic inhibition.

■ Digoxin has a narrow therapeutic margin. Its therapeutic trough levels in serum are between 0.5 and 0.9 ng/mL.

■ The primary indications for administration of digoxin in symptomatic heart failure caused by impairment of left ventricular systolic function and an underlying rhythm of atrial fibrillation are:
  – intolerance to beta-blockers, or
  – inadequate heart rate control despite the use of beta-blockers (given in combination with a beta-blocker).

■ Digoxin is not used to convert recent-onset atrial fibrillation (ineffective) or supraventricular paroxysmal tachycardias (delayed onset of action, less effective than adenosine). It is also not used to prevent episodes of atrial fibrillation (ineffective).

19

Digoxin toxicity

Digoxin or digitalis toxicity is a set of cardiac and extracardiac manifestations caused by the toxic effects of digoxin and generally associated with elevated serum levels of digoxin (usually >2 ng/mL). In recent years the incidence of digoxin toxicity has declined due to the decreased use of this drug along with the improved technology for monitoring digoxin levels and the increased awareness in drug-to-drug interactions.

Warning! Digoxin toxicity can develop even at therapeutic levels of digoxin when other conditions increase myocardial sensitivity to digoxin (Table 19.1).

Manifestations of digoxin toxicity

- Gastrointestinal disorders: nausea, anorexia, vomiting, diarrhea.
- Neurological manifestations: confusion, disorientation, color vision (yellow/green halo around lights), weakness, vertigo, etc.
- Arrhythmogenesis: ventricular (e.g. bigeminy) or atrial (e.g. atrial tachycardia) arrhythmias.
- Sinus bradycardia or atrioventricular (AV) conduction disturbances (1st, 2nd or 3rd degree) due to marked parasympathetic stimulation.
- A combination of AV conduction disturbances and arrhythmogenesis: atrial tachycardia with AV block, etc.

TABLE 19.1	Conditions that increase myocardial sensitivity to digoxin
1) Hypokalemia, hypomagnesemia	5) Acute myocardial infarction
2) Age >70 years	6) Acute myocarditis
3) Hypoxemia	7) Hypothyroidism
4) Acidosis	

Treatment of digoxin toxicity

1) Discontinue digoxin and drugs that increase the levels of digoxin, and take blood samples to check the levels of digoxin, sodium, potassium, magnesium and creatinine (to rule out renal failure). If acute myocardial ischemia is suspected, check cardiac troponin levels.

2) Continuous ECG monitoring.

3) In cases of acute digoxin overdose, **activated charcoal** (50-100 g) may be administered orally in order to prevent its absorption in the gastrointestinal tract. This measure is more effective when digoxin has been taken within the previous hour.

4) In cases of hypokalemia, administer **potassium** IV: the rate of infusion will depend on the severity of the hypokalemia. If 10 ml ampoules of 10% KCl are used, for severe hypokalemia 4 ampoules of KCl (4 x 13.5 = 54 mEq of potassium) are added to 500 mL of 0.9% NaCl (or 5% D/W for patients with heart failure) and administered at a rate of 100-150 mL/h (see Chapter 12). Hypokalemia potentiates the toxic effect of digoxin on the myocardium because it inhibits the sodium pump; furthermore, potassium levels <3.0 mEq/L decrease the renal excretion of digoxin.

5) In cases of hyperkalemia due to inhibition of the sodium pump (a predictor of a poor outcome), rapid correction is required (see Chapter 13). Avoid administering calcium chloride or gluconate because of the risk of provoking ventricular tachycardia or ventricular fibrillation (may enhance the arrhythmogenic effect of digoxin).

6) For potentially malignant ventricular arrhythmias, antiarrhythmics are administered only when digoxin-specific antibodies (the treatment of choice) are not available; antiarrhythmics are therefore given as bridging therapy until antibodies can be administered. The antiarrhythmic used most commonly is **magnesium sulfate,** which is considered more effective than those given in the past, i.e. lidocaine and phenytoin. It is administered at a dose of 2 g IV over 2 min and it is available in various concentrations, i.e., 25% in 10 mL ampoules (provides 2 mEq/mL of Mg), 50% in 10 mL ampoules (provides 4 mEq/mL of Mg), etc. It is also effective in the absence of hypomagnesemia because it indirectly antagonizes the effects of digoxin on the sodium pump.

Warning! Electrical cardioversion of ventricular tachycardia (without severe hemodynamic compromise) due to digoxin toxicity should be avoided because of the risk of precipitating ventricular fibrillation "refractory" to defibrillation, or ventricular asystole. If an electrical shock is given, low energy levels should be used (e.g. 10-25 J) and the prior administration of 100 mg of lidocaine IV is recommended.

7) In cases of symptomatic bradycardia: 0.5 mg of **atropine** IV, which may be repeated every 3-5 min up to a maximum dose of 3 mg. If there is no response, then **temporary pacing** is performed. Isoproterenol should be avoided because of the increased risk of arrhythmogenesis.
8) Administration of **digoxin-specific antibodies** (Digibind or DigiFab vials, which contain 38 or 40 mg, respectively, of digoxin-specific immune Fab [Fragment antigen-binding]) in the following cases:
   - Severe arrhythmia due to digoxin toxicity, e.g. ventricular tachycardia, symptomatic bradyarrhythmia not responsive to atropine, etc.
   - Hyperkalemia (serum potassium >5.0 to 5.5 mEq/L) in the setting of severe digoxin toxicity
   - Serum digoxin levels >10 ng/mL in acute or >6 ng/mL in chronic ingestion
   - Acute ingestion (intentional or accidental) of >10 mg of digoxin.

Each vial of Digibind or DigiFab can bind and inactivate ~0.5 mg of digoxin. The patient usually begins to improve >30 min. The mean dose of antibodies in patients who receive chronic treatment with digoxin and develop digoxin toxicity is 4-6 vials administered IV over 30 min. The antibody-digoxin complexes are excreted by the kidneys.

If the serum levels of digoxin are known, the following formula may be used to calculate the approximate antibody dose:

$$\text{Dose (in vials)} = \frac{\text{serum digoxin level (ng/mL) x weight (kg)}}{100}$$

If the acute dose taken is known (e.g. in a suicide attempt), then the following formula is used:

$$\text{Dose (in vials)} = \frac{\text{total amount of digoxin taken (mg) x 0.8*}}{0.5}$$

Measurements of digoxin levels are an unreliable indicator of therapeutic response, because total serum digoxin levels increase markedly after antibody administration, whereas most of the digoxin is inactive because it is bound to antibodies. The most important adverse effect of this treatment is hypokalemia, caused by restoration of sodium pump function.

---

*Approximately 80% of an oral dose of digoxin is absorbed.

9) Dialysis is not useful because it cannot remove digoxin effectively. Patients with renal failure and digoxin toxicity who receive digoxin-specific antibodies should also undergo plasmapheresis to remove the digoxin-antibody complexes.

 Key points

- Digoxin toxicity can develop even at therapeutic levels of digoxin, when other conditions increase myocardial sensitivity to digoxin; such conditions are hypokalemia, hypomagnesemia, age >70 years, hypoxemia, acidosis, acute myocardial infarction, acute myocarditis, or hypothyroidism.

- The manifestations of digoxin toxicity usually include gastrointestinal disorders, neurological manifestations, arrhythmias and AV conduction disorders.

- Indications for administration of digoxin-specific antibodies are:
  a. severe arrhythmias due to digoxin toxicity
  b. potassium levels >5.0 to 5.5 mEq/L in the setting of severe digoxin toxicity
  c. serum digoxin levels >10 ng/mL in acute or >6 ng/mL in chronic ingestion
  d. acute ingestion of >10 mg of digoxin.

- For potentially malignant ventricular arrhythmias, if digoxin-specific antibodies are not readily available, magnesium sulfate may be administered IV.

- Electrical cardioversion of ventricular tachycardia (without severe hemodynamic compromise) due to digoxin toxicity should be avoided because of the risk of precipitating ventricular fibrillation "refractory" to defibrillation, or ventricular asystole.

ALGORITHM FOR THE TREATMENT OF DIGOXIN TOXICITY

Weak elderly individual with bradycardia (usually), confusion or gastrointestinal disorders ± renal failure, receiving digoxin

Suspected DIGOXIN TOXICITY

Basic tests
1) Na, K, Mg, creatinine
2) Digoxin levels (usually >2 ng/mL)
3) ECG (usually bradycardia, atrioventricular conduction disorders, bigeminy)

Major conditions that increase the risk of digoxin toxicity
1) Hypokalemia
2) Age >70 years
3) Renal failure
4) Acute myocardial ischemia
5) Concurrent administration of amiodarone, quinidine, propafenone, verapamil, etc.

Therapeutic measures

With hypokalemia

With severe ventricular arrhythmia (if digoxin-specific antibodies are not available)

With symptomatic bradycardia

In case of
- Severe arrhythmia
- Potassium levels >5.0 to 5.5 mEq/L
- Digoxin levels >10 ng/mL in acute or >6 ng/mL in chronic ingestion
- Acute ingestion of >10 mg of digoxin

IV potassium solution (4 amps of 10% KCl in 500 mL of 0.9% NaCl at 100-150 mL/h)

Magnesium sulfate: 2 g IV over 2 min

0.5-3 mg of atropine IV

If unsuccessful

Temporary pacing (if digoxin-specific antibodies are not available)

Digoxin-specific antibodies IV (Digibind or DigiFab)

20

Treatment of hemorrhagic events and perioperative management of patients taking vitamin K antagonists

The two main classes of vitamin K antagonists (VKAs) are:

a) Coumarin derivatives:
- warfarin (Parwarfin, Coumadin, Coumarin) with a half-life ($t^1/_2$) of ~36-42 h. Warfarin is the most widely used VKA (USA, UK, Italy, Canada, etc.)
- acenocoumarol (Sintrom) with a $t^1/_2$ of 10-24 h
- phenprocoumon (Mancoumar) with a $t^1/_2$ of ~5 days, used mainly in Germany

b) Indanedione derivatives, such as fluindione (Previscan) with a $t^1/_2$ of ~30 h, used mainly in France.

The warfarin effect is achieved ~4-5 days after its administration begins because of the long $t^1/_2$ of factor II (prothrombin), which is ~60 h. Warfarin, is a racemic mixture of R- and S-enantiomers (the S-enantiomer is more potent than the R-enantiomer). It is completely absorbed after po administration and is highly bound to plasma proteins. It is metabolized by cytochrome P450 (CYP2C9 metabolizes S-warfarin) and vitamin K epoxide reductase complex-1 (VKORC-1) to inactive metabolites excreted mainly in urine. Variants of CYP2C9 and VKORC-1 genotypes are a major cause of interindividual differences in warfarin effectiveness.

Table 20.1 lists the major indications for VKA administration.

Complications of VKAs

The most important complication of VKA use is hemorrhage, usually from the gastrointestinal and urinary tracts; the most dangerous site is cerebral hemorrhage. The risk of hemorrhagic complications is greater

TABLE 20.1	Major indications for vitamin K antagonist use

1) Atrial fibrillation (see Chapter 14)

2) Mechanical prosthetic heart valves; with bioprosthetic heart valves, VKAs are indicated for the first 3 months after valve replacement.

3) Deep vein thrombosis

4) Pulmonary embolism

5) Mitral valve stenosis of rheumatic etiology and sinus rhythm, when one or more of the following exist:
   – History of systemic embolism or paroxysmal atrial fibrillation
   – Presence of a thrombus or marked spontaneous echo contrast in the left atrium
   – Large left atrium (>55 mm)

6) Elective cardioversion of atrial fibrillation or flutter that has lasted ≥48 h (administered for 3 weeks before and at least 4 weeks after cardioversion)

when the international normalized ratio (INR) is increased (especially to levels >5.0), in persons older than 70 years, in patients with a history of cerebrovascular accident (CVA) or gastrointestinal bleeding, in cases of renal failure, in alcoholics, and with concomitant administration of nonsteroidal antiinflammatory drugs (NSAIDs). The annual rate of major hemorrhages, i.e. those that require blood transfusion or are life-threatening (e.g. cerebral hemorrhage), is ~2%. Very rarely, skin necrosis may occur (on the 3rd-8th day after administration) because of thrombosis of subcutaneous capillaries. Individuals with protein C or protein S deficiency are more susceptible to this complication.

Main contraindications to VKA therapy

Severe uncontrolled arterial hypertension (>180/100 mmHg), history of cerebral hemorrhage, active peptic ulcer, history of gastrointestinal hemorrhage during the previous 6 months, acute pericarditis, hepatic cirrhosis, thrombocytopenia (platelets <100,000/mm^3), and pregnancy (especially in the first trimester, because of the risk of teratogenesis and 2 weeks before birth due to the risk of bleeding at the time of delivery). When VKA administration is considered necessary, the risk/benefit ratio should be assessed in each case.

VKAs are also contraindicated if the patient is unwilling or unable to comply with blood monitoring because of cognitive impairment, alcoholism, psychosis, or problems accessing services.

Regarding the history of gastric hemorrhage, if ulcer healing can be determined endoscopically and if the infection is eradicated from patients positive for *Helicobacter pylori,* then VKAs can be administered with caution as long as proton pump inhibitors (PPIs) [avoid omeprazole] are also given.

Practical instructions for the administration of VKAs

- The following tests must be requested before administration: complete blood count, activated partial thromboplastin time (aPTT), INR* and transaminases.
- The use of VKA loading doses (10 mg warfarin or 8 mg acenocoumarol) should be avoided, because they cause a rapid and substantial drop in the levels of protein C ($t^1/_2$ ~6 h), the most important natural coagulation inhibitor, before the levels of the other vitamin K-dependent clotting factors are significantly reduced. This can lead to paradoxical hypercoagulability during the first 48 h and, rarely, to complications involving skin necrosis (developing on the 3rd-8th day). Therefore, anticoagulation treatment usually starts with 5 mg of warfarin or 4 mg of acenocoumarol. Even lower starting doses are given to elderly patients.
- By omitting the loading dose, therapeutic levels (INR >2.0) are achieved after >4 days. If rapid anticoagulation is required, then heparin should be administered concurrently until the desired INR is achieved (for at least 4 days).
- During the first week of VKA administration, the INR is usually measured every 2-3 days. For the following 2 weeks it is measured twice weekly, and after the INR has stabilized within the therapeutic range measurements are usually made monthly.
- VKAs are preferably administered in the evening (6 pm) so that the dose can be adjusted depending on the INR levels in the morning measurements.
- Foods rich in vitamin K should be consumed in small amounts because of the risk of weakening the effectiveness of the VKA. Such foods are listed in Table 20.2; green leafy vegetables figure prominently in this list. Specifically, the highest vitamin K levels among vegetables are found in parsley (fresh) [~1600 µg/100 g], kale (raw) [~700 µg/100 g], cress (raw) [540 µg/100 g) and spinach (raw) [~480 µg/100 g], followed by turnip greens (raw) [~250 µg/100 g], Brussels sprouts (raw) [~175 µg/100 g], lettuce (raw) [~125 µg/100 g] and broccoli (raw) [~100 µg/100 g]. Most important, however, is that the patient should adhere to a steady and unvarying diet for such foods. A steady diet, even one with moderate quantities of vitamin K, will lead to an adjustment of the VKA dose to a higher

*Normal level of INR <1.2

TABLE 20.2	Foods with high vitamin K content (≥50 µg/100 g)	
50-100 µg/100 g	**100-250 µg/100 g**	**>400 µg/100 g**
Olive oil	Turnip greens (raw)	Parsley (fresh)
Cabbage (raw)	Brussels sprouts (raw)	Kale (raw)
Canola oil	Soybean oil	Cress (raw)
Asparagus (raw)	Lettuce (raw, green leafs)	Spinach (raw)
Avocado (raw)	Broccoli (raw)	
Cauliflower (raw)		

Source: USDA Nutrient Database, http://ndb.nal.usda.gov/

level so as to ensure therapeutic INR values. It is estimated that for each increase in 100 µg of vitamin K intake, the INR will be reduced by 0.2. In addition, the ingestion of alcohol should be minimal and the attending physician should be informed of any new drugs taken.

- A patient under VKA treatment should be aware of some common foods that contain low levels of vitamin K. This includes most fruit — e.g. orange (<0.01 µg/100 g), banana (0.5 µg/100 g), apple (~2.0 µg/100 g), peach (~2.5 µg/100 g) — and most animal products (meat and dairy). Tomatoes and peeled cucumbers also have a relatively low vitamin K content (~8 µg and ~7 µg/100 g, respectively) and can be used in salads to replace green vegetables. Note that the recommended daily allowance of vitamin K for the general population is ~1.0 µg/kg.

- The anticoagulation effect is best evaluated by determining the INR. This is more reliable than prothrombin time, since it corrects for any differences caused by the use of different thromboplastin reagents.

Warning! When cooked in olive oil (has high content in vitamin K [~60 µg/100 g]), foods with low vitamin K content can become significant sources of vitamin K uptake. Furthermore, elderly people often take multivitamin nutritional supplements rich in vitamin K.

- The bleeding risk seems to be higher when warfarin is coadministered with clopidogrel than when it is coadministered with aspirin (Keeling D, et al. Br J Haematol 2011;154:311-24).

- In patients with stable coronary artery disease who are taking VKAs (e.g. atrial fibrillation with CHA_2DS_2-VASc score ≥2) and undergo intracoronary stenting, a bare-metal stent (BMS) should be preferred over a drug-eluting stent (DES). After BMS implantation, dual antiplatelet therapy (DAPT)+VKA needs to be administered for at least one month (as opposed to 3-6 months in the case of DES), followed by VKA coadministered with aspirin (75-100 mg/day) or clopidogrel (75 mg/day) for a further 11 months. After the first year, treatment continues with VKAs alone. The latest European Guidelines on Myocardial Revascularization (Windecker S, et al. Eur Heart J 2014;35:2541-619) suggest that the new-generation DES (i.e. everolimus-eluting stents [Xience-V, Promus] and zotarolimus-eluting stents [Endeavor, Resolute]) should be preferred over BMS in patients requiring VKAs if the bleeding risk score is low (HAS-BLED ≤2). With the new-generation DES, the initial triple therapy of DAPT+VKA should be considered for a duration of at least one month, followed by VKAs+aspirin (75-100 mg/day) or clopidogrel (75 mg/day) continued up to 12 months.

- In patients with acute coronary syndrome (with or without stent implantation) at low bleeding risk (HAS-BLED ≤2) who are taking VKAs (e.g. atrial fibrillation with CHA_2DS_2-VASc score ≥2), the administration of triple antithrombotic medication should be limited to a period of 6 months, irrespective of stent type, followed by coadministration of VKA with aspirin (75-100 mg/day) or clopidogrel (75 mg/day) until the completion of the first year, after which treatment continues with VKAs alone.
- In patients at high bleeding risk (HAS-BLED ≥3) who are taking VKAs (e.g. atrial fibrillation with CHA_2DS_2-VASc score ≥2), triple antithrombotic therapy [VKA + aspirin (75–100 mg/day) + clopidogrel (75 mg/day)] should be considered for a duration of one month followed by VKA and aspirin (75–100 mg/day) or clopidogrel (75 mg/day) irrespective of clinical setting (stable coronary artery disease or acute coronary syndrome) and stent type (BMS or new-generation DES) until the completion of the first year. After the first year, treatment continues with VKAs alone.
- The use of ticagrelor and prasugrel (instead of clopidogrel) is not recommended as part of triple antithrombotic therapy.
- When VKAs are given in combination with clopidogrel ± aspirin in patients with atrial fibrillation, the desired INR should be in the range of 2.0–2.5.
- Gastric protection with PPIs should be considered in patients with VKAs and concurrent antiplatelet therapy, particularly DAPT.

Causes of elevated INR

Table 20.3 presents the major causes that increase the risk of hemorrhage when taking VKAs, especially due to INR elevation. It should be stressed that concurrent administration of VKAs with NSAIDs increases the

TABLE 20.3	Causes of increased hemorrhagic risk when taking vitamin K antagonists (VKAs)

1) VKA overdose

2) Alcohol consumption

3) Hyperthyroidism

4) Hepatic or renal failure

5) Interaction with other substances (nonsteroidal antiinflammatory drugs, amiodarone, etc.)
   See Table 20.4

6) Concurrent administration of $P2Y_{12}$ receptor inhibitors (clopidogrel, prasugrel, etc.)

7) Advanced age

8) Febrile illness

risk of hemorrhagic events without necessarily increasing the INR. Table 20.4 lists substances that increase or decrease the effect of VKAs.

Treatment of hemorrhagic events in patients taking VKAs

1) In serious and life-threatening bleeding (i.e. cerebral hemorrhage) at any elevation of INR:
   - Immediate discontinuation of the VKA.
   - Four-factor prothrombin complex concentrate (4F-PCC) [contains factors II, VII, IX, and X, as well as proteins C and S] at a dose of 25-50 U/kg IV. The exact dose depends on the pretreatment INR levels, i.e. 25 U/kg if INR is 2.0-3.9 (max dose 2500 U), 35 U/Kg if INR is 4.0-6.0 (max dose 3500 U), and 50 U/Kg if INR is >6.0 (max dose 5000 U). Note that the dosage is expressed in units of factor IX activity. 4F-PCC (Kcentra, Beriplex) has been approved by the FDA (2013) for urgent VKA reversal. It is infused within 10-20 min, has a rapid onset of action (significant INR decline within 10 min) and its effect lasts ~6-8 h. If 4F-PCC is not available then fresh frozen plasma (FFP) can be used, but it should be noted that it produces suboptimal anticoagulation reversal, its effect is more delayed compared to 4F-PCC, and very large volumes of plasma (15-30 mL/kg) have to be infused rapidly. This can lead to fluid overload in patients with compromised cardiac or renal function. Although recombinant factor VIIa (rFVIIa) [NovoSeven] rapidly corrects the INR, its effectiveness for stopping bleeding is unclear and it is not recommended for emergency anticoagulation reversal (Keeling D, et al. Br J Haematol 2011;154:311-24).

TABLE 20.4	Substances that enhance or weaken the effect of vitamin K antagonists (VKAs)

1) Substances that enhance the effect of VKAs

Alcohol
Allopurinol
Aminoglycosides
Amiodarone
Ampicillin
Anabolic steroids
Aspirin
Cephalosporins
Chloramphenicol
Cimetidine
Dipyridamole
Erythromycin
Fenoprofen
Fibrates
Fluconazole
Ibuprofen
Indomethacin
Isoniazid
Itraconazole
Ketoconazole
Ketoprofen
Mefenamic acid
Methotrexate
Metronidazole
Naproxen
Neomycin
Niflumic acid
Omeprazol
Penicillin (at high IV doses)
Phenytoin
Piroxicam
Propafenone
Propranolol
Propylthiouracil
Quinidine
Quinolones
Statins
Sulfonamides
Tamoxifen
Tetracyclins
Thyroxin
Tricyclic antidepressants
Trimethoprim-sulfamethoxazole
Verapamil

2) Substances that weaken the effect of VKAs

Barbiturates
Carbamazepine
Carbimazole
Cholestyramine
Cyclosporin
Estrogens
Griseofulvin
Phenytoin (can also enhance anticoagulation effect)
Rifampicin
Thiouracil
Vitamin K

- Vitamin K_1 (phytomenadione) in a dose of 5-10 mg IV within 30 min after dissolution in 50 mL of 0.9% NaCl or 5% D/W. It is always administered with 4F-PCC to maintain coagulation factor levels once the effect of 4F-PCC has diminished. Note that the full effect of vitamin K_1 is delayed by 8-12 h, the time required for the liver to synthesize coagulation factors. On rare occasions, IV administration of vitamin K_1 can be complicated by anaphylactoid reactions.

2) If INR ≥9.0, with or without mild hemorrhage (e.g. nosebleeds, hematuria):
   - Discontinue VKA for 1-2 days
   - Administer vitamin K_1 at a dose of 2.5-5.0 mg po.

   If the patient is at high risk for a hemorrhagic complication (age >70 years, uncontroled hypertension, concurrent use of an antiplatelet agent, renal or hepatic failure), it is preferable to keep them under observation for at least 12 h (short-term care unit) and discharge them when the INR drops below 5.0.

3) If INR ≥5.0 but <9.0, with or without mild hemorrhage: discontinue VKA for 1-2 days and monitor the INR. Consider giving vitamin K_1 po (1.0-2.5 mg) for patients at high risk of bleeding, i.e. advanced age, decompensated heart failure, active malignancy.

Warning! In patients with a mechanical heart valve and bleeding due to pathologically prolonged INR, administration of vitamin K_1 is contraindicated because of the risk of valve thrombosis, unless the patient's life is in danger, in which case a dose of 1 mg may be administered by slow IV infusion. Furthermore, this administration makes them resistant to reaching therapeutic INR levels for 2 weeks after the VKA is restarted (concurrent administration of heparin will be required for a short time).

4) For INR above therapeutic levels but <5.0, with or without mild hemorrhage: reduce or omit usually one dose of the VKA.

5) In case of bleeding at therapeutic INR levels, organic causes of bleeding such as possible malignancy (e.g. bladder, renal tract, or large intestine malignancy) must be ruled out.

Warning! Patients on VKA presenting to the Emergency Room with a head injury should have their INR measured urgently and a head computed tomography (CT) scan should be performed at a lower threshold, because they are prone to develop intracranial bleeding, even with minor head injuries. This is more likely with elderly patients.

Target INR for various conditions
- Atrial fibrillation: INR=2.0-3.0.
- Mechanical heart valves: 2.5-3.5. Specifically, for a mechanical mitral

valve the target INR is 3.0-3.5 whereas for a mechanical aortic valve it is 2.5-3.0. An exception are older mechanical heart valves (Starr-Edwards, Bjork-Shiley), where an INR of 3.0-4.5 is sought.
• Deep vein thrombosis or pulmonary embolism: INR=2.0-3.0.

Perioperative management of patients who are taking VKAs and undergo elective surgery with high or moderate bleeding risk

The need for discontinuation of VKAs perioperatively in order to reduce the risk of hemorrhagic complications, and for bridging anticoagulation with heparin, depends on the type of surgery and the patient's thromboembolic risk. Table 20.5 describes the stratification by perioperative risk for a thromboembolic episode. The CHADS$_2$ scoring system assesses thromboembolic risk in atrial fibrillation and includes the scores of 5 risk factors: Congestive heart failure, Hypertension, Age ≥75 years, Diabetes mellitus, and previous Stroke or transient ischemic attack. Each factor is given 1 point except for the last one, which is given 2 points.

For surgery with a high (coronary artery bypass surgery, heart valve replacement, major orthopedic surgery, surgery involving the blood vessels, the prostate, the kidneys, malignant tumors, the spine or the brain) or moderate (intestinal polyp excision, prostate or liver biopsy, pacemaker or defibrillator implantation, etc.) risk of hemorrhagic complications, VKAs should be discontinued so that the patient may be brought to the operating room with an INR <1.5. For patients with high or moderate thromboembolic risk, bridging anticoagulation with heparin (preferably low-molecular-weight heparin, LMWH) should be administered at the same time, as described below.

Most literature references involve patients under warfarin treatment, since that is the most widely used VKA in the world. So, for such patients with high or moderate thromboembolic risk (Table 20.6):

1) **Before surgery:** Warfarin is discontinued 5 days before surgery, so that the patient will be brought to the operating theater with an INR <1.5. Over the following days, the INR is checked daily and, if it falls below the lower therapeutic limit (usually in 2 days), e.g. INR <2.0 in cases of atrial fibrillation or <2.5 in patients with mechanical aortic valve, LMWHs are started.

For patients at high thromboembolic risk LMWHs are given at therapeutic dose, e.g. enoxaparin (Lovenox, Clexane) 1 mg/kg x 2/day or 1.5 mg/kg x 1/day, tinzaparin (Innohep) 175 U/Kg x 1/day or dalteparin (Fragmin) 100 U/kg x 2/day or 200 U/kg x 1/day, subcutaneously. The LMWH is discontinued 24 h before surgery (i.e. the last dose is given 24 h before the operation) so as to reduce the chances of residual anticoagulation activity during surgery. If the patient was

TABLE 20.5	Suggested patient risk stratification for perioperative thromboembolism (Spyropoulos AC, et al. Blood 2012;120:2954-62)		
Risk stratum	**Mechanical heart valve**	**Atrial fibrillation**	**VTE**
High (>10% /year risk for ATE or >10% /month risk for VTE)	• Any mechanical mitral valve • Older (caged-ball or tilting disc) aortic valve prosthesis • Recent (<6 months) stroke or transient ischemic attack	• CHADS$_2$ score of 5 or 6 • Recent (<3 months) stroke or transient ischemic attack • Rheumatic valvular heart disease	• Recent (<3 months) VTE • Severe thrombophilia (e.g. deficiency of protein C, protein S or antithrombin, antiphospholipid antibodies, or multiple thrombophilias)
Moderate (4-10% /year risk for ATE or 4-10% /month risk for VTE)	Bileaflet aortic valve prosthesis and one of the following: atrial fibrillation, prior stroke or transient ischemic attack, hypertension, diabetes, congestive heart failure, age >75 years	CHADS$_2$ score of 3 or 4	• VTE within the past 3 to 12 months • Non-severe thrombophilic conditions (e.g. factor V Leiden, heterozygous factor II mutation) • Recurrent VTE • Active cancer (treated within 6 months or palliative)
Low (<4% /year risk for ATE or <4% /month risk for VTE)	Bileaflet aortic valve prosthesis without atrial fibrillation and no other risk factors for stroke	CHADS$_2$ score of 0 to 2 (and no prior stroke or transient ischemic attack)	Single VTE occurred >12 months ago and no other risk factors

*CHADS$_2$ = Congestive heart failure - Hypertension - Age - Diabetes - Stroke.
ATE: arterial thromboembolism, VTE: venous thromboembolism

taking tinzaparin, then only half of the daily dose is given 24 h before the operation. Alternatively, unfractionated heparin (UFH) may be given by continuous IV infusion that is stopped 4 h before surgery. Of course, the use of IV UFH has the drawback of requiring admission to the hospital, which is why LMWHs are preferred.

TABLE 20.6	Perioperative management of patients with high or moderate thromboembolic risk under long-term warfarin treatment, who are undergoing surgery with high or moderate bleeding risk

Day before/after surgery

-5	Discontinue warfarin (last dose on day -6)
-4	No anticoagulation
-3	± LMWH (depending on INR levels)
-2	LMWH
-1	LMWH (only morning dose)
0 (Day of surgery)	Warfarin (12-24 h after surgery)
+1	Warfarin ± LMWH (24-72 h after surgery)
+2	Warfarin + LMWH
+3	Warfarin + LMWH
+4	Warfarin ± LMWH (depending on INR levels)
+5	Warfarin ± LMWH (depending on INR levels)
+6	Warfarin

LMWH: low-molecular-weight heparin

For patients at moderate thromboembolic risk the bridging or no bridging approach can be chosen based on patients' characteristics and the type of surgery.

Lastly, for patients at low thromboembolic risk bridging anticoagulation therapy is not recommended during interruption of VKA therapy.

It should be mentioned, that the previously recommended practice is based on weak evidence. Recently, the BRIDGE trial (Douketis JD, et al. N Engl J Med 2015;373:823-33) reported that perioperative bridging with LMWH in patients with atrial fibrillation was noninferior for the prevention of arterial thromboembolism compared to interruption of warfarin and no perioperative bridging and was associated with lower risk of major bleeding. In this study patients with a mechanical heart valve or recent stoke/transient ischemic attack had been excluded.

Warning! If a patient on VKA needs to undergo emergency surgery, then 4F-PCC (25-50 U/kg IV) must be administered for the rapid reversal of VKA anticoagulation (+ 5-10 mg IV of vitamin K_1 to maintain the VKA effect reversal >12 h).

2) **After surgery:** Warfarin is administered 12-24 h after surgery, i.e. in the afternoon of the operation day or the next morning.

For patients at high thromboembolic risk the LMWH is usually restarted 24 h after surgery and is continued until the INR becomes ≥2.0 (usually 4-5 days). If, however, the risk of postoperative bleeding is high and effective hemostasis cannot be achieved, then the LMWH may be delayed for 48-72 h. Note that the LMWH anticoagulant effect peaks 3-5 h after the first dose, whereas VKAs need at least 48 h to start showing even mild anticoagulation (INR >1.5). Ideally, the INR should be measured daily until therapeutic levels are achieved. If UFH is preferred, then its infusion begins 24-72 h after surgery and continues for ~4-5 days.

For patients at moderate thromboembolic risk the postoperative administration of LMWH is determined by patients' characteristics and surgery-related criteria, while for patients at low thromboembolic risk postoperative administration of LMWH is not required.

For patients taking acenocoumarol, because of its shorter half-life and therefore shorter duration of action, the management described for warfarin is slightly modified. Therefore, for patients at high thromboembolic risk the drug is discontinued 3-4 days before surgery and LMWH administration can

TABLE 20.7	Perioperative management of patients with high or moderate thromboembolic risk under long-term acenocoumarol treatment, who are undergoing surgery with high or moderate bleeding risk
Day before/after surgery	
-4	Discontinue acenocoumarol (last dose on day -5)
-3	± LMWH (depending on INR levels)
-2	LMWH
-1	LMWH (only morning dose)
0 (Day of surgery)	Acenocoumarol (12-24 h after surgery)
+1	Acenocoumarol ± LMWH (24-72 h after surgery)
+2	Acenocoumarol + LMWH
+3	Acenocoumarol ± LMWH (depending on INR levels)
+4	Acenocoumarol ± LMWH (depending on INR levels)
+5	Acenocoumarol

LMWH: low-molecular-weight heparin

begin 1 or 2 days after the discontinuation of acenocumarol, depending on the INR (Table 20.7). After surgery, the period of concurrent LMWH administration is shorter than with warfarin (usually 3-4 days). In patients with low thromboembolic risk, acenocoumarol can be discontinued 3-4 days before surgery and restarted 12-24 h after surgery, with no need for heparin.

Figure 20.1 shows a simplified form of the protocol for bridging anticoagulation in patients taking warfarin, who have high or moderate thromboembolic risk and are undergoing surgery with high or moderate risk of bleeding.

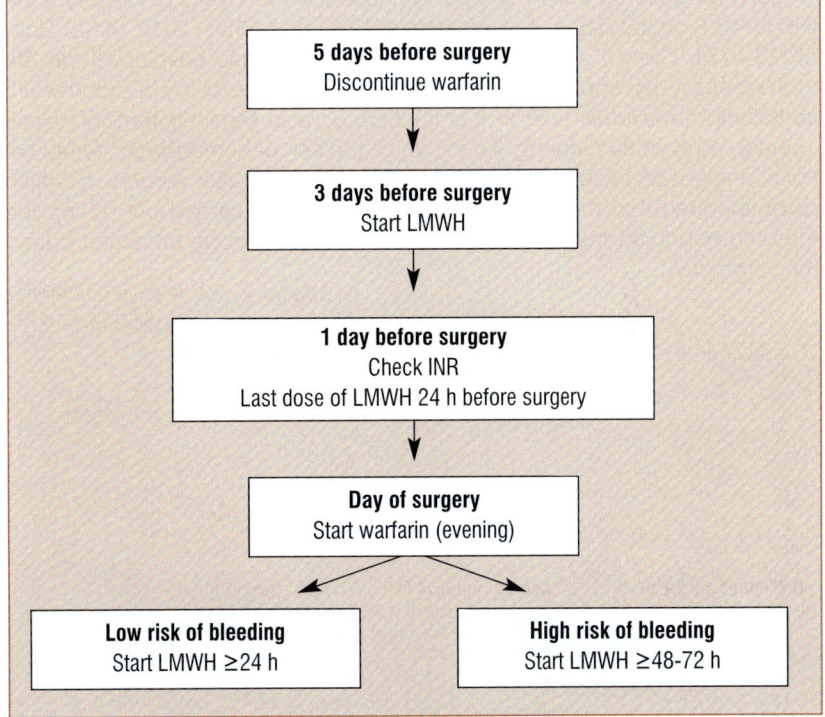

Figure 20.1. Simplified protocol for bridging anticoagulation in patients taking warfarin who have high or moderate thromboembolic risk and are undergoing surgery with high or moderate risk of bleeding. *LMWH: low-molecular-weight heparin*

Perioperative management of patients who are taking VKAs and undergo surgery with a low risk of bleeding

Patients undergoing surgery with a low risk of bleeding do not need to discontinue the VKA, provided their INR is <3.0 on the day of surgery. In general, it is wise to keep INR levels in the lower therapeutic range.

Low bleeding risk operations are:

1) Minor dental procedures: extraction of one or more teeth and root canal. However, when more than 3 teeth need to be extracted staged visits may be most appropriate.
2) Minor dermatology procedures: excision of basal and squamous cell carcinomas, actinic keratoses and malignant or premalignant nevi.
3) Minor ophthalmological procedures: cataract surgery.

We emphasize here that for minor dental procedures, a common type of surgery, no dose reduction or discontinuation of the VKA is necessary if the INR is <3.0 on the day of surgery [Guyatt GH, et al. Chest 2012;141(2)(Suppl):7S-47S]. Even if a hemorrhagic complication does develop, it can be treated easily by applying local pressure with gauze or by a mouthwash containing tranexamic acid or ε-aminocaproic acid (Amicar) [antifibrinolytic agents], or even by suturing. To minimize the risk of hemorrhagic complications, analgesics such as NSAIDs should be avoided after surgery. It is also recommended that the dental procedure should be carried out during the morning hours, so that any bleeding complication can be managed during the same day.

Key points

- Achieving therapeutic INR levels through administration of VKAs requires excellent collaboration between the patient and the attending physician.

- When starting treatment with VKAs, loading doses (10 mg of warfarin or 8 mg of acenocoumarol) are avoided because of the risk of paradoxical hypercoagulability.

- A patient taking a VKA and presenting hematuria or gastrointestinal bleeding must be investigated for possible organic conditions. The need is greater when INR levels are therapeutic or only slightly prolonged.

- In a patient taking a VKA and undergoing elective surgery, with high or moderate bleeding risk, perioperative discontinuation of the VKA should be considered in order to reduce the risk of hemorrhagic complications. At the same time, the need to administer bridging anticoagulation with heparin should be evaluated in order to reduce the risk of thromboembolism. As a result, the management of such patients will depend on the type of surgery and the degree of thromboembolic risk.

- Patients with high thromboembolic risk undergoing surgery with high or moderate risk of bleeding should discontinue warfarin 5 days, or acenocoumarol 3-4 days, before surgery (INR target <1.5 on the day of the operation) and should receive a LMWH that will be discontinued 24 h before surgery. The VKA will be restarted 12-24 h and the LMWH 24-72 h after surgery. The LMWH is given until therapeutic INR levels are achieved.

- For a tooth extraction, VKAs do not need to be discontinued provided the INR is <3.0 on the day of the procedure and local hemostatic measures are used.

- In addition to the temporary interruption of the VKA, a patient with INR ≥9.0 ± mild bleeding must also receive vitamin K_1 po (2.5-5.0 mg).

- When rapid reversal of the effect of a VKA is required because of severe bleeding (e.g. cerebral hemorrhage, retroperitoneal hematoma) and prolonged INR, 4F-PCC (25-50 U/kg IV), or if not available, FFP (15-30 mL/kg), should be given together with vitamin K_1 (5-10 mg) by slow IV infusion.

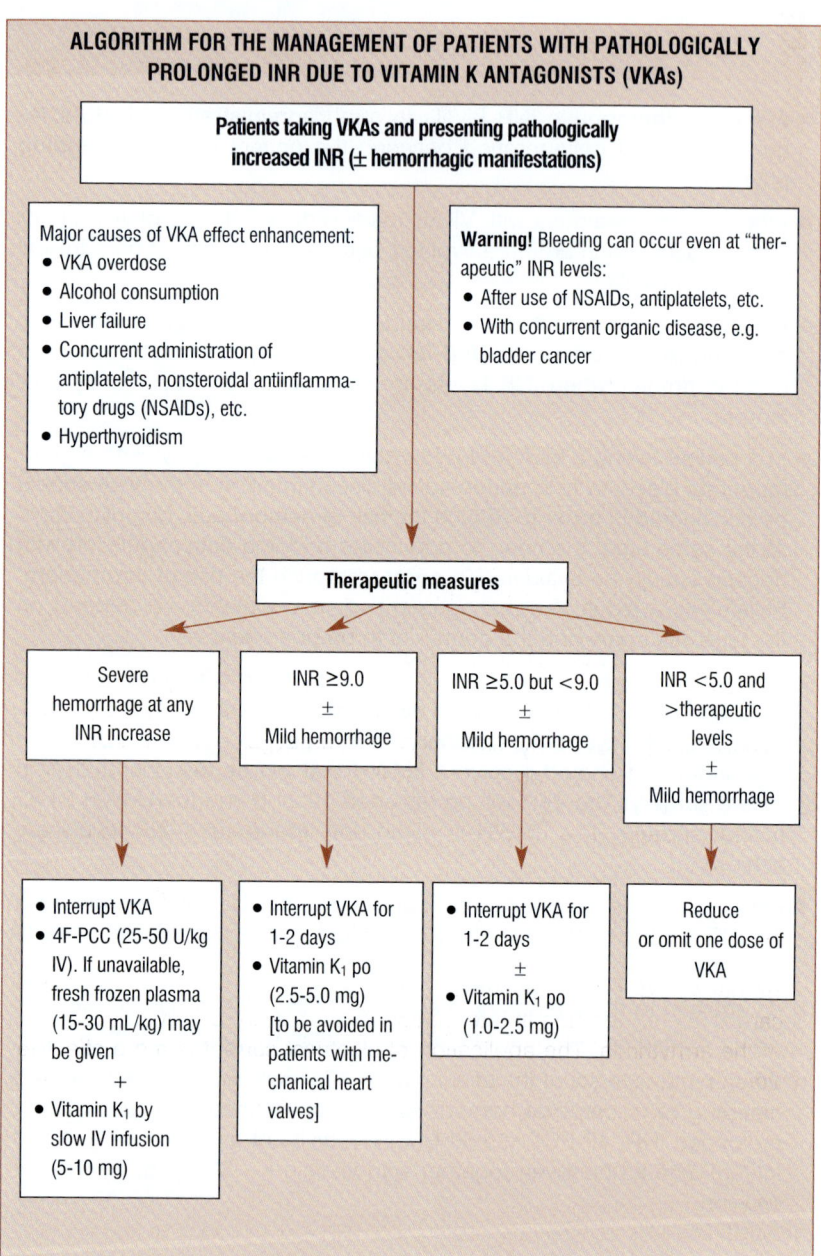

ALGORITHM FOR THE MANAGEMENT OF PATIENTS WITH PATHOLOGICALLY PROLONGED INR DUE TO VITAMIN K ANTAGONISTS (VKAs)

Patients taking VKAs and presenting pathologically increased INR (± hemorrhagic manifestations)

Major causes of VKA effect enhancement:
- VKA overdose
- Alcohol consumption
- Liver failure
- Concurrent administration of antiplatelets, nonsteroidal antiinflammatory drugs (NSAIDs), etc.
- Hyperthyroidism

Warning! Bleeding can occur even at "therapeutic" INR levels:
- After use of NSAIDs, antiplatelets, etc.
- With concurrent organic disease, e.g. bladder cancer

Therapeutic measures

Severe hemorrhage at any INR increase	INR ≥9.0 ± Mild hemorrhage	INR ≥5.0 but <9.0 ± Mild hemorrhage	INR <5.0 and >therapeutic levels ± Mild hemorrhage
• Interrupt VKA • 4F-PCC (25-50 U/kg IV). If unavailable, fresh frozen plasma (15-30 mL/kg) may be given + • Vitamin K_1 by slow IV infusion (5-10 mg)	• Interrupt VKA for 1-2 days • Vitamin K_1 po (2.5-5.0 mg) [to be avoided in patients with mechanical heart valves]	• Interrupt VKA for 1-2 days ± • Vitamin K_1 po (1.0-2.5 mg)	Reduce or omit one dose of VKA

INR: international normalized ratio, 4F-PCC: Four-factor prothrombin complex concentrate

21

Electrical cardioversion and defibrillation

Electrical cardioversion and defibrillation involve the application of electric current for the restoration of sinus rhythm in certain cardiac arrhythmias. More specifically, we distinguish between:

- **Cardioversion,** when the discharge (shock) is delivered in synchrony with the R wave on the patient's ECG, such as in atrial fibrillation, atrial flutter, ventricular tachycardia (VT), etc. An exception is pulseless VT, when defibrillation is applied to avoid losing time before energy is delivered.
- **Defibrillation,** when the shock is given asynchronously with the R wave of the patient's ECG, such as in ventricular fibrillation (VF) or pulseless VT. The only contraindication is the prior expression by the patient (or patient's surrogate) of an informed wish not to be resuscitated.

The delivery of shock causes the simultaneous depolarization of all the myocardial fibers, resulting in interruption of the reentry circuit and termination of the arrhythmia. The application of electrical current is more effective (conversion rate 70-95%) in tachyarrhythmias that are due to a reentry mechanism. Table 21.1 shows the contraindications for electrical cardioversion.

Technique

Application of electrical current may be required either as an emergency, in situations where the arrhythmia leads to severe hemodynamic compro-

TABLE 21.1	Contraindications for electrical cardioversion

1) Tachyarrhythmias due to increased automaticity (e.g. multifocal atrial tachycardia): ineffective

2) Tachyarrhythmias on a substrate of digitalis toxicity, provided there is no severe hemodynamic compromise: risk of causing difficult-to-treat ventricular tachycardia or ventricular fibrillation (if cardioversion is applied use a low initial energy setting of the order of 10-25 J, with prior administration of 100 mg IV lidocaine)

3) Tachyarrhythmias on a substrate of severe electrolyte disturbances, provided there is no severe hemodynamic compromise: risk of causing ventricular fibrillation

4) Atrial fibrillation or flutter of duration >48 h, unless 3 weeks' prior anticoagulant medication has been administered or transoesophageal echocardiography has been performed to rule out thrombus in the left atrium: risk of causing embolism

5) Atrial fibrillation due to hyperthyroidism: ineffective

mise (acute pulmonary edema, angina, drop in blood pressure or loss of consciousness), or as an elective procedure. The conscious patient should be sedated in advance, so as not to be aware of this painful procedure.

In the case of elective electrical cardioversion, the following steps should be taken:

- Informed consent form should be obtained from the patient.
- The patient should fast for 6 h and electrolyte levels should be determined to rule out hypokalemia. When a shock is applied to a patient with hypokalemia there is a risk of causing VT or VF.
- Placement of a peripheral line and confirmation of availability of cardiopulmonary resuscitation in the cardioversion area. Cardioversion should preferably be performed in the coronary care unit.
- Twelve-lead ECG recording and continuous ECG monitoring.
- Placement of pulse oximeter for monitoring arterial blood oxygen saturation.
- Clinical examination of the patient, with emphasis on the palpation of peripheral pulses to check for any peripheral thromboembolic episodes following cardioversion.
- Placement of defibrillator patches on the patient and selection of the lead that shows a distinct R wave, without artifacts.

Warning! If high T waves appear on the defibrillator screen there is a risk of these waves being detected as R waves, leading to asynchronous shock with a risk of VF. In consequence, a lead should be selected where the R waves are significantly higher than the T waves.

- Placement of the defibrillator electrodes (self-adhesive pads or paddles) on the chest. If paddles are used, gel should be spread in the area where they will be placed in order to reduce the resistance. The electrodes may be placed in:
  - Anteroapical position: one electrode is placed parasternally on the right, below the clavicle, and the other over the apex of the heart (fifth intercostal space in the anterior axillary line avoiding the breast).
  - Left anteroposterior position: the anterior electrode is placed in a low left parasternal position and the posterior electrode just inferior to the left scapula. Anteroposterior placement is easier to perform when self-adhesive pads are used.
- Confirmation that the defibrillator has been set to the "SYNCH" position and that on the screen a dot appears on the R wave of ECG (and not on the T wave).
- Cardioversion should be preceded by the administration of oxygen for 5-15 min via nasal cannulas or mask, continued for at least 15 min after conversion. During the shock delivery the oxygen source should be moved away from the patient.
- Sedation of the patient through IV administration of a short-acting benzodiazepine, e.g. 2-5 mg midazolam (Dormicum) and additional IV administration of an opioid analgesic, e.g. 0.05-0.1 mg fentanyl (Fentanyl citrate, Sublimaze). Antidotes to these drugs should always be available:
  - for midazolam → flumazenil (Anexate) in a dose of 0.2-1 mg IV
  - for fentanyl → naloxone (Narcan, Evzio) in a dose of 0.4-1.2 mg IV.
- Once the patient is sedated, the electrodes are applied firmly (if paddles are used) to the chest, the desired level of energy is chosen and charged, the operator issues a warning and checks that nobody is in direct or indirect contact with the patient, and the shock is then delivered. If the first shock has no result, it is repeated with a higher energy (Table 21.2). The interval between two successive shocks should not be <1 min. If the maximum shock of 360 J is unsuccessful, the same shock may be repeated; there is a chance that it will be successful because of a reduction in transthoracic impedance after the previous discharge. Another option is to reposition the electrodes, i.e. if initially the electrodes had been placed in anteroapical position, the shocks can be repeated with left anteroposterior electrode placement, since this is consider more effective. It is worth noting that <10% of the energy delivered actually reaches the heart.
- If cardioversion of atrial fibrillation fails, the procedure may be repeated after pretreatment with ibutilide (1 mg IV) since it has been shown to increase the likelihood of successful cardioversion.
- Apart from VF and pulseless VT, where a specific algorithm is fol-

TABLE 21.2	Energy delivered to treat arrhythmias with a monophasic defibrillator*
Arrhythmia	**Energy delivery sequence**
Atrial fibrillation	200 J → 360 J → 360 J
Atrial flutter	50 or 100 J → 200 J → 360 J
Ventricular tachycardia (not pulseless)	50 or 100 J → 200 J → 360 J
Ventricular fibrillation or pulseless ventricular tachycardia	360 J (1st shock) → CPR x 2 min → 360 J (2nd shock) → CPR x 2 min → 360 J (3rd shock) + adrenaline + amiodarone → CPR x 2 min → (see Chapter 10)

If biphasic current is used, smaller quantities of energy are needed, about half those delivered with monophasic current: e.g. in ventricular fibrillation or pulseless ventricular tachycardia we start with 150-200 J.

CPR: cardiopulmonary resuscitation (compressions:breaths = 30:2 in a nonintubated patient or 100-120:10 /min in an intubated patient).

lowed, during elective cardioversion of other arrhythmias, a sequence of up to 3 shocks is usually applied. If these are unsuccessful, the attempt at electrical cardioversion is usually stopped.
- The patient usually remains in hospital for 24 h after the cardioversion procedure.

Observations
- Before elective cardioversion of atrial fibrillation, hyperthyroidism must be ruled out. Cardioversion should be performed when the patient is in a normothyroid (euthyroid) state.
- Before the delivery of current, any self-adhesive drug patches should be removed from the chest.
- After the energy delivery, apart from the expected increase in creatine kinase (CK) from the destruction of musculoskeletal cells, a small increase in cardiac troponins may be observed.
- If there is suspicion of sick sinus syndrome, a temporary transvenous pacemaker should be placed before the procedure as a precaution against asystole or severe bradycardia.
- If the patient has a permanent pacemaker or an implantable cardioverter defibrillator (ICD), the electrodes should be placed at least 8 cm away from the pacemaker or ICD generator (anteroposterior position is preferred). After the cardioversion the device should be checked, because of the risk of causing complications such as movement of the leads, or an

increase in the pacing threshold due to conduction of current along the electrodes and injury to the myocardium.

- In the rare cases where electric shock needs to be delivered to a pregnant woman for the conversion of arrhythmias, it should be noted that this is safe for the fetus. However it is recommended to use the smallest effective amount of energy, the fetus should be outside the electrode discharge path, and the fetal heart rate should be checked after the shock delivery. The mother should not be in a supine position in order to avoid compression of the inferior vena cava by the gravid uterus, which could lead to hypotension. For this reason cardioversion in a pregnant woman should be performed with the patient in the left lateral position (e.g. support placed under the right hip).
- Biphasic, if available, should be preferred over monophasic current because it is more effective and a lower amount of energy is required for cardioversion/defibrillation.

Main complications
- In the case of cardioversion of atrial fibrillation of >48 h duration, without any prior anticoagulant medication, there is a 1-7% risk of causing thromboembolic episodes. In these cases, if anticoagulation is given for three weeks before cardioversion, the risk drops to <1%.
- After cardioversion, early ventricular or supraventricular extrasystoles may appear, and more rarely transient sinus pause or atrioventricular block. The risk of development of malignant arrhythmias is increased in digitalis toxicity or severe hypokalemia.
- Skin burns. This side effect may be reduced by the use of gel and the selection of the smallest possible quantities of energy for cardioversion of the arrhythmia.
- Rarely, after the successful cardioversion of atrial fibrillation or atrial flutter, acute pulmonary edema may occur. This is due to a transient atrial dysfunction (stunning) that is more apparent in the left than in the right atrium.

Management of the patient who comes to the Emergency Room reporting ICD shock(s)
Because of the increasing number of patients who have an ICD, is not unusual for a patient to come to the Emergency Room to report that their device has delivered one or more shocks. The management of patients with ICD shocks, whether **appropriate** (triggered by VF or very rapid VT) or **inappropriate** (triggered by supraventricular tachycardia, signal misinterpretation, or electromagnetic interference), depends mainly on their hemodynamic condition, on the number of shocks, and on the history of previous similar episodes. Specifically,

1) If the patient shows hemodynamic compromise because of recurrent arrhythmia that is also the cause of the shocks, the treatment should be according to the type of underlying arrhythmia and the patient should be admitted.

2) If the patient is in good general condition, without any concomitant palpitations (the ECG shows no sign of arrhythmias), dyspnea, or chest pain:
   - If the patient has received 1-2 ICD shocks within seconds or a few minutes admission is usually not required, provided that electrolyte disturbances have been ruled out (check potassium and magnesium levels) and there is the possibility of a check-up the next working day in the ICD clinic to determine if the shocks were appropriate or inappropriate (interrogation of the defibrillator). Even though this approach is recommended in an expert consensus document (Braunschweig F. Europace 2010;12:1673-90), in our own clinical practice these patients are usually admitted to the clinic. Another factor that also supports the admission of these patients is their extremely high stress level, especially if they have experienced no previous shocks in the past, which reduces the threshold for triggering arrhythmias. In these cases, benzodiazepines should be added to their medication.
   - If the patient has received >2 ICD shocks within minutes or hours, admission is always necessary so that, apart from interrogation of the defibrillator, electrolyte and metabolic disturbances should be ruled out, together with myocardial ischemia, and modification of the antiarrhythmic medication can be considered.

3) If the patient has received repetitive ICD shocks or the ICD is still delivering shocks in the absence of tachyarrhythmia (inappropriate) or due to tachyarrhythmia (VT, i.e. electrical storm* or supraventricular tachycardia) that is hemodynamically well tolerated, the shocks are temporarily stopped by placing a magnet over the ICD device. While shocks are being suppressed, the patient's ECG should be continuously monitored for the appearance of potentially life-threatening ventricular tachyarrhythmias. It should be noted that the magnet does not affect the function of the ICD's antibradycardic pacing. In such cases admission is always required.

---

* Electrical storm is defined as the occurrence of ≥3 episodes of sustained VT, VF, or appropriate ICD interventions (shocks or antitachycardia pacing) within 24 h.

Key points

- Electrical cardioversion should always be performed in an area where cardiopulmonary resuscitation is available.

- If the underlying rhythm is VF, shock delivery must be asynchronous because lack of identifiable QRS complexes prevents a defibrillator in the synchronous mode from discharging.

- During shock delivery it is necessary to ensure that the procedure is painless for the patient and safe for the operator and bystanders.

- Avoid cardioversion of atrial fibrillation or flutter of >48 h duration, unless anticoagulation medication has been administered for 3 weeks, or transesophageal echocardiography is performed to rule out thrombus in the left atrium.

- When cardioversion is performed in a patient with a permanent pacemaker or an ICD, these devices should be checked afterwards.

- The management of patients who come to the Emergency Room reporting ICD shock(s), whether appropriate or inappropriate, depends mainly on their hemodynamic condition and on the number of shocks. If the patient:
  - shows hemodynamic compromise, or has received >2 ICD shocks within minutes or hours, admission is required.
  - has received 1-2 shocks within seconds or a few minutes and is asymptomatic, admission is usually not required, provided that electrolyte disturbances have been ruled out and the ICD can be checked on the following working day.
  - has received repetitive ICD shocks or the ICD is still delivering shocks (appropriate or inappropriate) without any hemodynamic compromise, a magnet should be placed over the device to inhibit further shock delivery. Admission is always required.

22 Common cardiology procedures

1) Catheterization of the subclavian vein

The subclavian vein is one of the most frequently catheterized of the large veins. The advantages of using this vein are the easy access and good tolerance by patients. Vein puncture should be avoided when the patient has a hemorrhagic disposition (e.g. platelets <50,000/mm^3 or an international normalized ratio [INR] >2.0), because it is not feasible to apply direct pressure to achieve good hemostasis if the subclavian artery is punctured by mistake. Other contraindications include the presence of infection over the puncture site and a distorted local anatomy (i.e. prior surgery, fracture of the ipsilateral clavicle). Table 22.1 shows the indications for subclavian vein catheterization.

Nowadays, the vascular access, i.e. the catheterization of subclavian or internal jugular vein, may be assisted by ultrasound guidance. This is particularly useful in high risk situations (e.g. critically ill patients with coagulopathy).

TABLE 22.1	Indications for subclavian vein catheterization

1) Administration of drugs that would irritate smaller vessels (e.g. prolonged administration of amiodarone to avoid superficial thrombophlebitis) or drugs whose extravasation needs to be minimized (e.g. dopamine).

2) Placement of a Swan–Ganz catheter for hemodynamic monitoring.

3) Placement of a temporary pacing electrode.

4) Inability to locate a peripheral vein for IV administration of fluids or drugs.

5) Simultaneous administration of multiple drugs where mixing in their administration line is not permitted. This can be achieved using triple lumen catheters.

Anatomical data

The subclavian vein runs below the middle third of the clavicle and above the first rib, meeting the internal jugular vein near the manubrium of the sternum to form the brachiocephalic or innominate vein. The subclavian artery runs slightly higher and deeper than the vein.

Technique (infraclavicular approach)

Once the landmarks have been located, puncturing is carried out using Seldinger's* technique. More specifically:

- The medical procedure is explained to the patient.
- The patient is placed in the Trendelenburg position with an inclination of 15-30° to ensure filling of the veins of the neck and reduce the risk of air embolism. Be aware that placing a rolled towel between the patient's shoulders or excessive turning of the head away from the catheterization side decreases the size of the vein. Puncture of the right subclavian vein is preferred, in order to avoid the very small risk of puncturing the thoracic duct, which drains into the left subclavian vein, near its junction with the left internal jugular vein.
- The region below the clavicle is cleaned with antiseptic solution and local anesthesia is applied. The area is usually infiltrated with 5-10 mL of 1% or 2% lidocaine solution, using a 10-mL syringe and a 21-gauge needle**. The needle is introduced 1 cm below the clavicle, at the boundary between its middle and medial third, and the region below the clavicle is infiltrated in the direction of the puncture that will ensue. Aspiration should always precede the infusion so as to avoid direct administration of the anesthetic into the circulation.

Warning! When lidocaine solution is used as local anesthetic for "cardiological" medical procedures, lidocaine solution containing adrenaline should be avoided (commonly used for dental procedures to reduce bleeding).

- To determine the landmarks for puncture, the physician's left index finger is placed in the suprasternal notch, with the thumb over the middle third of the clavicle (Figure 22.1). The introducer needle (usually

---

*Seldinger's technique includes: puncture of the vessel with the introducer needle → introduction of the flexible guidewire (J wire) through the needle → removal of the needle → "dilation" by introducing the dilator → removal of the dilator and introduction of the catheter (or sheath) over the guidewire → removal of the guidewire, leaving the catheter.

**Inner diameter of needle ~0.51 mm

Figure 22.1. Landmarks for puncturing the subclavian vein. The left index finger is placed in the suprasternal notch and the thumb over the middle third of the clavicle. The needle is introduced 1 cm below the clavicle at the junction between its middle and medial third and is moved horizontally towards the suprasternal notch. (From Current Emergency Diagnosis and Treatment by Mills T, Ho MT, Trunkey DD, edition 1983, p 686, with permission).

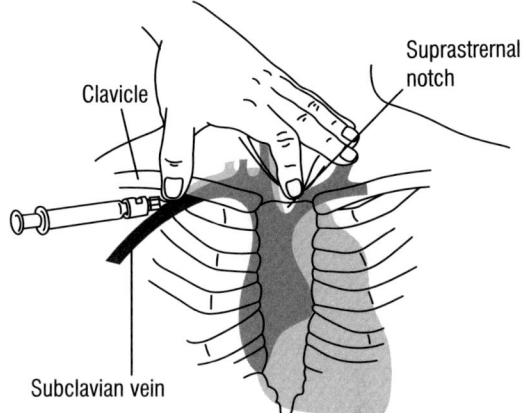

18-gauge*) is inserted 1 cm below the clavicle, at the border between its middle and medial third, and advanced horizontally in the direction of the suprasternal notch. The needle is advanced slowly, with constant negative pressure in the syringe, until venous blood is aspirated (usually at a depth of 3-4 cm). If resistance is encountered or air bubbles appear within the syringe, it should be withdrawn.

Warning! It is very important that the introducer needle follow a horizontal course, with no large changes in direction, so as to avoid damage to the subclavian artery or the pleura.

- Once the vein has been punctured, the syringe is removed from the needle and the J-tipped end of the flexible guidewire (J-wire) is introduced through the needle's lumen and advanced to a depth greater than the length of the needle (usually a depth of 20 cm). If resistance is encountered, the guidewire should be fully withdrawn, blood should be aspirated from the needle in order to confirm its position within the vein, and a new attempt should be made to advance the wire through the needle. It may be necessary to alter the angle of the needle slightly in order to achieve entry of the guidewire into the vein.

Warning! When the syringe is removed, the hub of the introducer needle should immediately be covered with a finger to prevent air entering the bloodstream and causing embolism.

---

*Inner diameter of needle ~0.84 mm

- After the introduction of the guidewire, the needle is removed (the guidewire remains within the vein) and a 1-2 mm nick is made in the skin with a scalpel at the guidewire's entry point.
- The dilator* is then introduced over the guidewire and advanced using a twisting motion. The introduction of the dilator is essential to facilitate the entry of the catheter (usually 7-French [Fr]), which is softer and runs the risk of "crimping" if it is introduced without any prior dilation. Note that 1 Fr corresponds to a catheter with an external diameter of 0.33 mm. Removal of the dilator is followed by the introduction of the catheter over the guidewire. Before the catheter is introduced, its lumen is flushed with normal saline. The correct placement of the catheter is confirmed by the aspiration of venous blood. Of course, during introduction of the dilator or catheter the external tip of the guidewire must be held and kept visible. Note that a catheter with the fewest lumens required should be used because the risk of infection increases with the number of lumens.
- Finally after placement of the catheter, the guidewire is removed, the catheter is stabilized by suturing to the skin, and its lumen is flushed with normal saline to preserve the patency, so that it may be used according to the indications for placement.

If the first attempt fails, a second attempt may be made, provided that the introducer needle has been rinsed to restore the patency of its lumen. After 2 failed attempts, it is better to ask for assistance from a more experienced physician, or to perform the puncture on the other side, once a chest X-ray has ruled out pneumothorax.

Main complications

- Pneumothorax (1.5-3%). After catheterization of the subclavian vein a chest X-ray should be performed to rule out pneumothorax and at the same time to check the position of the catheter.
- Puncture of the subclavian artery (<1%). This is usually indicated by bright red blood spurting out—evidence that may, however, be absent under conditions of shock. When the subclavian artery is punctured, the needle must be removed immediately and hemostatic pressure applied, although as stated above this has little value.

---

*In some types of puncture device, the dilator is introduced together with the catheter as a single unit, and the dilator is then removed together with the guidewire, leaving just the catheter.

2) Catheterization of the internal jugular vein

The indications and contraindications for internal jugular vein puncture are the same as those for the subclavian vein. Since it is possible to apply direct local pressure to the internal jugular, a hemorrhagic disposition is only a relative contraindication.

Anatomical data

It is necessary to locate the triangle formed by the heads of the sternocleidomastoid muscle (forming the sides of the triangle) and the medial third of the clavicle (forming the base of the triangle). The insertion points of the heads of the sternocleidomastoid muscle are in the mastoid process, while the origin of the clavicular head is the medial third of the clavicle (upper surface) and that of the sternal head is the front of the upper part of the manubrium sterni. The internal jugular courses along the imaginary straight line that connects the mastoid process with the clavicle at the origin of the clavicular head (inner margin). Within the triangle of the sternocleidomastoid muscle, the internal jugular vein runs laterally (on the outside) and in front of the common carotid artery, and joins the subclavian vein to form the brachiocephalic vein (Figure 22.2).

Technique

Once the landmarks have been located, namely the sternocleidomastoid muscle triangle, puncturing is performed using Seldinger's technique. Before it is started, the procedure must be explained to the patient. There are various techniques of approach, such as the anterior, the posterior, etc. Below we describe the anterior way of access. More specifically:

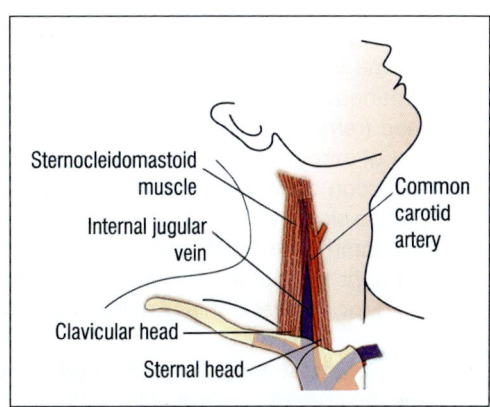

Figure 22.2. The course of the right internal jugular vein in the neck region within the sternocleidomastoid muscle triangle.

- The patient is placed in the Trendelenburg position with an inclination of 15-30°, with the head turned at a 45° angle away from the catheterization side (further turning should be avoided, because the vein becomes compressed and empties). Placing the patient in this position ensures filling of the veins of the neck and reduces the risk of air embolism. Usually, puncture of the right internal jugular vein is preferred, because the maneuvers are easier for right-handers and the possibility of thoracic duct injury is avoided. In addition, this vein has a direct course towards the superior vena cava and the right atrium, which facilitates the successful advancement of the catheter to the right atrium.

- Antiseptic is applied and local anesthetic is administered (usually 1% or 2% lidocaine solution) using a syringe with a 21-gauge needle (can be used as a **guiding needle** as described below). First, the common carotid artery is palpated with the fingers of the left hand (for right-handers) to locate its position and to avoid puncturing it. The entry of the needle is at the apex of the triangle formed by the sternocleidomastoid muscle, at an angle of 30° to the horizontal. Then, the skin and subcutaneous tissue are perfused, with the needle directed towards the ipsilateral nipple. Before the infusion of the drug, aspiration is always performed to avoid direct injection of the anesthetic into the circulation. Once the internal jugular vein has been punctured, the syringe is removed and the guiding needle is left in place so that the direction and depth of the subsequent puncture may be determined.

- The larger diameter **introducer needle** (18-gauge), through which the guidewire will be advanced, is inserted at an angle of 30° right beside the previous needle, which acts as a guide for safe puncture. The direction of its introduction is towards the ipsilateral nipple and the needle is advanced parallel to the guiding needle with continuous negative pressure applied to the syringe until venous blood is aspirated (usually at a depth of 2-4 cm).

- Once the vein has been punctured, the guiding needle is removed and the maneuvers described for subclavian vein catheterization are performed (removal of syringe, introduction of flexible guidewire (J-wire), removal of introducer needle, nick in the skin at the guidewire entry point, introduction of dilator, removal of dilator, insertion of catheter and suturing to the skin).

- If the common carotid artery is punctured by mistake (spurting blood with bright red color), the needle must be removed and local pressure applied for at least 5 min. Another vein should then be chosen for puncture.

- Finally, a chest X-ray is performed to rule out pneumothorax and to check the correct position of the catheter.

Main complications

The same as those reported for subclavian vein catheterization, but with different incidences. Pneumothorax occurs more rarely (0.1-0.2%), while puncture of the common carotid artery is more frequent (~3%). The incidence of catheter infection during internal jugular vein catheterization is 8-9 cases per 1000 catheter-days, compared to 4 cases for subclavian vein catheterization.

3) Placement of temporary pacemaker

The placement of a temporary pacemaker is a common medical procedure in emergency cardiological practice. Table 22.2 shows the indications for temporary pacing. We will refer to 2 types of temporary pacing: transvenous and transcutaneous. The latter is applied in emergency situations, usually as a bridge to transvenous pacing.

Warning! Before puncture we must confirm that the size of the sheath is the same size or at most one size larger than that of the temporary pacing electrode, which is usually 5 or 6 Fr. Consequently, the sheath should have a size of 5 or 6 Fr when a 5 Fr electrode is used, or a size of 6 or 7 Fr when a 6 Fr electrode is used.

A) Transvenous placement of temporary pacemaker

Technique

1) If the procedure is elective, peripheral intravenous access should be obtained before the start of catheterization to give drugs if necessary.
2) Usually, catheterization of the right internal jugular or the right subclavian vein is preferred. The choice of the right internal jugular vein has the advantage of providing a direct route for the electrode (lead) to the right atrium. When the subclavian vein is chosen, the right is preferred, so that if permanent pacing is subsequently needed the left subclavian vein will be free for the introduction of the pacing electrode. The catheterization is performed using Seldinger's technique under strictly aseptic conditions, and after infiltrating the skin and subcutaneous tissue with a 1% or 2% lidocaine solution. In the case of hemorrhagic disposition, e.g. because of previous fibrinolysis, the femoral venous access is preferred, bacause hemostasis can be achieved by applying direct pressure if there is hemorrhage at the puncture site. It is obvious that if the pacing wire is advanced via the femoral vein, this must always be done under fluoroscopic guidance.

TABLE 22.2	Indications for temporary transvenous pacing

A) Acute myocardial infarction (AMI)

  1) Symptomatic bradycardia (sinus bradycardia or Mobitz type I AV block not responsive to atropine)
  2) New bifascicular block (RBBB + LPH or RBBB + LPH) in anterior or lateral AMI
  3) Alternating RBBB and LBBB
  4) New LBBB + first degree AV block (alternatively, transcutaneous pacing pads can be applied for potential use)*
  5) Mobitz type II AV block or third-degree AV block in anterior or lateral AMI. In inferior AMI, transvenous pacing is rarely required (prophylactic placement of transcutaneous pacing pads is reasonable)

B) Without acute myocardial infarction:

  1) Symptomatic bradycardia, bradyarrhythmia, second- or third-degree AV block from causes (drugs or electrolyte disturbances) whose elimination will lead to restoration of rhythm, or as a bridge to permanent pacing
  2) Polymorphic ventricular tachycardia on a substrate of a long QT interval, if resulting from bradycardia or pauses
  3) Prophylactic perioperatively:
    – bifascicular block + syncope
    – asymptomatic trifascicular block (no consensus about this indication)
  4) Overdrive pacing for termination of persistent tachyarrhythmia, e.g. typical atrial flutter
  5) In patients undergoing:
    – cardioversion in the setting of sick sinus syndrome
    – right heart catheterization ± myocardial biopsy in the setting of LBBB
    – alcohol septal ablation for hypertrophic cardiomyopathy

*The choice of pacing system (transvenous versus transcutaneous) varies across centers (O'Gara PT, et al. Circulation 2013;123:e362-e425).
AV: atrioventricular; RBBB: right bundle branch block; LBBB: left bundle branch block; LAH: left anterior hemiblock; LPH: left posterior hemiblock.

3) The patient is connected to a continuous ECG monitoring device and e-quipment for cardiopulmonary resuscitation should be at hand.

4a) If fluoroscopy is not available, a balloon-tipped bipolar pacing electrode (flow-directed) is used. In this case access is through the subclavian or internal jugular vein. Before the introduction of the pacing electrode, we check whether the balloon inflates (with 1-1.5 mL of air) and deflates quickly. Then, the pacing electrode is advanced through the lumen of the sheath. When it is judged that the tip of the electrode has emerged from the sheath the balloon is inflated and the electrode is advanced to the right atrium and subsequently through the tricuspid valve to the apex of the right ventricle. It usually needs to be advanced ~35-40 cm from the puncture point. During entry to the right ventricle, ventricular extrasystoles are usually observed. When the electrode is judged to be in the desired position (right ventricular apex; Figure 22.3), the balloon is deflated, and the two poles (external ends) of the pacing electrode are connected to the pacemaker device as follows (sometimes crocodile clips are used): the **pacemaker's anode (+) [red] is connected to the proximal pole** and the **pacemaker's cathode (-) [black] to the distal pole** of the pacing electrode, respectively. If the poles are inadvertently reversed, the pacing threshold will be significantly higher. The criterion for the correct placement of the electrode is the recording on the ECG of pacing complexes that show left bundle branch block (LBBB) with left-axis deviation.

4b) If puncture of the femoral vein is preferred (lies medial to the femoral artery), fluoroscopic monitoring must be available. Once the sheath is placed in the femoral vein (Seldinger's technique), the pacing electrode is introduced via the sheath and advanced, aiming towards the right atrium (the fluoroscopy is performed in the anteroposterior position). If the

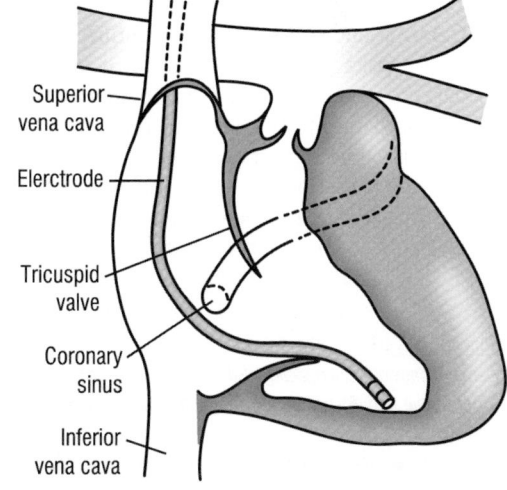

Figure 22.3. Correct position of the electrode in the right ventricular apex during temporary ventricular pacing. (From Acute Medicine: A Practical Guide to the Management of Medical Emergencies by Sprigings DC, Chambers JB, 3rd edition, 2001, Wiley-Blackwell, Figure 55.3a, with permission).

Superior vena cava

Elerctrode

Tricuspid valve

Coronary sinus

Inferior vena cava

electrode deviates to the left a little before the level of the diaphragm, it has most likely entered the hepatic vein, in which case it should be withdrawn and advanced again with its tip turned towards the right. During entry to the right atrium, the right lateral fluoroscopic view is preferred. If difficulty is encountered in passing through the tricuspid valve, the electrode is formed into a loop within the right atrium and is then turned towards the interatrial septum and advanced, after which it usually protrudes through the tricuspid valve. After emerging from the tricuspid valve it is advanced towards the right ventricular apex and then connected with the pacemaker device.

Warning! After the pacing electrode has entered the heart, it is advanced using gentle motions in order to minimize the risk of injuring or perforating the myocardium. This risk is greater with these electrodes, since they are more inflexible than the balloon-tipped pacing electrodes. If resistance is encountered, the electrode is withdrawn and a new attempt is made to advance it.

5) Pacing: the pacemaker (pulse generator) is switched on and the pacing indicator is set to the "demand*" position, initially selecting a rate ~20 beats/min faster than the patient's intrinsic rate, or a rate of 70-80 beats/min in the case of extreme bradycardia. The pacing output is set at 3 V. If there is no pacing rhythm (capture**), a better pacing site is sought. Each time the balloon-tipped pacing electrode is withdrawn we ensure that the balloon is deflated, while each time it is advanced it is inflated.

6) Determination of **pacing threshold:** to find the pacing threshold the stimulus voltage is reduced progressively until pacing stops (absence of capture, meaning that the pacing spikes are not followed by ventricular depolarization). The voltage reading at this point is the threshold (i.e. the lowest voltage that achieves pacing). An acceptable threshold is <1 V. If the threshold is higher, an attempt is made to improve it by changing the site of the electrode. Generally, a larger threshold can be acceptable in the case of a large myocardial infarction (acute or old), or

---

*Demand pacing means pacing at the selected rate (e.g. 60 beats/min) unless the patient's intrinsic rate exceeds that (e.g. 65 beats/min), in which case the pacemaker "senses" the patient's intrinsic rhythm and is inhibited.

*"Capture means that the pacing spike stimulates the ventricle and is followed by a wide QRS complex and T wave.

when the patient is taking antiarrhythmic medication (e.g. amiodarone). The output voltage is then adjusted to 3 V, or 3 x the threshold if it is >1 V. This is essential, as the threshold will increase over the following days because of the local inflammatory reaction.

7) Check of **sensing threshold:** to check the pacemaker sensing threshold, namely the lowest intraventricular potential that is sensed, the pacing rate is set lower than the intrinsic rate so that the patient's native rhythm takes over. The sensitivity of the external pacing system is then gradually increased (e.g. 1→ 2→ 3 mV → ...), so that the pacemaker becomes less sensitive in the detection of intraventricular potentials. The sensitivity setting at the point where pacing beats appear is the sensing threshold and the pacemaker is usually set at one-half the sensing threshold. This means that the pacemaker is only sensing impulses that generates potentials above the sensing threshold.

8) Check of electrode stability: the patient is asked to cough heavily and the ECG is monitored for any failure of capture. In the case of capture failure a better electrode site is sought.

9) Adjustment of pacing rate: in atrioventricular block or bradycardia the pacing rate is set to 70-80 beats/min, whereas in cardiogenic shock it is set to 90-100 beats/min.

10) The pacing lead is then sutured to the skin near to the entry point and the rest of the lead is stabilized on the skin using adhesive tape. It is very important to ensure a stable connection between the external ends of the electrode and the pacemaker device.

Warning! Deaths have been reported as a consequence of disconnection of the external ends (poles) of the pacing electrode from the pacemaker.

11) A chest X-ray is always performed to confirm the position of the electrode (the tip should be directed towards the right ventricular apex, if it is directed leftwards and upwards it is probably within the coronary sinus) and to rule out pneumothorax in the case of subclavian or internal jugular vein puncture. In addition, a complete ECG recording is made (if the electrode is placed correctly and there is pacing rhythm, this shows LBBB with left-axis deviation) and the pacing threshold is checked daily. Finally, the patient's intrinsic rhythm should be checked on a daily basis, by gradually reducing the pacing rate until pacing does not occur.

Complications
1) Myocardial perforation. The risk of perforation is greater in the case of a-

cute right ventricular infarction. Perforation should be suspected if there is:
- Pain of pericardial type.
- Signs of cardiac tamponade (rare manifestation).
- Capture failure.

In these cases an emergency echocardiographic examination should be performed to confirm the diagnosis.

2) Pneumothorax. This is a rare complication arising from puncture of the subclavian or internal jugular vein.

3) Infection. This is usually due to contamination of the puncture site by *Staphylococcus epidermidis* or *Staphylococcus aureus*. The risk of infection is greater for femoral vein puncture than for the other veins (femoral > internal jugular > subclavian vein).

B) Transcutaneous (external) temporary pacing

This type of pacing may prove life-saving for the patient when there is an immediate need for pacing. It functions as a bridge to the placement of a temporary pacemaker. The advantages of transcutaneous pacing are its very rapid, easy (minimal training), and noninvasive method of use.

Technique

The external transcutaneous pacing device has two large self-adhesive electrodes. Most pacing devices also have the capability of defibrillation through the same electrodes. Before attaching the electrodes, it is necessary to ensure the skin is dry. The electrodes are usually attached one below the right clavicle and the other on the outside of the left nipple (Figure 22.4). Alternatively, anteroposterior placement is possible. Then, demand pacing and the pacing rate are selected. Note that the duration of the pacing stimulus is long (20-40 ms). The strength of the stimulus is then increased progressively, under ECG monitoring, until capture is achieved (usually at 50-100 mA), i.e. the pacing stimulus (spike) is followed by a wide QRS complex and a T wave. If the QRS complex after the pacing stimulus is not followed by a T wave, then the recorded waveform does not represent ventricular depolarization. In addition, palpation of the pulse is a clinical criterion to confirm the presence of effective cardiac contraction.

The main disadvantage of this technique is that it is painful, because it causes strong contraction of the skeletal muscles; for this reason, analgesia or sedation (e.g. midazolam IV) of the conscious patient is required. Finally, if despite the increasing strength of the delivered stimulus there is no palpable pulse or capture on the ECG, then this means that there is no viable myocardium.

Figure 22.4. Placement of electrodes for transcutaneous pacing in the anterolateral pacing position.

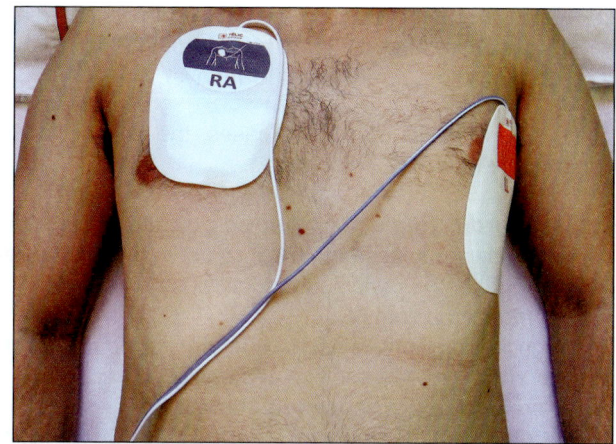

4) Pericardiocentesis

Pericardiocentesis is usually performed to improve the hemodynamics of patients who exhibit cardiac tamponade. At the same time, it will contribute to the identification of the cause of pericardial fluid accumulation, if unknown, through examination of the fluid itself.

Relative contraindications

- Platelet count <50,000/mm^3.
- Use of vitamin K antagonists with INR >1.8. If the pericardiocentesis is emergent, rapid INR reduction can be achieved with the administration of four-factor prothrombin complex concentrate (Beriplex, Kcentra) [reconstituted solution from a lyophilized powder] prior to the procedure.
- Typically, hemopericardium secondary to type A acute aortic dissection is treated with emergent surgery (pericardiocentesis may lead to exsanguination). However, in situations where circulatory collapse is imminent and the patient cannot survive until surgery, small volume pericardiocentesis (usually 20-40 mL) should be considered as a means of temporarily stabilizing patients before surgery (maintain systolic blood pressure at ~90 mmHg).

Techniques

There are three pericardiocentesis techniques:

- Echocardiographically guided at the patient's bedside (usually performed in the coronary care unit).
- Fluoroscopically guided (usually performed in the cardiac catheteriza-

tion laboratory). In this case a portable echocardiograph may be of assistance in determining the best route for pericardiocentesis.
- ECG-guided (rarely used nowadays).

Of course, in all the above cases, the pericardiocentesis is performed under continuous ECG monitoring.

A) Echocardiographically guided pericardiocentesis
1) The patient is placed at 30-45° to draw the pericardial fluid inferiorly.
2) If the patient is conscious, a low dose of sedation is administered (e.g. 2-3 mg midazolam IV).
3) Echocardiography is used to determine the region of the pericardial sac that shows the largest fluid accumulation and is also easily accessible. It is preferable to choose the shortest route that the pericardiocentesis needle needs to cover in order to enter the pericardial sac. The three usual locations of pericardiocentesis are the apical (sixth or seventh left intercostal space, on the anterior axillary line), the paraxiphoid subcostal (to the left of the xiphoid process and below the left costal margin) and the parasternal (fifth left intercostal space, just lateral to the sternum). More specifically, the site chosen for pericardiocentesis should ideally contain a significant quantity of fluid, so the distance between the two pericardial laminae at this point during diastole should be ≥20 mm. It is also of great importance for the doctor performing the pericardiocentesis to remember the orientation of the ultrasound beam during the determination of the best route, so that it can be followed during the pericardiocentesis procedure. If the pericardiocentesis is performed at an intercostal space, the upper surface of the lower rib should be preferred, so as to avoid damage to the intercostal artery, which runs along the lower surface of the upper rib.
4) Under strictly sterile conditions, and after the induction of local anesthesia with a 1% or 2% lidocaine solution, a long pericardiocentesis needle (15 cm long and 18-gauge in diameter) is introduced along the same line as the ultrasound beam that indicated the shortest route. This needle is connected to a 10 mL syringe containing a lidocaine solution. The needle is advanced slowly, with periodic infusion of small quantities of local anesthetic, while continuous aspiration is performed at the same time. When the needle enters the pericardial sac (usually at a distance of 6-8 cm, indicated by the aspiration of serous, serosanguineous, or sanguineous fluid), the syringe is removed from the needle and the flexible guidewire is introduced through the needle's lumen and advanced.
5) When there is doubt as to the position of the needle, before the guidewire is introduced, an injection of agitated normal saline is per-

formed and the bubbles are detected echocardiographically; alternatively, a contrast agent may be injected. If the bubbles or contrast agent appear inside the pericardial sac, this confirms the correct position of the needle, whereas if they appear within the cardiac cavities it is an indication of penetration of the cardiac wall and the needle must be withdrawn immediately.

6) When the fluid aspirated is hemorrhagic, it is necessary to rule out the possibility of hemopericardium from injury to a coronary artery, or the possibility of the needle entering one of the cardiac cavities. This is done by placing a small quantity of hemorrhagic fluid in a test-tube without anticoagulants. If the fluid clots, then it comes from the cardiac cavities or there has been damage to a coronary artery resulting in hemopericardium. If the fluid is sanguineous in the context of pericardial accumulation – e.g. idiopathic pericarditis, which is often accompanied by sanguineous fluid – then it does not clot. If doubts still remain, then a sample of the aspirated fluid can be sent for emergency hematocrit determination and comparison with the hematocrit of a venous sample from the patient.

7) After the introduction of the guidewire, the needle is removed, leaving the guidewire in place, and a nick is made with a scalpel in the skin at the entry point of the guidewire.

8) If the dilator is independent of the sheath (i.e. it is not combined with the sheath in a single unit, in which case it is removed together with the wire) it is advanced over the wire in order to create nominal conditions for the introduction of the sheath.

9) The dilator is removed and the sheath is advanced over the wire.

10) Using the sheath as an entry port, a pigtail catheter* is introduced and fluid is withdrawn. Immediate clinical improvement may be observed after the removal of as little as 50-100 mL of fluid. It is prudent to avoid the immediate removal of >1 liter of fluid, since there is a risk of acute dilation of the right ventricle. Samples of the fluid aspirated are sent for testing according to the clinical suspicion (Table 22.3).

11) The catheter usually remains open for 6-12 h to continue gravity drainage of the pericardial fluid. Subsequently it is heparinized, closed, and aspiration of any newly accumulating fluid is performed every 6-12 h. The catheter is left in place until fluid drainage is <25 mL/day. It has been shown that extended (for several days) pericardial catheter drainage is associated with reduced recurrence rates of the effusion.

---

*A catheter with multiple holes on the sides of its circular distal tip

12) After the pericardiocentesis, a chest X-ray must be performed to rule out pneumothorax.

B) Fluoroscopically guided pericardiocentesis

The subxiphoid approach is preferred (Figure 22.5), since the risk of puncturing the pleura, the coronary arteries, or the internal mammary arteries is very small. The patient's head and chest are placed in a 30-45° reclining position so that the fluid will accumulate in the lower part of the heart. The pericardiocentesis needle is inserted at the angle formed by the xiphoid process and the left costal margin, inclined at an angle of ~30° to the patient's abdominal surface, and is advanced in the direction of the left shoulder under fluoroscopic control. The correct position of the needle may be checked by injection of contrast agent. The remaining maneuvers are the same as those in echocardiographically guided pericardiocentesis.

The subxiphoid approach is usually preferred in emergency cases where pericardiocentesis must be performed "blind".

C) ECG guided pericardiocentesis

Here again the subxiphoid access route is usually preferred. The pericardiocentesis needle is connected with crocodile clips to lead V_1 of the ECG. The maneuvers used are similar to those in the techniques described above. When ST-segment elevation or ventricular extrasystoles are recorded on the ECG, this indicates puncture of the right ventricular wall, while de-

TABLE 22.3	Tests performed on pericardial fluid samples

1) Biochemical tests: specific gravity*, glucose, protein, lactate dehydrogenase (LDH), cholesterol (elevated in severe hypothyroidism).

2) Microscopic examination for cell count and differential.

3) Carcinoembryonic antigen and cytology for neoplastic cells (if malignancy is suspected).

4) Cultures for aerobic and anaerobic bacteria (if bacterial infection is suspected).

5) Ziehl–Nielsen stain for *Mycobacterium tuberculosis* (if tuberculosis is suspected).

6) Adenosine deaminase (ADA) [high levels suggest tubercular pericarditis] and polymerase chain reaction (PCR) for detection of mycobacterial DNA (if tuberculosis is suspected).

The following are indicative of exudate: specific gravity >1.015, protein >3.0 g/dL, pericardial fluid protein/serum protein >0.5, serum albumin - pericardial fluid albumin <1.2 g/dL, LDH >200 IU/L, pericardial fluid LDH/serum LDH >0.6.

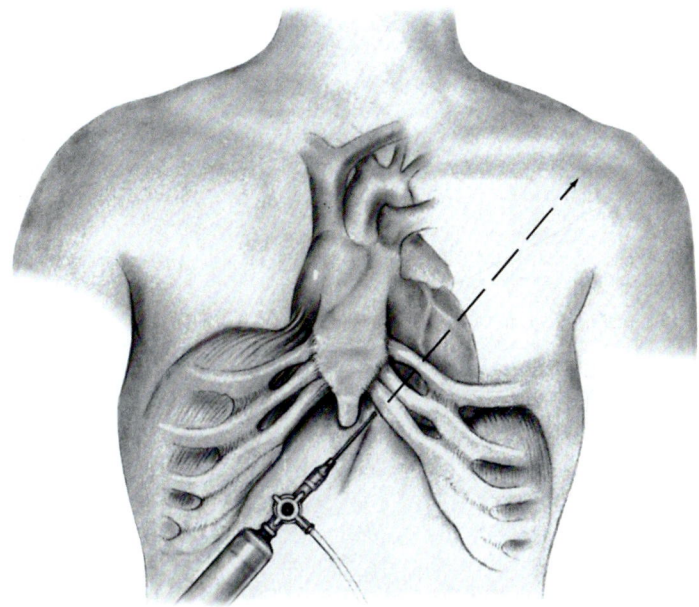

Figure 22.5. Position and direction of pericardiocentesis using the subxiphoid (more precisely, paraxiphoid subcostal) approach. The pericardiocentesis needle is inserted ~1 cm to the left of the xiphoid process and ~1 cm below the left costal margin, at an angle of ~30° to the patient's abdominal surface, and is advanced towards the left shoulder. (From Intensive Care Medicine by Rippe JM, Irwin RS, Alpert JS, Fink MP, 2nd edition, 1991, Little, Brown and Company, p 290, with permission).

pression of the PR interval and supraventricular extrasystoles are indicative of puncture of the right atrium. Obviously, in both these cases the pericardiocentesis needle must be withdrawn.

Complications

The main complications (<5%) that may be observed during pericardiocentesis are a vasovagal reaction, arrhythmias, puncture or perforation of the right ventricular wall, coronary artery injury, pneumothorax, liver injury, and infection. Echocardiographic guidance is considered to be the safest technique for pericardiocentesis.

23
Most common intravenous drugs in emergency cardiology

1) Nitroglycerin

Mechanism of action

Nitroglycerin is an exogenous source of nitric oxide (NO), which activates guanylate cyclase to produce cyclic guanosine monophosphate (cGMP). cGMP causes relaxation of the vascular smooth muscle cells, hence vasodilation of the veins and, to a lesser degree, of the arteries (including the coronaries, particularly the large epicardial and arterioles with >100 μm diameter). Venous vasodilation reduces preload and left ventricular diastolic wall stress, resulting in decreased oxygen demand, while arterial vasodilation reduces afterload and left ventricular systolic wall stress, also leading to reduced oxygen demand. In addition, coronary artery vasodilation increases oxygen supply to the heart. When nitroglycerin is administered IV, its effect begins within 2-5 min and its plasma half-life is ~3 min.

Indications
- Non ST-segment elevation acute coronary syndrome for pain relief. It is also beneficial in patients with heart failure or hypertension.
- ST-segment elevation myocardial infarction (STEMI) in patients with heart failure or hypertension. Note that the routine use is not recommended.
- Acute pulmonary edema (cardiogenic).
- Coronary artery spasm.
- Perioperative hypertension.

319

Contraindications

- Inferior STEMI with right ventricular involvement (risk of precipitous drop in blood pressure [BP] because of reduced preload).
- Hypotension (systolic BP <90 mmHg) and hypovolemia.
- Use of selective phosphodiesterase type 5 inhibitors during the preceding 24 h in the case of sildenafil (Viagra or Revatio) or vardenafil (Levitra), or the preceding 48 h for tadalafil (Cialis). There is a risk of precipitous drop in BP is such cases.
- Hypertrophic obstructive cardiomyopathy and severe valve stenosis.
- Constrictive pericarditis.
- Increased intracranial pressure.

Precautions

- Discontinue administration if the systolic BP falls to <90 mmHg or the diastolic BP falls to <60 mmHg. When the systolic BP rises again to >90 mmHg, nitroglycerin is restarted at low dosage.
- When a case of STEMI is under hemodynamic monitoring, the pulmonary capillary wedge pressure must be maintained between 15 and 18 mmHg.
- The drug must be discontinued gradually.
- After prolonged administration (>48 h), tolerance may develop (weakening or loss of effect).
- In rare cases of prolonged administration at high dosages, cyanosis may develop due to increased methemoglobin levels (cyanosis despite normal partial pressure of oxygen [PO_2] in arterial blood gases).

Adverse effects

Hypotension, headaches, facial flushing and tachycardia.

Dosage

Begin administration at 5-10 µg/min and increase by 5-10 µg/min every 5-10 min until the therapeutic goal is achieved or the maximum dose of 200 µg/min is reached. The average dosage for most patients is ~25 µg/min.

Solution preparation and administration

Usually, 25 mg of nitroglycerin (Nitro-Bid, Tridil) are added to 250 mL of 5% D/W*. The resulting solution has a concentration of 0.1 mg/mL or 100

Generally, before adding a drug that comes in the form of an ampoule or vial and has a volume >10 mL (e.g. 20 mL) to a glucose or NaCl solution, an equal amount of solution (e.g. 20 mL) is removed, so that the final volume will remain unchanged.

µg/mL. Infusion begins at a rate of 3-6 mL/h (5-10 µg/min), which is increased by 3-6 mL/h (5-10 µg/min) every 5-10 min, depending on the patient's response. The maximum dosage is 120 mL/h (200 µg/min) and the average dosage is ~15 mL/h (25 µg/min).

Table 23.1 shows the method of administration of a nitroglycerin solution.

2) Sodium nitroprusside

Mechanism of action

Nitroprusside causes an immediate (within a few seconds) drop in BP,

TABLE 23.1	Administration of 250 mL of a 100 µg/mL nitroglycerin solution (25 mg of nitroglycerin in 250 mL of 5% D/W)	
Dose (µg/min)		**Infusion rate (mL/h)***
5		3
10		6
15		9
20		12
25		15
30		18
35		21
40		24
45		27
50		30
60		36
70		42
80		48
90		54
100		60
120		72
140		84
160		96
180		108
200		120

*mL/h = microdrops/min, where 1 mL = 60 microdrops.

by causing arterial and venous vasodilation (with equivalent effect on both arteries and veins), through the active metabolite NO. The drop in BP is accompanied by reflex tachycardia. Its hypotensive effect is lost 2-3 min after the infusion is stopped; this must be done gradually because of the risk of rebound hypertension when it is administered for a hypertensive crisis.

Indications
- Hypertensive crisis not responding to other, "easier" intravenous antihypertensives (e.g. nitroglycerin).
- Acute aortic dissection, in which case nitroprusside must be coadministered with beta-blockers if systolic BP remains >120 mmHg despite the initial administration of beta-blockers.
- Severe acute heart failure or cardiogenic shock, particularly when caused by acute mitral or aortic valve regurgitation (to increase cardiac output).

Contraindications
- Systolic BP <90 mmHg or diastolic BP <60 mmHg.
- Liver or kidney failure, because of the poor elimination of toxic nitroprusside metabolites (cyanides in the case of liver failure and thiocyanates in the case of kidney failure).
- Hypertrophic obstructive cardiomyopathy and severe valve stenosis.
- Hypothyroidism and malnutrition.
- Elevated intracranial pressure.
- Pregnancy.

Precautions
- During administration, the patient must be monitored closely (an electronic infusion device for accurate dosing and an arterial line for BP monitoring should be used).
- Avoid administration at maximum dosage (10 μg/kg/min) for >10 min (even if BP has not been adequately controlled) because of the risk of cyanide toxicity.

Warning! Because nitroprusside solutions are sensitive to light, the infusion device must be wrapped in aluminum foil or the solutions must be administered using a special, opaque device.

- The prepared solution, when adequately protected from light, is stable for 24 h.

Adverse effects

- Headache, nausea, eructations and abdominal pain.
- Cyanide toxicity: this occurs when high doses (>7 µg/kg/min) are administered for long periods of time (>48 h) or in cases of liver failure, due to the accumulation of cyanides (products of nitroprusside metabolism); these are toxic and cause lactic acidosis by inhibiting the cells' oxidative metabolism. In the liver, cyanides are converted to thiocyanates that are excreted by the kidneys. Cyanide toxicity is manifested by confusion, convulsions and abdominal pain. Lactic acidosis is an early finding in laboratory examinations. Antidotes to cyanide toxicity are:
  - sodium nitrite (10 mL of 3% solution within 3-5 min IV) and
  - sodium thiosulfate (12.5 g in 50 mL of 5% D/W over 10 min IV).
- Thiocyanate toxicity (toxic levels [>100 µg/mL] of thiocyanates in the blood): usually occurs in cases of kidney failure and manifests as nausea and mental disorders. Hemodialysis eliminates thiocyanates from the blood.

Dosage

The infusion begins with 0.25 µg/kg/min and gradually increases every 5 min by 0.2 µg/kg/min, depending on the therapeutic effect. The average dose is ~3 µg/kg/min (range: 0.25-10 µg/kg/min).

Solution preparation and administration

Usually, 50 mg of nitroprusside (Nitropress, Niptide) are added to 100 mL of 5% D/W to produce a 500 µg/mL solution. For a person weighing 70 kg, infusion begins at 2 mL/h (~0.25 µg/kg/min) and the dosage is then increased every 5 min by approximately 2 mL/h until a therapeutic effect is achieved. The average dose is ~25 mL/h (3 µg/kg/min). Table 23.2 gives the dosage per body weight in more detail.

3) Dobutamine

Mechanism of action

Dobutamine is a synthetic catecholamine that stimulates β_1 and, to a lesser degree, β_2 and α-receptors ($\beta_1 > \beta_2 > α$). Its inotropic effect is stronger that its chronotropic effect. This is due primarily to the combined stimulation of β_1 and α-receptors, since both of these have an inotropic effect, whereas only β_1-receptors have a chronotropic effect. Its relatively neutral effect on the BP is probably explained by the fact that the systemic vasoconstriction caused by α-receptor activation counteracts the vasodilator effect caused by β_2 stimulation. In cases of heart failure, it increases cardiac output and

Most common intravenous drugs in emergency cardiology

TABLE 23.2	Administration of 100 mL of a 500 µg/mL sodium nitroprusside solution (50 mg of nitroprusside in 100 mL of 5% D/W)										
Weight (kg)	50	55	60	65	70	75	80	85	90	95	100
(µg/kg/min)					Infusion rate (mL/h)						
0.25	1.5	1.6	1.8	2	2.1	2.2	2.4	2.5	2.7	2.8	3
0.5	3	3	4	4	4	4	5	5	5	6	6
1	6	7	7	8	8	9	10	10	11	11	12
1.5	9	10	11	12	13	13	14	15	16	17	18
2	12	13	14	16	17	18	19	20	22	23	24
2.5	15	16	18	19	21	22	24	25	27	28	30
3	18	20	22	23	25	27	29	31	32	34	36
3.5	21	23	25	27	29	31	34	36	38	40	42
4	24	26	29	31	34	36	38	41	43	46	48
4.5	27	30	32	35	38	40	43	46	49	51	54
5	30	33	36	39	42	45	48	51	54	57	60
5.5	33	36	40	43	46	49	53	56	59	63	66
6	36	40	43	47	50	54	58	61	65	68	72
6.5	39	43	47	51	55	58	62	66	70	74	78
7	42	46	50	55	59	63	67	71	76	80	84
7.5	45	49	54	58	63	67	72	76	81	85	90
8	48	53	58	62	67	72	77	82	86	91	96
10	60	66	72	78	84	90	96	102	108	114	120

For reasons of practicality, decimals have been rounded to the nearest integer, except for the infusion rate at the initial dose of 0.25 µg/kg/min where the decimal places are retained.

decreases systemic resistance and left ventricular filling pressure. When administered at a dose <20 µg/kg/min, the increase in cardiac output is not accompanied by any significant increase in heart rate. It has a half-life of ~2 min.

Indications
- Acute or decompensated chronic heart failure, not responding to vasodilators and diuretics, provided the systolic BP is >80 mmHg.

> **Warning!** If the systolic BP is <80 mmHg, dobutamine must be coadministered with dopamine at vasoconstriction doses.

- Cardiogenic shock (the same limitations with regard to BP apply).
- Beta-blocker overdose.

Contraindications
Hypertrophic obstructive cardiomyopathy, severe aortic valve stenosis, pheochromocytoma and hypersensitivity to dobutamine.

Precautions
- The prepared solution must be used within 24 h.
- Any hypovolemia must be corrected before administration.
- Administration must be stopped gradually.
- Serum potassium levels must be checked because hypokalemia might develop (β_2-receptor stimulation).

Adverse effects
At high doses (>20 µg/kg/min), tachycardia and arrhythmogenesis (to a lesser degree than dopamine).

Dosage
Between 2.5 and 10 µg/kg/min, or as high as 40 µg/kg/min in rare cases. The dose to be taken by an individual patient depends on the response (improvement in cardiac output). The average dose is usually ~5 µg/kg/min. However, a general rule when administering inotropic drugs, in order to minimize their side effects, is to prescribe the lowest possible dosage and for the shortest possible time in order to achieve the desired result.

Solution preparation and administration
Usually, 250 mg of dobutamine (Dobutrex, Dobutamine Hydrochloride) are added to 250 mL of 5% D/W to produce a 1000 µg/mL solution. For a person weighing 70 kg, the average dose is 5 µg/kg/min, which corresponds to an infusion rate of 21 mL/h for such a solution. Table 23.3 gives the dobutamine dosage per body weight in more detail.

4) Dopamine

Mechanism of action
Dopamine is a precursor of noradrenaline. It has a half-life of ~2 min. It stimulates:

TABLE 23.3	Administration of 250 mL of a 1000 µg/mL dobutamine solution (250 mg of dobutamine in 250 mL of 5% D/W)										
Weight (kg)	50	55	60	65	70	75	80	85	90	95	100
(µg/kg/min)	Infusion rate (mL/h)										
1	3	3	4	4	4	4	5	5	5	6	6
1.5	4	5	5	6	6	7	7	8	8	9	9
2	6	7	7	8	8	9	9	10	11	11	12
2.5	7	8	9	10	10	11	12	13	13	14	15
3	9	10	11	12	13	13	14	15	16	17	18
3.5	10	12	13	14	15	16	17	18	19	20	21
4	12	13	14	16	17	18	19	20	22	23	24
4.5	13	15	16	18	19	20	22	23	24	26	27
5	15	16	18	19	21	22	24	25	27	28	30
6	18	20	22	23	25	27	29	31	32	34	36
7	21	23	25	27	29	31	34	36	38	40	42
8	24	26	29	31	34	36	38	41	43	46	48
9	27	30	32	35	38	40	43	46	49	51	54
10	30	33	36	39	42	45	48	51	54	57	60
12	36	40	43	47	50	54	58	61	65	68	72
15	45	49	54	58	63	67	72	77	81	85	90
20	60	66	72	78	84	90	96	102	108	114	120

For reasons of practicality, decimals have been rounded to the nearest integer.

- D_1 dopaminergic receptors, causing vasodilation in the coronary, visceral and renal vasculature (improved renal perfusion and increased diuresis).
- D_2 dopaminergic receptors, preventing the release of noradrenaline and causing systemic vasodilation.
- β_1 and β_2-receptors, causing primarily increased cardiac output.
- α-receptors (at high doses), causing vasoconstriction.

Indications
- At renal doses (<3 µg/kg/min) to improve diuresis in oliguric patients with low cardiac output who do not respond to diuretics.
- At vasoconstriction doses for cardiogenic or septic shock.

Contraindications

Pheochromocytoma, ventricular arrhythmias, use of monoamine oxidase inhibitors (which enhance the effect of dopamine), etc. If monoamine oxidase inhibitors have been given within the preceding 2-3 weeks, the dopamine dosage is reduced to 1/10.

Precautions

- Administration into a central vein is preferred because of the risk of ischemic tissue necrosis in case of extravasation. Extravasation is treated by local infiltration with phentolamine (alpha-blocker) at a dose of 5-10 mg in 10-15 mL of 0.9% NaCl.
- Before administration, any hypovolemia should be corrected.
- Serum potassium levels must be checked because hypokalemia might develop (β_2-receptor stimulation).

Adverse effects

Arrhythmogenesis, tachycardia and nausea. The first two occur more commonly compared to dobutamine.

Dosage

Receptor stimulation, and therefore the effect of dopamine, is dose-dependent. Specifically:

- At low or renal doses (<3 µg/kg/min), selective stimulation of D_1 dopaminergic receptors predominates, leading to improved diuresis.
- At intermediate or inotropic doses (3-10 µg/kg/min), β-receptor stimulation predominates, producing improved cardiac output.
- At high or vasoconstriction doses (>10 µg/kg/min), α-receptor stimulation predominates, leading to vasoconstriction and increased BP. With the high dosage regimen, renal perfusion usually falls. In some patients, vasoconstriction is also observed at doses of 5-10 µg/kg/min.

Solution preparation and administration

In clinical practice, dopamine is used most commonly at renal or vasoconstriction doses. For a patient weighing 70 kg:

- For renal doses (e.g. 2 µg/kg/min): usually, 250 mg of dopamine (Intropin, Dopmin) are added to 500 mL of 5% D/W to produce a 500 µg/mL solution, which is administered at a rate of 17 mL/h.
- For vasoconstriction doses (e.g. 10-15 µg/kg/min): usually, 500 mg of dopamine are added to 250 mL of 5% D/W to produce a 2000 µg/mL solution, which is administered at a rate of 21-31 mL/h.

Table 23.4 shows the administration of a dopamine solution (800 µg/mL) per body weight.

Most common intravenous drugs in emergency cardiology

TABLE 23.4	Administration of 250 ml of an 800 µg/mL dopamine solution (200 mg of dopamine in 250 mL of 5% D/W)										
Weight (kg)	50	55	60	65	70	75	80	85	90	95	100
(µg/kg/min)					Infusion rate (mL/h)						
1	4	4	5	5	5	6	6	6	7	7	8
2	8	8	9	10	11	11	12	13	14	14	15
3	11	12	14	15	16	17	18	19	20	21	23
4	15	17	18	20	21	23	24	26	27	29	30
5	19	21	23	24	26	28	30	32	34	36	38
6	23	25	27	29	32	34	36	38	41	43	45
7	26	29	32	34	37	39	42	45	47	50	53
8	30	33	36	39	42	45	48	51	54	57	60
9	34	37	41	44	47	51	54	57	61	64	68
10	38	41	45	49	53	56	60	64	68	71	75
12	45	50	54	59	63	68	72	77	81	86	90
15	56	62	68	73	79	84	90	96	101	107	113

For reasons of practicality, decimals have been rounded to the nearest integer.

5) Noradrenaline (Norepinephrine)

Mechanism of action

Noradrenaline is a powerful vasoconstricting agent for all vascular systems, including the renal vasculature. Thus, it increases systolic and diastolic BP while also reducing blood flow to the kidneys. It primarily stimulates α and β_1-adrenergic receptors and, to a lesser degree, β_2-receptors. Compared to adrenaline, it has a greater effect on α-adrenergic receptors and a smaller effect on β_2-adrenergic receptors. Consequently, noradrenaline increases peripheral resistances and systolic and diastolic BP, whereas a-drenaline, because of its stronger stimulation of β_2-receptors (peripheral vasodilation), may lead to a reduction in peripheral resistances and diastolic BP. Noradrenaline has a half-life of ~3 min.

> **Warning!** As a brief memory guide to the comparative action of inotropes/vasopressors on receptors, note the following: noradrenaline $\alpha > \beta_1 > > \beta_2$, adrenaline $\beta_1 = \beta_2 > \alpha$, dobutamine $\beta_1 > \beta_2 > \alpha$, dopamine $D_1 = D_2 > \beta > \alpha$ (α stimulation at high doses), and isoproterenol $\beta_1 > \beta_2$.

Indications
- Septic shock (it is the vasoconstrictor of first choice and is superior to dopamine)
- Cardiogenic shock. In the setting of mechanical complications in STEMI patients, it is usually given as a complementary therapy to the intra-aortic balloon pump.

Contraindications
Hypersensitivity to the drug, use of monoamine oxidase inhibitors (risk of severe hypertensive episodes), pregnancy (risk of uterine contractions), etc.

Adverse effects
Headache, tachycardia, tremor and occasionally bradycardia (reflex parasympathetic activation) that can be treated with atropine.

Precautions
- Any hypovolemia should be corrected. Administration to hypovolemic patients can cause a reduction in cardiac output and tissue hypoxia.
- The infusion should be stopped gradually.
- Administration into a central vein is preferred because of the risk of ischemic tissue necrosis in case of extravasation. Extravasation is treated by local infiltration with phentolamine.

Dosage
The infusion begins with 8-12 µg/min and is titrated according to patient's response (desired systolic BP between 80-100 mmHg). The usual maintenance dose ranges between 2-4 µg/min but it should be mentioned that there is a great variation in the dose required to maintain an adequate BP. In septic shock, higher doses are usually necessary (up to 3 µg/kg/min).

Solution preparation and administration
Usually 8 mg of noradrenaline base (supplied as Levophed or Levophed Bitartrate ampoules which contain 4 mg of noradrenaline base/4 mL) are added to 250 mL of 5% D/W to produce a 32 µg/mL solution. Note that while ampoules are labeled in terms of the noradrenaline bitartrate or acid tartrate, doses are expressed in terms of the base (2 mg noradrenaline bitartrate = 1 mg noradrenaline base). Table 23.5 shows the infusion rate in more detail.

6) Esmolol
Esmolol is an ultra-short-acting cardioselective beta1-blocker with a half-life of 9 min. Its effect begins within 1-2 min and lasts 10-30 min after admin-

TABLE 23.5	Administration of 250 mL of a 32 µg/mL noradrenaline solution (8 mg of noradrenaline base in 250 mL of 5% D/W)	
Dose (µg/min)	Infusion rate (mL/h)	
4	7	
5	9	
6	11	
7	13	
8	15	
9	17	
10	19	
11	21	
12	22	
15	28	
20	37	

For reasons of practicality, decimals have been rounded to the nearest integer.

istration is terminated. It is metabolized by erythrocyte esterases and therefore its half-life is prolonged in patients with anemia.

Indications
- Acute aortic dissection.
- Perioperative hypertension (except for pheochromocytoma crises).
- Acute coronary syndrome when relative contraindications to beta-blockers exist.
- Supraventricular paroxysmal tachycardia (atrioventricular nodal reentrant tachycardia, atrioventricular reentrant tachycardia) where adenosine treatment has failed.
- Atrial fibrillation and atrial flutter (heart rate control).

Contraindications
The primary contraindications are low BP, bronchial asthma, severe bradycardia and second or third degree atrioventricular block. For acute conditions, e.g. acute aortic dissection, it may be administered on a trial basis even if the presence of a contraindication to beta-blockers is suspected, because its short half-life means that its effect will fade rapidly if administration is terminated because of side effects.

Extravasation of the administered solution must be avoided because of the risk of skin necrosis.

TABLE 23.6	Administration of 250 mL of a ready-to-use 0.9% NaCl solution of 10 mg/mL esmolol (Brevibloc)										
Weight (kg)	50	55	60	65	70	75	80	85	90	95	100
µg/kg/min					Infusion rate (mL/h)						
50	15	16	18	19	21	22	24	25	27	28	30
100	30	33	36	39	42	45	48	51	54	57	60
150	45	49	54	58	63	67	72	76	81	85	90
200	60	66	72	78	84	90	96	102	108	114	120
250	75	82	90	97	105	112	120	127	135	142	150
300	90	99	108	117	126	135	144	153	162	171	180

For reasons of practicality, decimals have been rounded to the nearest integer.

Dosage

It is administered at an initial loading dose of 500 µg/kg IV over one minute, followed by continuous infusion at a maintenance dose of 50 µg/kg/min for 4 min. If the desired result is not achieved, the loading dose is repeated and the maintenance dose is increased to 100 µg/kg/min for another 4 min. If the desired result is still not achieved, the loading dose is repeated and the maintenance dose is increased to 150 µg/kg/min for another 4 min. If this fails again, the same titration process may be repeated up to a final maximum maintenance dose of 300 µg/kg/min. Table 23.6 shows the method of continuous IV administration of the ready-to-use esmolol solution by body weight.

Specifically in the case of perioperative hypertension, esmolol is given at a greater dosage (1 mg/kg over 30 s followed by continuous infusion at 150-300 µg/kg/min until hypertension resolves fully).

Solution preparation and administration

Esmolol (Brevibloc) is available in:
- 10 mL vials (10 mg/mL)
- premixed 250 mL (10 mg/mL) and 100 mL (20 mg/mL) ready-to-use bags (0.9% NaCl solutions).

Table 23.7 summarizes the average IV infusion rate for the most common drugs used in emergency cardiology.

Most common intravenous drugs in emergency cardiology

TABLE 23.7	Indicative average infusion rates for some emergency cardiology drugs			
Drug	**Brand name(s)**	**Solution**	**Average dose**	**Average infusion rate (mL/h)**
Nitroglycerin	Nitro-Bid, Tridil	25 mg in 250 mL 5% D/W	25 µg/min	15
Nitroprusside	Nitropress, Niptide	50 mg in 100 mL 5% D/W	3 µg/kg/min	25
Dobutamine	Dobutrex, Dobutamine Hydrochloride	250 mg in 250 mL 5% D/W	5 µg/kg/min	21
Dopamine	Intropin, Dopmin	• Renal dose: 250 mg in 500 mL 5% D/W • Vasoconstriction dose: 500 mg in 250 mL 5% D/W	• 2 µg/kg/min • 10-15 µg/kg/min	17 21-31
Noradrenaline	Levophed	8 mg of noradrenaline base in 250 mL 5% D/W	8-12 µg/min (initial dose)	15-22

Index